Sacred Ground, The Psychological Cost of 21st Century War

A Collection of True Stories

Robert S. Brown, MD, PhD

Robert S Brown, MD, PhD
COL, Medical Corps, USAR, (Ret.)
Visiting Professor
Psychiatry and Neurobehavioral Sciences
School of Medicine
University of Virginia
Charlottesville

Copyright © 2014 Robert S. Brown, MD, PhD
All rights reserved.

ISBN: 1501060228
ISBN 13: 9781501060229
Library of Congress Control Number: 2014916622
CreateSpace Independent Publishing Platform
North Charleston, South Carolina

Table of Contents

Part One	Beginning	v
	Acknowledgements and Appreciation	vii
	Preface: The Author tells Soldiers' Stories and His Own Story	ix
	Foreword	
	The Purpose of <u>Sacred Ground</u>	xv
Disclaimer	Confidentiality and Privilege	xxix
Chapter One	War on Sleep	1
Chapter Two	The Best Decisions	27
Chapter Three	War on Mothers	53
Chapter Four	War on Soldiers as People	83
Chapter Five	Little Bobby Brown	117
Chapter Six	War on Memory	149
Chapter Seven	A Soldier Suit for Christmas	177
Chapter Eight	War on Intimacy	199
Chapter Nine	Mondays and Tuesdays	227
Part Two	Middle	253
Chapter Ten	War on Spirit	257
Chapter Eleven	Kitty Garnett	279
Chapter Twelve	War on Self	305
Chapter Thirteen	The University	339

Chapter Fourteen	War on Temperament	365
Chapter Fifteen	Picking Up the Pieces	391
Chapter Sixteen	War on Trust	423
Part Three	**The End**	451
Chapter Seventeen	The Pieces in Place	453
Chapter Eighteen	War on Relationships	483
Chapter Nineteen	Who Could Ask for Anything More	507
Chapter Twenty	No End in Sight	531
Chapter Twenty One	Suffering: A Handbook on Understanding PTSD	553
Chapter Twenty Two	The Burden of Uncertainty	581
Chapter Twenty Three	An After Word: How You can Help	597
Chapter Twenty Four	Bringing it Together	617
Appendix	**Military Acronyms**	647

Part One
Beginning

Acknowledgements and Appreciation

As each chapter of **Sacred Ground** was written, I read it to my wife, Dottie, whose support kept me writing. The creative gift of Clinton, our youngest son, brought energy to the project: he put the manuscript on-line and on compact discs so that Soldiers could read what was written about them and make corrections where necessary. He also brought life to the cover design. The cover photograph is by Kevin Koehler.

An article about the Florence Smith Medical School Scholarships' first recipients attracted the attention of a gifted journalist whose intuitive knack for discovering and writing a story, led Gary Ruegsegger, Virginia Beach, to me. This began a friendship that I treasure. No person, other than my mother, encouraged me more than Gary. In addition, he painstakingly edited each line of Sacred Ground, putting aside his own tasks, sensing the importance of this work, but refusing to be identified as its co-author, saying, "this is your story, and you must tell it."

Bobby Trent, PhD, is a good friend from high school whose wife was my "wife" in the senior class play. At his invitation, Dottie and I joined All Saints Anglican Church. Bobby, retired Associate Executive Vice President and Professor Emeritus, University of Virginia, read the manuscript and identified with the author. "Our stories are very much alike," he said. "Let me help you get it published." His active efforts to assist in getting Sacred Ground in print are not to be forgotten. John Sanderson, PhD, Education Consultant, Judge Advocate General's School and Associate Professor Emeritus in the Curry School of Education, University of Virginia, was surprised by the length of <u>Sacred Ground</u>, but he read it thoughtfully, made recommendations that I followed, and compared me favorably to Garrison Keillor whose writing he admires.

Finally, Sarah Marshall, Charlottesville, Virginia, one of the world's most talented "proof readers," examined <u>Sacred Ground's</u> 192,000 words as Sherlock Holmes investigated the clues left by London's notorious criminals. The hours required by the task were enormous. "Why," I asked Sarah Marshall, "will you not permit me to pay you for your work?" She replied, "I'm an American, too." Most of all, indisputably, I appreciate Soldiers, the men and women who serve our country in all its uniformed services. Permitting me to hear their true stories is a privilege and honor that is surpassed only by their willingness to have their stories shared with you. Often, these Soldiers and their stories created a sense of the sacred, the importance of which sent me on a mission to tell their stories so that you, like me, will respect and cherish them and their families. These are our best people.

Preface: The Author Tells Soldiers' Stories and His Own Story

This book is about Soldiers. It is not about politics.

I am the story-teller of the Soldiers' stories. As their story-teller, in every other chapter, I tell the story of my own life.

Cobbling my story between the Soldiers' stories is two-fold. The reader deserves to know the story-teller in order to perceptively understand the Soldiers' stories. In addition, my story is offered as a respite or relief from the intensity of some of the emotionally gripping stories shared by Soldiers.

The rich resource upon which the book is based is the 12,500 doctor-patient encounters I was privileged to have, and continue to have, with these Soldiers. I consider myself the most indebted student of these master teachers, Soldiers, formed from "the finest gold… refined in the hottest furnaces."

During Operation Desert Storm, 1991, I served on active duty as an Army medical officer, first at Walter Reed Army Medical Center and then at an Army hospital near Washington, DC. From 2005 to the present, I have been employed by the Department of Defense as a staff psychiatrist, a contractor, at the same Army hospital in which I served on active duty during Operation Desert Storm.

In <u>Sacred Ground, the Psychological Cost of 21st Century War, a Collection of True Stories</u>, Soldiers tell their stories, in their own words, of the reality of combat in Afghanistan and Iraq. Its emphasis, however, is upon their struggle with coming home. One Soldier put it this way, "War is easy. Coming home is Hell." His perception is a pervasive theme of <u>Sacred Ground</u>.

Foremost, <u>Sacred Ground</u> is an accurate account of the stories Soldiers told to me, their psychiatrist and group psychotherapist.

<u>Sacred Ground</u> is about the psychological impact of 21st Century war. The psychological cost of combat while in the heat of battle is unimaginable. Hardly less stressful are the psychological symptoms, long after returning home, that imprison our Soldiers cognitively and sadden them and their loved ones.

Listening to these factual stories is compelling. Their impact is lingering.

War changes people. Fighting terrorists changes people uniquely.

I refer to the Soldier's identity sculpted by combat as the **post-traumatic self**. Families of Soldiers returning from the War on Terror often tell Soldiers they are "different." "I want back my son, the one I knew before combat," is the prayer of many mothers. "You are not the Soldier I married," many spouses lament.

Soldiers grieve for the loss of their **pre-traumatic self**. Regrettably, too often their grief becomes an unidentified disturbing background noise for the Soldiers with **Posttraumatic Stress Disorder (PTSD)**. These pages will reveal the nature of combat-induced PTSD, informing the reader as never before.

Fortunately, as <u>Sacred Ground</u> confidently reveals, there is good news. Attachment between Soldiers in combat is the most significant of human bonds. Survival depended, to a large extent, upon healthy, secure attachments between Soldiers. Healthy, secure attachments foster survival and healing.

<u>Sacred Ground</u> tells how attachment between Soldiers can be used as scaffolding to nurture attachment between therapist and Soldier in Cognitive Therapy. Attachment is equally effective when renewed between Soldiers, previously unknown to each other, in Cognitive Group Therapy.

The table of contents depicts the comprehensive approach of <u>Sacred Ground</u> to understand the effects of the War on Terror upon every aspect of the Soldier's life from intimacy to uncertainty.

These true stories are told with one objective in mind. Our nation needs to hear what psychological price our Soldiers have paid, and continue to pay, in the longest war in the history of the United States.

The psychological cost has been high.

Nothing in the Soldiers' stories has been exaggerated. Nothing has been omitted.

Our nation has risen in the past to identify its challenges and to master its enemies. Our nation is near another crisis now, however, one that it fails to recognize, one whose consequences may be incalculable: we have become indifferent, uncaring, uninterested and ignorant of the sacrifices required of our Soldiers by 21st Century war. This is the current crisis. It must be resolved without further delay.

The war has been interminable.

Little is published about the good our Soldiers have done to help the Afghan and Iraqi people.

There is no "victory" of the kind ordinarily associated with warfare. There is little cause for "celebration" as was the case in World War II. There is no surrender. There is no truce. Perhaps it cannot be otherwise, but there is no discernible end to this war. Sadly and understandably, there is no visible end to the war within our Soldiers who return to us with combat-induced PTSD; yet we are hopeful.

<u>Sacred Ground</u> encourages America to examine its conscience. It enlightens our nation about the psychological suffering our Army, comprised of less than one-per cent of our population, endures on our behalf. Our Soldiers are worth getting to know. They are worthy of our admiration.

Neither the nation nor their family need fear Soldiers with combat-induced PTSD. These are peace-loving, peace-seeking, non-violent men and women.

<u>Sacred Ground</u> is not a self-help book. It is written to educate the American public about Soldiers.

We must not continue to be indifferent to our Soldiers who protect and defend our freedom. We cannot disregard the sacrifices willingly made by Soldiers and their families. Now is the time to recognize and assure them of our unending respect and trust.

Chapters 1-9 examine the effect of 21st Century war on Soldiers upon returning home. Its alternating chapters give the reader a view of the story-teller's early life and the influence of his love for the Army.

Chapters 10-16 address the impact of 21st Century War on the spiritual domain, temperament and trust. The story-teller's high school substitute teacher enters his life and remains there. He enters the University. A shattered life finds failure to be a masterful teacher. His bride is Heaven-sent.

Chapters 17-24 describe the war's influence on relationships, on suffering and on uncertainty. The story-teller perceives that life was abundantly doubly blessed when he became a doctor to Soldiers.

Foreword
The Purpose of <u>Sacred Ground</u>

MOST NATIONS SUPPORT their military. America has a long history of supporting its military; however, Americans know little about the psychological effort, emotional expenditure and prolonged suffering that are the consequences of its 21st Century War on Terror.

I believe the public wants to know more about the impact of our War on Terror on the well-being of our Soldiers. They want to know this without bias, polemics or hidden agendas of any form. The gory details, unnecessary and unwelcomed as they are, are less important than the influence of war on what our Soldiers think and feel and how they function in combat and upon returning home.

What is it like to endure the nearly constant threat of death over protracted periods of time on frequent deployments? What is it like to return from war to a home that is changed? What is it like to come home only to be told "you are changed…you are not the person I knew before you were deployed?" What is it like to have Posttraumatic Stress Disorder, also called PTSD? In fact, what is PTSD?

I want people to know the truth of the psychological impact on our Soldiers who fight for us in this Century. I want people to hear what our Soldiers tell me, their psychiatrist, about the war in combat and the war they bring home locked in the vault of their mind. The truth has to be told if people are going to understand the psychological cost of War on Terror. If the psychological injuries inflicted upon our Soldiers are going to heal, it will be the result of an informed and grateful nation who cares because it wants to understand.

Sacred Ground provides a forum, like no other, in which Soldiers tell their stories in their own words. These are not "war stories." These are love stories. Yes, these are stories of love. Repeated for emphasis, no human relationship is more intense than that between Soldiers in combat. Survival in combat and mission success depends most upon attachment between Soldiers.

One of the highest psychological costs of war is PTSD. To understand PTSD, however, we must first understand the horror of war.

I do not know war

Like most Americans, I never served my country in combat. I have not seen war with my own eyes, smelled war, heard war, touched war, or tasted war. For the past nine years, however, I've had the privilege as a physician to look into the faces of Soldiers who know war. These men and women are helping me to help them understand events that are nearly beyond the limits of human comprehension: IEDs (Improvised Explosive Devices), HME (Home Made Explosives), RPGs (Rocket Propelled Grenades), VBIEDs (Vehicle Borne IED), suicide bombers, roadside bombs, mortar rounds, the unique stench of burning human beings, atrocities perpetrated by men, women, and children who are not dressed as enemy Soldiers but as anonymous enemies who kill with radical religious fervor, and who give map co-ordinates to fellow enemies to destroy the targets at night in which they worked as "trusted" paid employees during the day. The list of repulsions seems to be without limit.

Danger is everywhere in war. There are no front lines, only 360 degrees of danger. Our Soldiers are trained and prepared to fight or die, to expect the unexpected, and to care for each other. Only a combat Soldier can know and understand another combat Soldier. They cover each other's back ("I've got your six" (Six O'clock)). Sleep in war is elusive, grabbed as naps and made possible only by fellow Soldiers standing guard. "Incoming" (rockets/mortars) sounds are unlike "outgoing" (weapons fired by our Soldiers) sounds. Knowing the difference between "incoming" and "outgoing" means the difference between life and death, between continuing to brush your teeth at night and scampering to a bunker.

The tympanic membrane (ear drum), stretched by the tiny bones inside the ear, magnifies even the tiny distant sounds of war. Hyperacusis, marked sensitivity to sound, like many physiological responses to stress, occurs automatically, like a reflex, often outside the sphere of awareness. It does not subside easily. This is why Soldiers with PTSD are made uncomfortable by noise even while sitting in the safety and comfort of their own home following deployment. Unexpected noise may cause escape behavior that results in extreme discomfort and embarrassment as bystanders stare in amazement. Extreme reflexes for extreme situations are extremely slow to calm down.

The memories of war, buried deep in the part of the mind that knows no sense of time, vividly override awareness during the waking state as realistic re-experiencing of an unimaginable life-threatening event. The flashback is precisely like the original event: sudden, unexpected, and all-consuming, near totally devastating. The message from the brain is meant to help the Soldier survive: ceaselessly, the brain says "don't forget this! I will keep reminding you of it in order to keep you safe." Any element of the original scene, in learning theory called an "identical element," may become a "trigger" that invokes a disturbing reenactment of the original scene. The season of the year, for example, hot weather or time of day, the dark of night or public gatherings can trigger or start a rapid reduction in emotional self-control. Often a trigger explodes into a panic attack, the very worst kind of anxiety.

Sacred Ground will answer the following questions:

What is combat-induced PTSD and how is it different from noncombat-induced PTSD? What are its causes? How is the diagnosis made? How is it treated? How many Soldiers have it? What is TBI (Traumatic Brain Injury) and how is it related to PTSD? How can PTSD be prevented? What can family members do for PTSD? What is "resilience"? What is the military doing for PTSD?

I am a witness to the agony of Soldiers described in their own words. As their messenger, their stories are from their soul to yours with enthusiastic hope that you will be strengthened to understand and help reduce their torment.

What is PTSD?

What is combat-induced PTSD and how is it different from PTSD? What are its causes? How is the diagnosis made?

Combat-induced PTSD is a term I use to describe Posttraumatic Stress Disorder caused by combat. Combat is warfare. Combat is engagement with the enemy. Going "out of the wire" expresses the state of increased danger of combat: getting shot at, bombed, ambushed, and becoming the target of explosions. Convoys, trucks and personnel transporting fuel and other necessary supplies for war, even humanitarian supplies, are all vulnerable to enemy attack. Mortars and rocket propelled grenades, of course, also crash into buildings and tents inside the wire and into "green zones," or areas alleged to be "safe."

Injuries from the War on Terror may be visible, invisible or both visible and invisible.

Traumatic brain injury (TBI), the signature injury of this war, may be invisible. PTSD, another invisible injury, is three times more likely to occur if TBI is present. Fortunately, 80 to 85% of cases of TBI are mild and its symptoms are expected to resolve within six to twelve months. Mild TBI is the result of damage to brain cells and their connections caused by the blast or physical force created by an explosion. "Explosion injuries" that lead to

TBI cause an altered state of consciousness such as "seeing stars," feeling "dazed" or being "confused," even momentarily. TBI symptoms include problems with balance, hearing loss, headaches, trouble concentrating, or memory loss. Polytrauma is a term used to describe a Soldier with multiple physical and psychological or visible and invisible wounds.

"Sir, what is a Disorder?"

The Tuesday Morning Post-Deployment Psychotherapy Group, one of my favorite groups, one I look forward to meeting with each week, was facing a crisis. All nine members of this group have Posttraumatic Stress Disorder (PTSD) from combat in Iraq and or Afghanistan. Several members of the group are medically retired because of PTSD, several are in the MEB (Medical Evaluation Board) process, and several continue on Active Duty.

Ordinarily, once retired, medically or non-medically, Soldiers who are no longer on Active Duty are ineligible for Behavioral Health Treatment at our MTF (Medical Treatment Facility). Our Chief of Behavioral Health, however, to our good fortune, permits all Soldiers who began group therapy at our MTF before retirement to continue to receive group psychotherapy after retirement. Individual therapy and or medication, if required after retirement, are provided at the near-by Veterans Administration Medical Center. Continuity of care is thus preserved to an important degree.

The policy to continue group therapy at our MTF is perceived by some members of the Tuesday Morning Group as "tentative." Not infrequently, for example, members of the Tuesday Morning Group tell me, "Sir, we are afraid this group will be canceled when you leave." Reassurance, even to the sensitive ears of brave Soldiers, goes unheard, despite its repetitive promise. Any change for Soldiers with PTSD, even changes, no matter how minimal, especially in treatment, is perceived as stressful. A change in therapy was announced, anxiety rose, resistance to the change was mounted by the Tuesday Morning Group and soon a crisis loomed. The change in this case is the Behavioral Health Data Portal (BHDP), a recently mandated Army-wide survey the details of which I will describe below.

Adam Douglas, a divorced 41-year-old African-American man, is a tall, once strong, once erect, once a responsible 1SG (First Sergeant), but now his broad shoulders droop with the combined weight of PTSD and unremitting depression, the residuals with which he returned from multiple combat deployments.

Last year, when all his physical and medical records were reviewed, 1SG Douglas was granted temporary disability compensation with ratings or percentages that he considered fair and just. However, the MEB process was arduous, lengthy and stressful. Until his award is determined to be based on conditions considered to be permanent and unlikely to improve, the MEB process must be reviewed annually.

1SG Douglas and I recently met, reviewed his PTSD and depression symptoms, and at his request I wrote a Memorandum for Record in which I stated, based upon a reasonable degree of medical certainty, that it is my professional opinion that his Posttraumatic Stress Disorder and his Chronic Major Depression were both likely to have reached the maximum level of clinical improvement and that his gloomy prognosis was resistant to change.

With tears in his eyes as I read the Memorandum for Record to 1SG Douglas, he thanked me and left the office. Weeks after our individual meeting, in the Tuesday Morning Group, 1SG Douglas asked, "Sir, what is a disorder?"

1SG Douglas understood that PTSD means "post" or after or following a "trauma." He said he knew what "trauma" meant because he had experienced many traumas or traumatic events in his multiple combat deployments. He understood the meaning of "stress." What he did not understand, he said, was the "disorder" part of Posttraumatic Stress Disorder.

The Tuesday Morning Group, already anxious over the BHDP survey, a recent change in the treatment procedure, stopped in its tracks to hear the definition of a "disorder" as it may pertain to their own conditions.

Thanking 1SG Douglas for his good question, I went to the blackboard and wrote in large black letters, "DSM-5." Saying no more, I took my seat. Writing this vignette a week after it occurred, I wonder if what I did was a not a cop-out.

"Disorder," a term I use many times every day, had become so common place that its actual meaning never dawned on me until 1SG Douglas asked for its definition. If one googles "disorder," as I did, one may find six pages of its definitions. Bottom-line, as used diagnostically, "disorder" is an "illness or health problem." Let me quickly add, however, that when I first began my study of psychology and psychiatry, "disorder" was not employed in the diagnostic nomenclature; "reaction" was the appropriate term. There were no mood disorders in the late 1950s, only mood reactions. Furthermore, PTSD was a late arrival in the classification system. It made its entry in 1983, significantly influenced by the undeniable crippling effects on the minds of our Soldiers returning from the war in Vietnam.

"Dr. Brown, What is DSM-5?"

DSM-5 is the <u>Diagnostic and Statistical Manual of Mental Disorders, Fifth Edition</u>. It was published in 2013. Its fascinating history, briefly described in the manual itself, is traced back to the 1840 Census, "the first official attempt to gather information about mental health in the United States."

Over the years, the DSM came to include more than statistical information, becoming more descriptive of the many different mental disorders.

At times, the <u>Diagnostic and Statistical Manual (DSM)</u> has been the subject of controversy. Ever ready to make necessary corrections, sometimes at the behest of strong social pressure, its editors and many contributors have tried to be intellectually honest, fair and reasonable. The DSM is the accepted authority on matters of diagnostic criteria of mental disorders. Its primary relevance to the Soldiers in <u>Sacred Ground</u> is this simple fact: in order for a Soldier to be diagnosed with PTSD and its co-morbid disorders (Panic Disorder, Major Depression, Substance Use Disorders), the Soldier's symptoms must meet the diagnostic criteria as described for PTSD and, if present, the PTSD co-morbidities must also meet the diagnostic criteria in DSM-5.

"What is a Mental Disorder?"

DSM-5 tells us that a mental disorder is "characterized by a clinically significant disturbance in an individual's cognition, emotion regulation, or behavior that reflects a dysfunction in the psychological, biological, or developmental processes underlying mental functioning. Mental disorders are usually associated with significant distress or disability in social, occupational, or other important activities…" The definition excludes socially acceptable reactions to loss, such as death. It further excludes socially deviant behavior (political, religious, or sexual) and conflicts that are primarily between the individual and society "unless the deviance or conflict results from a dysfunction in the individual as described above." See page 20, <u>Diagnostic and Statistical Manual of Mental Disorders, Fifth Edition</u>, 2013.

"What is the BHDP (Behavioral Health Data Portal) Survey?"

Behavioral Health Data Portal (BHDP) is a computerized survey developed by the Army Medical Command. Self-administered prior to each clinical interview, BHDP addresses the level of general distress, suicide risk factors, anxiety, depression, Posttraumatic Stress Disorder, and alcohol ingestion.

BHDP results are graphically displayed in the electronic medical record, readily assisting the clinician to follow the Soldier's response to treatment over time and may serve to help fashion treatment goals.

It is unlikely that a clinician's diagnosis of a behavioral health disorder is made on the basis of the BHDP responses alone; nonetheless, it is useful in identifying inconsistencies between computer responses and clinical presentation. For example, a Soldier indicated on the BHDP that he was having suicidal thoughts with a method or plan to carry out his thoughts, ominous risk factors for suicide. This response, coupled with additional evidence of worsening of his clinical condition, a TDO or Temporary Detention Order (a legal necessity to have one taken to a hospital to be evaluated by a judge) was requested. The patient suffered from PTSD and depression, lived alone, and was ingesting more ethanol. The patient told the evaluator for the TDO, "I pushed the wrong button on the BHDP; I don't have a method or plan to end my life." Using a narrow interpretation of the law, the professional evaluating the patient for the TDO refused to issue a TDO. It took an additional one-hour session with the Soldier, his Commanding Officer and his 1SG, before it was jointly decided that his risk of committing suicide was not imminent. The Soldier was thus permitted to leave the clinic to return the following day.

"What is a Psychiatric Disorder?"

Technically, there are no "psychiatric disorders." In the complex and challenging taxonomy or classification of things that go wrong with the mind, there are only "mental disorders." To be even more precise, try defining what is meant by the word, "the mind." It is used universally but, regrettably, lacking a widely agreed upon definition.

Where does this leave serious Soldiers like 1SG Adam Douglas, and his fellow Tuesday Morning Group members? 1SG Douglas and the Tuesday Morning Group just want to understand the labels or terms used by professionals communicating with them and with fellow professionals about them.

How I make a Combat-induced PTSD Diagnosis

This is how I make a PTSD diagnosis: (1) Soldiers come to my office from several distinct referral sources (a) self-referred, least likely, (b) family, in particular spouse, or friend, (c) command, or (d) Post Deployment Health Risk Assessment (PDHRA), a post-deployment mandated survey; or (e) from fellow providers and colleagues, or (f) former patients. (2) The newly referred Soldier is asked to go to one of the large maps on my office wall and to point out where he or she served in combat, often enlightening because, as some Soldiers state, "it is like looking at a map of my home town"; (3) The Soldier is asked to describe his or her primary duties in combat; (4) The Soldier is asked to tell me, if sufficiently comfortable, the worst combat traumas he or she endured. The traumas are often multiple and Soldiers may have difficulty selecting one trauma that was the worst. If the trauma(s) meets the diagnostic criteria for PTSD in severity and if the Soldier's response to the trauma(s) suggests its severity, I then proceed to inquire about the Soldier's PTSD symptoms: intrusion symptoms; avoidance symptoms; cognition and mood symptoms; arousal and reactivity symptoms; reckless or self-destructive behavior. If the symptoms have persisted for more than one month, I ask the Soldier for examples of how the PTSD symptoms have impaired his or her social, occupational, or other important areas of functioning.

An interview of the Soldier with his or her spouse often proves informative; it adds a dimension that may otherwise make the assessment less than complete. Their interaction as well as their information often provides observation that proves invaluable.

How Soldiers Respond to being told their Diagnosis is PTSD

Most Soldiers do not want a PTSD diagnosis. Mistakenly, undoubtedly influenced by societal misinformation, Soldiers too often believe, "PTSD means I'm weak…if I had been stronger in combat, I would not have PTSD." A PTSD diagnosis may thus confirm one's self-doubts, perhaps long-standing, about failing to tolerate pressure. Regrettably, Soldiers underestimate the degree of combat stress, unwilling to acknowledge that some levels of stress are intolerable and incompatible with normality for anyone.

Soldiers who have received financial compensation for PTSD tell me, "All the money in the world is not as important to me or to my family as my health. I would give every penny back to the government if I could get back my health." Some Soldiers mistakenly believe, "I will lose my security clearance," or "I can never buy a gun," or "I can never get a good job." None of this is true. Security clearance is based, among other factors, upon whether the subject is a risk to the U.S. government. Having PTSD does not, in and of itself, increase one's risk to our government. Investigators have sought my professional opinion on many occasions regarding Soldiers under my care for the treatment of combat-induced PTSD. Up to this time, none of my patients with PTSD, in my professional opinion, based upon a reasonable degree of medical certainty, has proven untrustworthy or at increased risk or danger to the security of the US.

Combat-induced PTSD does not result from mental, moral or physical weakness. The "stress" or "S" component of PTSD derives from the field of engineering. It determines the amount of force a physical structure can tolerate before it collapses. "Exposure to actual or threatened death, or serious injury…," language from the DSM-5 Diagnostic Criteria for PTSD, could not more vividly describe the "force" upon which our Soldiers continually operate combating terrorism. It is remarkable that merely 15-20% of our Soldiers are inflicted with PTSD, every one a brave Soldier to whom the Army is dedicated to nurture back to health.

I am privileged to enter into the suffering of these Soldiers, men and women, with combat-induced PTSD, a task more rewarding than imaginable. You are going to be privileged and incredibly educated, to hear the stories they have permitted me to share with you. If the goal of imparting their stories to you is achieved, your understanding of PTSD will be increased. Your intolerance of misinformation about Soldiers with PTSD will be sharpened, and you will seek opportunities to calm the storms of our Soldiers, the best in the history of the world.

How is Combat-induced PTSD Treated?

The Department of Defense and the Veterans Administration recognize four forms of treatment for PTSD: Cognitive Therapy; Cognitive Reprocessing Therapy; Continuous or Prolonged Exposure Therapy; and Eye Movement Desensitization Recall (EMDR) Therapy. In addition, the Food and Drug Administration (FDA) has approved two antidepressants, Zoloft and Paxil, for PTSD. Many clinicians also use Prazosin (Minipress), one of the older antihypertensive medications, serendipitously discovered to be effective in the management of nightmares. As a Fellow of the American Academy of Cognitive Therapy, I have been extensively trained in Cognitive Therapy. I have also been trained in Cognitive Reprocessing Therapy and Continuous or Prolonged Exposure Therapy. Attachment Theory and Object Relations Theory, explained later in the text, significantly inform my treatment of Soldiers with combat-induced PTSD.

The treatment of combat-induced PTSD is arduous, challenging and slow. It is like teaching someone to swim who, for very good reasons, is afraid of the water. It requires trust and hope when both have been broken.

The special relationship between patient and therapist is called the "therapeutic alliance." It is built on mutual respect and trust, adheres to strict confidentiality and requires collaboration in achieving specific goals to help the patient. The therapeutic alliance in treating Soldiers with PTSD is critically important. Although Soldiers with PTSD avoid the pain of discussing their trauma, they will do so with a qualified listener: a professional with education, training and experience who can be trusted to listen, who is available when needed and who cares that the Soldier is suffering.

A qualified listener assesses the Soldier's capacity and readiness to recall the traumas of combat. Sufficient detailed memories of the traumas are necessary in order to bring them into cognitive awareness. Distortions can be reduced, accurate appraisals of the traumas can be made, and the Soldier's resources to cope with them are strengthened when the truth of the trauma is identified.

What is meant by the phrase, "the truth of the trauma?" you may well ask.

Foundational in Cognitive Therapy is the premise, "It is not what happens to us that primarily affects us. It is the meaning we give to what happens to us that determines its effects upon us."

In Cognitive Therapy with Soldiers with PTSD, upon hearing the detailed description of the combat trauma, I listen for the meaning it is given by the Soldier. Then the Soldier and I search for distortions of its meaning to the Soldier. When the distortions are minimized, the truth of the trauma takes on the ring of truth which is almost immediately liberating. Examples are given throughout the text, beginning in Chapter One, found in the subsection entitled, "Doctor, I haven't slept for three months."

Combining individual therapy with weekly group cognitive therapy is well received by Soldiers, utilizes the strength of close attachments that were often life-saving in combat, and informs Soldiers that their PTSD symptoms are also experienced by others and can be understood and successfully controlled. Individual therapy without group therapy is deemed appropriate for some Soldiers. Family therapy is also a strong addition to individual and group therapy.

"Timing is everything" is an applicable phrase in the treatment of PTSD. Readiness is a term used to depict "timing." The therapeutic alliance is the foundation upon which the healing of PTSSD begins. The therapist's interactions with the Soldier will provide clues about readiness. Every wound, as Shakespeare reminds us, heals by degree. The healing process will appear to be slow; however, the most unbearable traumas are buried outside awareness in a part of the mind where timelessness prevails. When trauma memories break into awareness, they are accompanied by a distortion of the sense of time, thus convincing the Soldier they will last forever. It is comparable to the feeling of being trapped in a claustrophobic nightmare from which there is no escape and no end…but it is just a feeling; it is not the truth.

Understood in these terms, a Soldier's psychological defenses against recalling combat traumas are natural and entrenched. "Once the trauma is out, Sir," another Soldier said, "anything can set it off…then it keeps coming up. You can be having a good day…out with your wife and son to buy an ice cream cone…you pass a vehicle and you flash into a panic. It's a constant thing. It never goes away. There are always constant reminders of the war."

This mistaken perception is widespread among Soldiers with PTSD. It prevents Soldiers from directly confronting their traumas. It permits distortions of the traumas to control the Soldier's thoughts. It blocks the rational, logical functions of the mind from reasoning and recognizing the truth of his or her situation. A child learning to swim does not hesitate to jump into the deep water in which his or her father stands with out-stretched hands. Recovering from PTSD begins with a similar leap of trust.

Research into the best practices for the treatment of PTSD is ongoing. A treatment team of psychiatrists, psychologists, psychiatric nurse practitioners, social workers and substance abuse counselors work together for the common good of the Soldiers at the Military Treatment Facility (MTF) I have called home since 2005. Most fortunately, all the approved treatments for PTSD are available at our MTF.

Disclaimer
Confidentiality and Privilege

I am a clinician. It is my duty to keep confidential what is said to me by a patient. All the Soldiers whose stories are told in <u>Sacred Ground</u> have been my patients. It is the patient's privilege to have their medical records protected from unauthorized disclosure.

The names and personal details of specific Soldiers described in this work have been altered to avoid the unintended revelation of their identity; however, where possible, every Soldier discussed here has also personally read and approved the references made to them. One Soldier, interestingly, petitioned me to use his actual name and rank. His request was granted.

This book, dedicated to men and women who have served, as well as those now serving in our armed forces, is intended to honor them and their families by telling some of their stories in order that our nation may come to know and love them just as I have.

In a number of important ways, these Soldiers and their stories have become intertwined with my own personal story. My professional life as a retired military psychiatrist has been enriched by these Soldiers. For most of the last decade, I have been honored and privileged to treat thousands of active duty Soldiers serving in our current and recent military operations throughout the world.

The views expressed in this book are exclusively those of the author.

My views do not reflect the views or opinions of the Department of Defense, the Department of the Army, the Office of the Surgeon General of the Army, the Department of the Navy, Air Force, Coast Guards, or Marines, nor do they represent the views or opinions of the National Guard, our Reserve Forces or any governmental agency. Neither do they represent the views of the University of Virginia.

The accuracy of the reporting of the stories told to me by these remarkable Soldiers is assured by the proof-reading done by the Soldiers themselves. I was impressed by the degree of seriousness with which they willingly approached the task. No fact was too trivially incorrect to escape their attention. I was impressed, but I was not surprised, because their survival in combat depended upon constant attention to detail and to the truth.

Unfortunately, for many returning Soldiers, the burden of attention to detail, now called "hypervigilance," is exhausting. It preoccupies their awareness. It leaves little energy or time for relationships. It leads to an avoidant, constricted life-style. It interferes with sleep. It erodes basic trust. It presumes their world is not safe. Too often, their doubts and fears are confirmed, making it difficult to hope for a brighter future.

Thankfully, when treatment is successful, these valued Soldiers to whom we are so indebted are able to flourish. Witnessing the Soldier's journey back to health is more rewarding than one can imagine.

1

War on Sleep

"Doctor, I haven't slept for three months"

The Behavioral Health Clinic closes at 1630. I was busily completing my office notes describing the diagnosis and treatment of each patient I had treated that autumn day in October 2008.

Margaret, a tall, strong, caring middle-aged office assistant with prematurely graying-hair, stuck her head in my door at 1700. In her thick rural dialect, Margaret said, "I think you better see this one. He said, 'It can't wait until we open at 0730 tomorrow.'" Without much enthusiasm, I nodded approval.

The Captain, dressed in the camouflage green Army Combat Uniform (ACU), looked penetratingly at me through his dark eyes, emphasized by his thick black eye brows. With the facial expression of deep depression, he spoke just above a whisper and with a raspy voice. Almost excessively politely, he said, "Sir, I haven't slept for three months."

The Captain's demeanor, his manners, his obvious physical exhaustion, immediately reminded me of Jimmy Stewart in the movie, "Mr. Smith Goes to Washington." After a successful filibuster during which Jimmy Stewart stood up on his feet all night and into the next morning, he too was the picture of total exhaustion. Jimmy Stewart, however, had missed only one night of sleep.

"Thank you for seeing me, Sir. I know it's after closing time."

Almost every Soldier finds it difficult to seek mental health, now called behavioral health, treatment. Acknowledging that one needs help, in his or her mind, mistakenly is acknowledging weakness. It is a multifaceted, challenging dilemma. This subject requires and is receiving more attention than I am able to emphasize in this writing.

Senior noncommissioned enlisted and commissioned officers are the least likely to come in our doors. Sadly, more Soldiers would accept psychological treatment if they observed their leaders benefiting from counseling. Soldiers who step into my office never darken it. They brighten me and my surroundings.

"Let me thank you for coming to see us," I replied genuinely. "It's an honor and a privilege to talk with you. Take your time. We are in no hurry. I have nothing more important to do than to listen to you. Can you tell me why you can't sleep, Captain?"

He was a handsome man, even though he was highly distressed.

His military bearing was his most evident physical feature. His athletically-trained physique was carried by a man of medium build. His olive complexion was blemish-free. He held up his broad shoulders, I suspect, with great effort owing to his persistent, painful insomnia.

"What is the picture?"

The Captain's eyes, previously fixed on my face, instantly looked away from me when I repeated my question, "Captain, why can't you sleep?"

Nervously, he replied, "A picture comes into my mind when I try to sleep, Sir."

"What is the picture," I inquired

"I can't tell you the picture without crying, Sir."

"Do you need permission to cry?"

"An officer cannot cry in front of his men, Sir."

"You don't have to tell me now, Captain, if you don't want to," I said to help reduce his tension.

"I have to tell you now, Sir."

"Captain, what is the picture," I said in a calm voice.

"My wife is talking about leaving me, Sir."

"What is the picture?"

A host of things must be muddling his thoughts… half-formed thoughts… lacking the clarity that only restful sleep could straighten, I imagined. He painfully weighed the merits of disclosing to me, a stranger unknown to him fifteen minutes earlier. A haunting visual image from combat forces its entry into his consciousness. His sleep is stolen from the Captain.

This detested nocturnal thief comes to his bedside as regularly as night follows day. Like other Soldiers changed by combat, he prayed for the day to end. At the end of the day he then dreaded sleep because he felt helplessly vulnerable to whatever apparitions would invade his disturbed sleep at night.

He perceived that I was not judgmental, impatient, or preoccupied. I was not "just checking the boxes." I was not just going through the motions.

This time when I asked about the picture that kept him awake for the three months since he returned from Iraq, the Captain described the picture.

"We had a very good day. It was very hot, of course. I was covered with mud and sand, but we had lost no one and none of my Soldiers were injured. That is always a good day. I turned in my vehicle at the Motor Pool and took a short-cut across the FOB (forward operating base) to my CHU (Container Housing Unit).

Two young Soldiers walked up towards me just as I was walking past the Medical Aid Station. They were shouting 'Save our brother…Save our brother,' mistaking me for a medical officer.

I looked down as they approached me. I froze for a moment. The Soldier they were dragging between them, their "brother," had a very bad head wound."

The dreaded tears drenched his face. We sat in silence. He was about to pass the baton to me. Could I accept the baton, not drop it, and continue the race with him beside me?

"I could see brain matter protruding out of the side of their brother's head. That's the picture."

"What happened next, Captain?"

There was another period of silence. This was his first telling of his story. Instead of the sense of relief I expected to observe, however, he was more saddened, more regretful. With shame, the Captain covered his face. He wept.

More silence followed. The Captain's earlier reference to himself, "I froze for a moment," rang in the ears of my mind. Is this the key to unlock the entry into the Captain's self-doubt, his crisis of guilt that has cut off his emotional underpinnings? I wondered to myself.

"What happened next, Captain?"

"Funny you should ask me that, Sir," he replied. "In some ways it seems strange to me what happened next. The two Soldiers who asked me to help save their battle buddy would not leave me."

"How was it they would not leave you," I asked.

"After the medics took away their battle buddy, Sir, they just stayed with me for the rest of the evening. Their commander told them to move on, but they stayed with me. Later my commander told me to move on, but I told her I could not leave the two Soldiers."

"What did you and the two young Soldiers do?"

"They talked about their friend, Sir. He must have been a wonderful person. He was only nineteen years old. He had a girlfriend back home. He wanted to work on a farm. They told me his whole story."

"Did you think you were there to save the injured Soldier?"

"That's what I have been thinking, Sir."

"Ten of the best neurosurgeons in the world," I said, "could not have saved him, Captain."

The Captain's half-shut eyes opened widely. Speechless, the Captain was stunned.

"Could you have been there for some other reason?"

"Like what, Sir?"

"You tell me, Captain."

"Could I have been there for those two young Soldiers, Sir?"

"They will never forget you," I replied with complete assurance.

Until now, the Captain thought they may never forgive him for "freezing for a moment" and thus not saving their friend's life.

The Captain's invisible burden lifted. He no longer appeared totally exhausted. He corrected his misunderstanding. His irrational guilt, typical of the horrific trauma of combat, disappeared like the sudden, surprising, clearing of an early morning fog.

The Captain's facial muscles relaxed.

The Captain slept that night for the first time in three months. The Captain slept because he discovered the truth of the situation in which he had been placed at the end of a good day.

The Captain discovered the good he had done for two young Soldiers.

The Captain discovered he had done no wrong.

The Captain discovered that the good day he thought he had been having, in a sad but important way, was still a good day.

Refreshed by restorative sleep, the Captain returned the next morning. It took a while to repair the damage to his marriage, the result of his sleep deprived irritability and impatience. Weekly group therapy, supplemented by occasional individual Cognitive Behavioral Therapy, led quickly to the return of his normal sense of himself. Eventually, he required no medications of any type, came less frequently to the clinic, and no longer needed psychological assistance.

"How are you doing, Sir?"

Several months later I saw the Captain at the gym pumping iron in the weight room. Sweat poured from the Captain's muscular body, biceps bulging in his upper arms, his back erect as he sat upright on a bench viewing his world in the large mirrors that formed an entire wall, rhythmically raising and lowering several hundred pounds.

The heavy breathing of his strenuous exercise became louder as I walked nearer to him from the rear.

He first recognized my greeting, and then, looking up, he saw my reflection in the mirror.

"How are you doing, Sir," he warmly responded without missing a single repetition of his weights rising up and down effortlessly.

As he continued to pump iron, I thought I could detect a smile in his voice. As usual, the weight room was busily occupied by men of all stages of physical fitness, some chatting to each other, some seriously and solemnly invested in the machines on which they were exercising or the weights they were straining to lift.

I lowered my voice as I spoke to the Captain, not wanting to violate his trust or his confidentiality. Almost whispering, I said, "How are you doing, Captain?"

The Captain replied in what seemed to me to be a booming, self-confident voice, if not a cheer or yell, still pumping iron: "I'm doing fine, Sir."

To my surprise, the other exercising soldiers paid no attention to our conversation.

"Can you tell me, Captain, what helped you the most?"

He replied without hesitation, still pumping iron, still sweating, still speaking in a loud voice, more like a reflex than from deep, thoughtful contemplation.

"I got my thinking straight, got my sleep back, and I got back into exercise, Sir."

I perceived that the Captain felt joy and relief. An unbearable trouble was gone. A distorted picture in his mind had been corrected. I thought of the paralytic man in the Bible who, healed by Jesus, took up his mat and miraculously walked for the first time in his life.

I imagined his joy. He was no longer crippled, no longer dependent upon others to pick him up and carry him from place to place. He was no longer paralyzed and no longer fearful.

I slowly walked back to my locker. I experienced a precious feeling of thanksgiving and inner peace for the Captain. Suddenly I turned and walked again to the weight room, neither of us ever looking face to face at each other, only at each other's reflection in the huge mirror. "How is your marriage, Captain?"

Over the clanging sounds of weights and the buzz typical of weight rooms, unashamedly loud and still methodically pumping iron, the Captain replied stoutly, "My marriage is fine, Sir."

He had other things on his mind now. I could see that he was physically fit and self-confident. It was my last encounter with the Captain who had not slept for three months.

I will never forget him, his profound suffering, his horrifying "picture" that prevented sleep, his gift of meaningful comfort as a Captain to two young enlisted men far from home mourning the loss of their "brother," and his return to health.

Gunnery SGT Seth Johnson, USMC

GYSGT (Gunnery Sergeant) Seth Johnson, 47 year old, light-brown balding hair line, caring blue eyes, round face, average height, and slightly bulging midriff, is noticeably gentle, even kind. He is a soft-spoken man, with a slow, southern drawl.

Things had not gone well for GYSGT Seth Johnson. Marines don't talk about feelings. It's not because they don't have feelings. They have the same feelings we all have. Marines have a strict code of military conduct limiting the expression of feelings.

GYSGT Johnson had 5 combat deployments to Iraq and Afghanistan. No one knows what he experienced during his combat deployments. He will take those secrets to his grave.

He successfully denies the symptoms of PTSD during the day, but he cannot hide them while he sleeps.

His wife of 20 years witnesses his groaning restlessness throughout the night. His two teenage children are accustomed to his sudden bursts of anger during the day and his terrifying screaming in the late hours of the night.

Yes, there have been periods of domestic discord. At times, his teenagers have openly defied him. He is familiar with feelings of humiliation in his own home where he has felt out of place, even unwelcomed.

He loves his wife and children. He has been generous to them. He wants the best for them, but he cannot be his best for them.

Sleep-deprivation, chronic irritability, stress at work, and unhappiness at home proved fertile soil for clinical depression.

"Dr. Brown, I don't enjoy anything any more.

I'm always exhausted. I wake up in the morning just as tired as I was when I went to bed.

My nightmares are getting worse and more frequent.

I'm easily annoyed. I fly off the handle over the least thing.

No one wants to be around me. To a degree, that's alright with me because I prefer to be alone."

"Tell me," I said, "do you snore, GYSGT Johnson?"

Smiling, the GYSGT said, "Ask my neighbors. I bet you they can tell I snore. My wife and kids tell me I sound like a locomotive. My wife says I even stop breathing and gasp for breath."

The GYSGT met the clinical diagnosis of Sleep Apnea, stopping breathing many times during sleep. This was confirmed by a sleep study. He was fitted with a special mask supplying air forcefully into his nose when he stops breathing during sleep.

He got more sleep, but his nightmares 3 or 4 times a week persisted. He is awakened in a frightened state with his heart pounding, profuse sweating, and breathing so rapidly it felt like he had been running for miles.

Months passed, but his depression did not lift.

"I never looked at it that way, Sir"

GYSGT Johnson wanted to surprise his daughter Nancy with a special gift for her fourteenth birthday. Their relationship had been rocky. Nancy loved her father, but hated his unpredictable disposition.

"What's wrong with dad?" Nancy often asked her mother.

"You will have to ask him," her mother invariably replied, hiding her tears.

GYSGT Johnson's family was never told he suffered from PTSD (Posttraumatic Stress Disorder) because he was too proud. "A Marine is too strong to get messed-up in the head," he told me when he first came to the Department of Behavioral Health, 5 months earlier.

"Are Marines too strong to get Pneumonia," I asked GYSGT Johnson? "Are Marines too strong to take Shrapnel? Are Marines too strong to get a Purple Heart for a combat injury?"

"I never looked at it that way, Sir. Is PTSD an injury?"

My answer to GYSGT Johnson's question will affect him the rest of his life. He is asking me if he is weak. He is asking me if he is a failure. He is asking me if he is a coward. He is asking me if his 20 years in the US Marine Corps was a sham.

His eyes were pleading for the truth about himself as a person. His kind face was finally, but silently, asking for the dreaded reality, "If I tried harder, Sir, would I have never gotten PTSD?"

This was a sacred moment.

I felt very close to him. I felt very close to his children, although I had never met them. I felt very close to his wife whose suffering had been shared in several joint therapy sessions with her husband.

Addressing GYSGT Johnson, I told him his question was a good one, an important one.

"GYSGT Johnson," I said, "PTSD and mild TBI (Traumatic Brain Injury) from exposure to blasts in combat, are the two 'signature injuries' of the war in Iraq and Afghanistan."

His sense of relief filled my office.

He was injured.

He was not weak.

He was not a coward.

There was nothing wrong with him as a person.

Nancy's Birthday Present

The Johnsons love animals.

"I went to the Pound on Post," said GYSGT Johnson. "I wanted to find a dog for Nancy. She's good with animals. I was thinking it would be a present she would love.

There were a lot of good dogs to choose from. One dog caught my eye right away. I went right to the manager and asked about the dog.

A family had brought their dog to the Pound. They were going overseas and could not take him along. He was already named.

I had an automatic connection with 'Reaves' in the Pound at our first meeting.

Nancy was so pleased with Reaves she hugged me around the neck. I believe it was my first real hug from Nancy in a long time. It made me feel real good.

I can't explain it, but Reaves and I clicked. He followed me everywhere. Nancy didn't seem to mind.

Then something started to happen that I think is strange. I don't understand it.

Reaves sleeps with me at night.

Reaves gets up on the bed and sleeps on my feet. He is there all night.

The strangest thing about Reaves sleeping on my feet is something I cannot explain.

My nightmares have gone away completely!

I have not had a nightmare since Reaves started sleeping on my feet. With my Sleep Apnea mask on my face and Reaves on my feet, I sleep like a baby, Sir. Of course, I feel better and I treat my family better.

Once or twice, Reaves has gone down the hall to sleep with my son. When Reaves is not sleeping on my feet, the nightmares return.

If I get upset, Reaves will jump up in my lap."

"GYSGT Johnson," I said, "tell me about this remarkable birthday present for Nancy."

"He is a miniature Schnauzer, Dr. Brown. He only weighs 15 pounds and he is 6-8 inches tall."

"I wonder where Reaves studied Psychiatry," I said. "I'm sure he was the best student in his class. He knows you well, Gunnery SGT Johnson. He gives you something we all need. Reaves has a noble, caring heart and he knows how to soothe."

CPT Jack Scott

CPT (Captain) Jack Scott, born and reared in Montana, stands 6-feet-3 inches tall. His blond hair has been shaved off, leaving a shiny scalp, an appealing face with a broad smile and probing blue eyes.

He is physically fit. A college Lacrosse coach would immediately spot him as a potentially good prospect. He would be sized up as scrappy, fast and strong.

The Captain was burdened with an unforgettably disturbing combat memory, one haunting him by day and plaguing him at night. His unrefreshing sleep is fractured by the reenactment of the cause of his lingering fear.

CPT Scott's speech was articulate and serious.

"Fear is the worst! It encompasses everything. I try not to feel the fear. I try not to show it. We are required to control it in combat.

I don't want that feeling again. I was crying on the floor of my room. I never want to feel like that again.

One day before we were scheduled to come home from Iraq, we got extended, sent to Baghdad for an additional 4 months.

I was tired. I was tired of my job. I kept a knot in my stomach. At night, I couldn't stand the stress. I would start crying.

My grandparents died one month apart. They raised me. I was not there for them."

CPT Scott's Fear

In the Tuesday Morning Post-Deployment Psychotherapy group, CPT Scott asked, "How can one get over the horrible feeling that a mistake he made cost the life of someone else?"

The 7 fellow group members saw tears in the Captain's eyes. The question was not unfamiliar to anyone present. Each Soldier had asked himself the same question many times.

No one spoke.

CPT Scott's "fear," the fear that cast him in tears upon the floor of his room in Iraq, that placed a lingering knot in his stomach, was uniquely selfless. It was the fear and regret of causing harm to others.

I believe CPT Scott's fear was an entirely altruistic fear.

"May I go to the board and draw a diagram of an intersection in Iraq, Dr. Brown?"

I nodded approval.

In the upper left-hand corner of the intersection, CPT Scott drew a large school building. Directly to the right of the intersection, one of CPT Scott's Strykers, an 8-wheeled armored vehicle, was stuck in the mud.

CPT Scott placed one of his Strykers on a 45-degree angle. It projected into the intersection to block traffic. He placed his own Stryker in front of the stuck vehicle, blocking traffic from entering from that direction.

With his translator, CPT Scott walked back to the intersection to advise the children to stop throwing rocks at the vehicle parked in the middle of the intersection. He was concerned that "rocks could soon turn into rockets."

To be stalled at an intersection was one of the most vulnerable positions in combat in Iraq, 2005-2006.

Twelve of CPT Scott's Soldiers were involved in the operation.

"I had a sudden instinctive feeling there was danger, that I should not step into the intersection. At that moment, standing helplessly, I heard the crack of a sniper's rifle.

I was talking to SGT Rodriguez. He was standing up in the gun turret of his Stryker, the one blocking traffic in the middle of the intersection. He was struck right in the head and neck. He was killed instantly. His blood nearly filled the inside of the Stryker."

CPT Scott wept.

"The nation is uncaring. They don't have a clue"

CPT Scott continued.

"The word got out. 'They got Rod today.' Whether you know them or don't know them, it doesn't make any difference. The feeling is the same when a Soldier is killed in combat…it's family. It feels like I lost my brother.

It could be me. It's a very personal loss. Even if you don't know them you know them. They know some of the people you know. We are really a small family. There is not that many of us.

Whether you go to Bragg or Polk or Germany or Iraq or Afghanistan, you see Soldiers you have seen before.

Who do I fight for? I fight for the guy in the bunk next to me. I went to war for the people who went to war in 1941, Korea, Vietnam.

If we don't do it, who will?

The nation is uncaring. They don't have a clue.

You are loyal to those with whom you serve.

Awards…what are they worth in a pawn shop?

PTSD is a very personal form of grief."

"The unthinkable task…"

The group was fully present with the Captain because they had been there with their own combat brothers. His words created a sad song. Silently, the group hummed the familiar tune, some visibly, respectfully nodding their heads knowingly. Intuitively, I knew that healing was present in their mutual understanding.

CPT Scott continued.

"Two men took an inventory of everything our fallen brother possessed at his CHU (Container Housing Unit). They cleaned up the area. They didn't leave a trace of SGT Rodriguez. All painful reminders were removed.

Some units get Soldiers unknown to the fallen Soldier to clean out the vehicle. If the unit is small, the unthinkable task is assigned to those who lived and worked beside him.

Every drop of blood collects in the bottom of the Stryker. When SGT Rodriguez was shot, KBR (KBR, Inc., formerly Kellogg Brown & Root, a Global Engineering, Construction and Services Company) cleaned out his vehicle. It was a blessing to us. It was 120 degrees in Baghdad.

When we got back from the mission, they had cold Kool Aid ready for us." CPT Scott cried recalling this tender deed.

"And his vehicle was cleaned.

They took us off the road for a couple of days."

Later, CPT Scott would learn that his tears, the tears of an officer in front of Soldiers, gave courage to other Soldiers in the Tuesday Morning Group to follow his leadership.

CPT Scott's Guilt

"There are two things I could have done to have prevented SGT Rodriguez's death.

That morning, SGT Rodriguez put on a pair of Oakley tinted sun glasses. I warned him about the sun reflecting off his glasses, making him a target. He replied that the reflecting sun would blind a would-be sniper.

I also felt bad about not stepping into the intersection. Maybe I would have been the sniper's target if I had not stopped."

Fellow group members tried to console the Captain.

"You cannot plague yourself for the rest of your life with 'what if' questions. There are no answers to 'what if' questions. There are 3 things used by the devil to cause pain, guilt and shame. Those 3 things are doubt, fear and uncertainty."

Another Soldier said the Captain did all he could to protect the Soldier that was killed.

"You also saved the lives of 11 other Soldiers in that situation who otherwise would have been ambushed and destroyed by rocket-propelled grenades."

CPT Scott thanked the group.

"Before I came to the group there was no one to talk to. I felt alone. I feel better coming here because I kept things bottled up inside myself.

I can't tell you how many nights I have relived the death of SGT Rodriguez. I always wake up in a start. I check the doors and windows, always feeling insecure."

CPT Scott's Improvement

Faithfully, CPT Scott attended weekly Post-Deployment Group Therapy and biweekly individual therapy sessions. Gradually, more along a jagged edge than a straight upward slope, the Captain improved.

"In class today the instructor mentioned Mortuary Affairs. Immediately, my mind went back to Iraq, recalling the times I had to go identify the body of my Soldiers killed in combat. But I was better this time.

I didn't completely withdraw. I didn't lose the instructor's train of thought. It lasted for a short while. In the past, I would completely shut down. If I was at home and saw something on TV about the war that upset me I would go to bed, hopefully to sleep or just lie there alone and think.

Today, in class I decided I would try to get in touch with one of my buddies. I had PTSD on the monitor. One of the other officers saw what I had on the monitor and said, 'You got PTSD?' I didn't answer him. He said, 'I have it. You go to a shrink and they give you medication and you are so sleepy you can't think about it.'

I was unwilling to speak to the fellow Soldier. People don't understand. Even my wife does not understand. She thinks you say it once and then you are okay.

I keep it to myself. People are not worthy to hear my problems. They don't have respect enough for me to have confidence in them. I don't know what they will do with the information. They could help or hurt you."

CPT Scott, much improved after becoming securely attached, first in a trusting way to me and then equally attached to the group, rides his bicycle 50-100 miles each week. He still experiences traumatic memories unexpectedly, but he reacts to these memories in more adaptive ways. He is less disturbed by them, less shocked, and their effect lasts minutes, not days.

If CPT Scott has a nightmare, it is not frequent. Its negative impact is brief. It becomes raw material out of which we make clearer our understanding of the irrational elements of his guilt. It may reveal distortions in his conscious thinking that need correction.

CPT Scott never told me, despite our continuing relationship long after he moved on to another military Post and to promotion as Major, that his Stryker Brigade was awarded the Valorous Unit Award for their 16 month tour in Iraq.

"I don't want to be seen as weak"

It is troubling when a patient is a "No-Show," someone who neither cancels their appointment nor shows up.

I had a "No-Show." Our electronic medical records permit physicians and other providers to review a Soldier's medical record of treatment, wherever it is offered, including in "theatre" (combat).

The "No-Show" was a patient whose PTSD symptoms were minimally responding to treatment.

I reviewed his medical record. Like many Soldiers with PTSD, he dreaded his perception of its negative implications for his military career. "I don't want to be seen as weak. A weak Soldier is not good for the Army. He is not good for his family. He is not good for himself."

Sadly, these perceptions are wide-spread, incorrect, and difficult to change. It is these misconceptions that keep an estimated fifty-percent of Soldiers with PTSD from seeking and accepting treatment.

I made a "T-con" or telephone conference call to the patient. "I'm fine, Sir," he said. "How are you?"

The Soldier had a conflicting appointment, had rescheduled, but his name had not been removed from my schedule.

"I just wanted to make sure you are okay," I said.

The Soldier thanked me for my "concern." He rescheduled.

"There are 3 Soldiers I hope you can see, Dr. Brown"

John White, a good social worker, is embedded in our ADC (Active Duty Clinic).

John, in his mid-forties, is a quiet bald man. His large, round forgiving blue eyes are the most remarkable feature of his closely shaved light complexioned kind face.

His medium height and weight, with his slow southern drawl, combined with his non-imposing manner, create a non-threating counselor, patiently waiting to listen, to help.

The Army is attempting to reach Soldiers who need but avoid behavioral health treatment by placing behavioral health specialists in non-behavioral health settings. For example, in our MTF (Military Treatment Facility) we have well-trained behavioral health specialists in TMC (Troop Medical Clinics or "Sick Call"), Primary Care Clinic and Active Duty Clinic.

The Department of Behavioral Health is located on the fifth floor of the hospital. The Troop Medical Clinics, the Primary Care Clinic and the Active Duty Clinic are located in other buildings or on other floors. Soldiers watch which floor is selected on the elevator. "Reputations are ruined if you are seen on the fifth floor," they mistakenly judge.

John knocked softly on my door.

"Do you have a few minutes, Dr. Brown, to discuss something?"

I like seeing patients. This is the second or third time John has recently come to my office. He usually comes to refer patients that have PTSD. He comes prepared, knowing what I am going to ask him.

"There are 3 Soldiers I hope you can see, Dr. Brown. I believe they all have PTSD. They have high PCL (Posttraumatic Check List) scores.

Of course, they are resistant to being referred to behavioral health.

I'm very concerned about one of the patients. He is married. He has 2 small children. His wife is going to leave him if does not get help. He loves his kids."

John's Patient

John continued.

"My Soldier cannot sleep unless he barricades himself in his bedroom."

I wondered if he slept alone.

"He bolts the bedroom door. His wife and 2 small children spend the night in the same room with him.

He places his dog on a mat in front of the bedroom door. He sees the dog as an early warning informant. If the dog barks, he will have time to protect himself and his family.

He really doesn't sleep that much. He gets up all through the night, checking doors and windows.

He is very irritable. His marriage is on the rocks.

He also makes the family have safety drills.

In one of the safety drills, he trains his family to cut their seat belt should they become trapped in an accident.

All this comes from his multiple combat deployments."

Seeing John's visible concern for this Soldier, I reached for my appointment book. "John," I said, "I can work him in this week."

To my surprise, John said his patient had not consented to be referred to Behavioral Health.

"I've seen him twice. Each time I tell him that we have a physician who specializes in seeing patients with issues from deployment. I will see him again next week. If he agrees, I will have him call the front desk to make an appointment with you."

I gave John my cell number. I asked John to have his patient call me directly, thinking sooner is better than later for me to see his patient.

Wednesday Morning Post-Deployment Psychotherapy Group

Sitting in a semi-circle, 8 Soldiers garbed in ACUs (Army Combat Uniforms), came to share their thoughts.

Beneath the red, white and blue American flag patch on the right shoulder, a combat unit patch identifies these Soldiers as American citizens who know war. These Soldiers were in the heat of the war in the face of terror in Iraq and Afghanistan.

All these Soldiers wear an unseen patch. The unseen patch stretches from their heart to their soul.

They come for fellowship. They come with questions. They come for relief from unimaginable, unacceptable memories.

They come looking for "the old me."

They search for peace of mind.

They come looking for a good night's sleep.

It's been said that money can buy a bed, but it can't buy sleep. What is the cost of refreshing sleep for Soldiers robbed of trust?

I sit in the center, facing the semi-circle of Soldiers, honored by their honesty.

Poncho Liner

"If you want to know how I sleep, Dr. Brown, ask Janet. She is the one beaten up during the night. I swear, as God is my witness, I never put my hands on her in anger when I'm awake.

Ask Janet. I'm serious. She said that I kick her, choke her and move almost constantly in my sleep. I've never really hurt her. I have no memory of it. Some mornings, she shows me a bruise and asks me where it came from. I have no idea, Sir."

MSG (Master Sergeant) Keith L. Johnson's fellow group members hold him in high regard. They listened closely.

"I take power naps. From 0330 to 0500, I sleep like I'm in a coma. I go to the latrine first and then I go into my power nap."

SFC (Sergeant First Class) Guy Goodson, knowing Keith can be a heavy drinker, said, "That's when Jack and Jim go home . . . Jack Daniel and Jim Beam."

The group laughed.

"Don't forget his friend, Johnny. He goes home about then, too. I'm talking about Johnny Walker."

More laughter.

I love it when these Soldiers laugh.

Keith smiled. "I know I shouldn't drink, Dr. Brown, but it is the only way I keep nightmares away."

Calculating the amount of alcohol he consumes from arriving home after work to bedtime, I estimated for the group that alcohol's well known destruction of sleep's normal architecture would be ending just about the time of his trip to the latrine and his power nap.

"I can take a power nap almost anytime if I can cover myself with my poncho liner. It's the one I slept on in Iraq. I would not give it up for anything."

To Sleep

Guy Goodson, a recovering alcoholic, bright, caring 37-year-old SFC (Sergeant First Class) said, "It takes me 2-3 or even 4 hours to fall asleep. I can't slow my brain down. I get a thought in my brain and it gets stuck there."

Wes Franklin, 30-year-old SSG (Staff Sergeant), previously seriously wounded in combat but deployed twice since then, has severe Sleep Apnea. A surprisingly large number of Soldiers return from combat with this condition. They usually snore loudly. They cease breathing momentarily many times during the night.

Wes said, "I asked my wife who took my mask (C-PAP) off in the middle of the night? She said, 'You did. I watched you take it off, unplug the cord, and put in the dresser drawer.'

I do not remember it. The mask helps me sleep better, but I can't keep it on all night."

John said, "I can't sleep unless it is dead quiet."

Kevin said, "I can't sleep if it is quiet. I've got to turn on a fan. I need something that reminds me of the generators running all night in Iraq."

"Will we ever get over PTSD?" Wes asked. "I feel I will always have it."

Keith said, "I feel I'm too far gone. I can smell a dead animal in the woods and directly flash back to Iraq."

Guy said, "The world looks different to me when I drive now. The roads change color. They look orange. I remember that MSR (Main Supply Route) Tampa (road from Kuwait to Mosul in Iraq) was colored orange from the sand storms."

Terry is a new group member. This is his second session. He is a tall, large, quiet, dark Soldier who is depressed.

Terry said, "I have to cover my head with a pillow but it won't drown out the noise. Every time I close my eyes to sleep I hear bombs. My nightmares are real. I wake up. I look like somebody has thrown a bucket of water on me . . . drenched in sweat . . . and a bad headache. The fear of dying stays with me all the time. It goes through my head every day.

You hear one mortar hit. Then they walk them in. You don't know where the next one will land.

I just got back from Afghanistan. We are told now to lay down when you hear mortars coming in. We have to lay face down. We are told not to run to bunkers. According to this new policy, you are less likely to be injured by the blast and less likely to be hit by shrapnel if you hit the ground."

The New Me

SFC Ronnie Marks is a light-skinned, medium size man of 37 who looks much younger. There is something kind and delicate about him. He is sensitive. He takes things seriously. He worries a lot.

Ronnie spoke sadly. "I'm close to my family. I went to the family reunion last weekend. I told my family that I come to group. I told them I have PTSD. As soon as they heard me say I have PTSD, they made me feel alienated . . . like an alien to my own family.

They kept changing the subject.

Damn. I thought my family had my back!"

"They don't want to hear it," Byron said. "They want the old you."

Ronnie replied. "Are they waiting for the old me to come back?"

Wes stated, "My wife said, 'one day you will snap out of it.' It gives her a glimmer of hope. She wants the old me back."

I said that people fear what they don't know. They are frightened by the bad news depicted in the media.

In philosophy, I said, there is the fallacy of generalization. It means the mistake of judging everybody in a large group by the conduct of the few.

"The 'new me,'" said Wes, "fears the loss of my own control. My wife said, 'Don't hold it in. Let it out.' I said, 'No, you don't want to see me like that.' I don't want to explode. Sometimes, I can actually see myself…in my mind…hurting somebody. I don't want to ever do that…I have never done that.

They told us when we deployed to switch on the new me and to switch it off when we redeployed. Who can do it? Who can operate the switch?

My daughter turned 7 in March. I've only been home for one of her birthdays."

What hurt me the most?

The 35-year-old, Hispanic, married Soldier frowned chronically.

"I kept everything inside from 2003 till 2009.

It felt like a heavy granite block was on my chest.

A friend told me that I would ruin my career if I did not get treatment for PTSD. He had been for help and he felt better.

I kept it all inside for 7 years.

I left for Iraq on Christmas day, 2002, on a super supply ship to Kuwait. It took 3 weeks.

It was the beginning of the war. We met unexpected resistance. It was carnage. It really hurts to think about it.

Do you know what hurt me the most?

My mother visited us last year.

She saw my pills. I had not told anyone.

My mother confronted me.

'What happened to you?'

I was in shock.

I couldn't say anything.

To me, I felt normal. I felt others were wrong...but she noticed.

My mother said, 'in the past, you used to be happy and care-free. Now you are cold-hearted.

Why are you not smiling? Why are you not happy?'

Finally, I answered her, 'I don't know. This thing consumes me. I always think someone is watching me. I am always on guard.'"

The Soldier was deeply entrenched in a painful anxious depression over his PTSD.

He did not need information about what had consumed him.

He needed a comforting relationship.

"When I talk with you," I said, "I feel like I'm on sacred ground."

Like all Soldiers to whom I have honestly spoken these words, his eyes locked into mine.

"You have put your life on the line for me. I am putting my reputation on the line for you.

Here is my card." In large numbers, I wrote my cell phone number and assured him of my willingness to be called by him whenever it is needed.

Together, we mapped out a treatment plan.

What hurts our country the most?

We have neglected to understand the psychological cost of postmodern war.

We are frightened of Soldiers with combat-induced Posttraumatic Stress Disorder because we are too lazy to become informed about it, too indifferent to their suffering.

Our Soldiers with PTSD do not want to alarm others.

Our Soldiers want to be accepted for who they are.

Our Soldiers do not want pity. They want respect.

I have had 12,500 patient encounters with Soldiers who been deployed to combat. Most of these Soldiers have been repeatedly deployed. Nearly every one of these Soldiers I have been privileged to treat suffers from PTSD.

Thankfully, to the best of my knowledge, not a single one of these Soldiers has committed a violent act since returning home from combat.

I estimate that at least one-half of the Soldiers needing treatment for PTSD never come in to receive treatment. In a very large way, I hold our nation responsible for this fear of treatment.

With good reason, many Soldiers perceive they will be ostracized by society as a whole and in particular by their own families should the dreaded diagnosis of PTSD befall them.

Is this another variation of the concocted fear of witchcraft?

Soldiers with PTSD can be healed by secure attachment to qualified listeners who want to understand them and are consistently available to them.

Soldiers need attachment. Our country needs enthusiasm to rid itself of the unwarranted fear of Soldiers with combat-induced PTSD.

The opposite of fear is love.

Love these Soldiers back to "the old self." You will find little else, as I have, more rewarding and more fulfilling.

No reasonable person can do otherwise upon reading these Soldiers' stories.

A Nation Sleeps

We can sleep in peace because our Army never sleeps.
This is a wake-up call to a nation that slumbers and sleeps, drowsy and forgetful about the psychological cost of 21st Century war.

It is a sad irony that our Soldiers with PTSD and TBI from combat cannot rest while our nation snoozes and sleeps.

Awake or asleep, our psychologically injured Soldiers remain on high alert, expecting the unexpected, convinced that terrorists are prepared to strike again and again at the very heart of our nation. No recent terrorist attack on our nation has come unexpectedly to these men and women.

Our Soldiers face death daily by indistinct enemies who devalue life, wallow triumphantly in American blood and lust for our complete and total destruction.

The nightmares of our Soldiers with PTSD are our nightmares as well.

Wake up, America, to the suffering of our Soldiers. Listen as I listen to our Soldiers. Listen for their sake. Listen for your sake. Listen for the sake of our nation.

2

THE BEST DECISIONS

I HAVE CHOSEN to capitalize the word "Soldier" throughout this book as a personal and literary salute to the men and women in our armed forces.

I join all thoughtful Americans in expressing our heart-felt gratitude to our Soldiers past, present and future, in all branches of military service.

In this way, I entirely agree with 35th Army Chief of Staff of the United States Army, Gen. Peter J. Schoomaker (Ret.), who on 23 DEC 2003, decreed that all command information products, including base newspapers, capitalize the word "soldier" from now on.

"The change gives Soldiers the respect and importance they've always deserved, especially now in their fight against global terrorism," stated in an October Directive from the Office of the Chief of Public Affairs, Department of the Army. May God Bless our Soldiers and their families!

Two Needs

Two needs existed. One need arose from a depth and strength of which I was not fully aware.

I had always wanted to be a doctor.

Since childhood, I had always wanted to be a Soldier.

Thankfully, both of those dreams have come true.

Buried deep in my sub-consciousness, however, mingled with dreams and hopes from my childhood, remaining unknown to me, was one of my greatest needs.

I needed to be a doctor to Soldiers.

An exciting, emotionally-stirring thought entered my mind.

Is there anything more important than to be a doctor to Soldiers during a time of war?

Once the answer to this question entered my awareness, little could have prevented me from taking the necessary steps to act upon it.

The second need was more distinct.

The Army needed doctors to care for the psychiatric problems of courageous, brave Soldiers, whose combat in 21st Century War came with emotional consequences.

Few would not argue that our Soldiers' psychiatric problems are multiplied by the unique features of 21st Century War, by its duration . . . and by the world-wide spread of terror.

We are fighting a largely hidden enemy. This disguised enemy fights passively and aggressively.

It inflicts its most deadly effects by unmanned, unmanly, cowardly IEDs (Improvised Explosive Devices). The IED is the unseen enemy's signature weapon.

Our enemy takes pride in its uncommon warfare, in its unthinkable methods of human destruction.

Their ideas are born in evil.

Deputizing women, children and even animals, the enemy fashions a mob of heartless suicide bombers.

A Certainty

It was a beautiful day in Charlottesville in May 2005, but I was restless, sitting in my office staring out the window, waiting between patients.

Is "restless" the right word for an internal, troublesome feeling?

My thoughts fell into an inspired need to change the direction of my life.

My patients would not have observed a physically restless person before them. However, in a fleeting unguarded moment, my patients may have detected and accurately sensed a Nano second of distraction.

How this could be?

In the words of the songwriter, "How could anyone ask for anything more?"

I was surrounded by the comforts of fulfillment, blessed with a loving wife, three sons and a daughter and four fine grandchildren.

I had a successful medical practice and a notable career at one of America's leading universities.

It was an easy walk from my home to my office.

Leaving Charlottesville

Most of my previous years had been spent in Charlottesville, never very far from the University of Virginia. I was privileged to be educated and trained in Psychiatry at the University. I was a Clinical Professor of Psychiatry and Neurobehavioral Sciences.

Earlier, I was a Professor of Education teaching Mental Health. My large classes, averaging 500 students each semester, were made up primarily of undergraduate students in the College of Arts and Sciences at the University of Virginia, best known, as it is referred to here, as "The University."

In addition to my family, most of my good friends lived and worked nearby. My physicians, dentist, banker and my church were all nestled in Charlottesville.

Thomas Jefferson loved Charlottesville and its surrounding region, one of nature's most blessed. The nearby foothills are comforting. The hazy, beautiful Blue Ridge Mountains are inviting during the green spring and snow-capped in winter. Many come here for many reasons. Few of us ever leave.

The opening of my psychiatric practice in 1971 was part of a life-long dream that came true in Charlottesville.

However, something difficult to describe was happening to me.

It was partially outside my screen of awareness. A deep cognitive and spiritual nagging mumbled wordlessly to me.

Leaving Friends

Routines build a strong sense of security. In looking back, much of my life had become routine. One of my favorite routines was meeting with friends to exercise.

Each day between noon and 1400, I'd race to U Hall, a nick-name for University Hall, which housed the University of Virginia Athletic Department. The locker room was filled by "the gifted and the great" of the University.

My locker was adjacent to Dr. Frank Finger's, a retired Professor of Psychology, and a physically fit man in his 80s and a model for us all because he worked out daily. He was a highly successful competitive athlete.

Dennis Womack's locker was on the opposite wall. Dennis was the University of Virginia baseball coach for 26 years. He was the first to win the highly coveted ACC (Atlantic Coast Conference) Baseball Championship.

I never met a more humble or superb man than Dennis. A quiet man with a strong southern drawl, he recruited fine athletes. Many of the players he coached later played in major league baseball.

David Ibbeken's locker was to the right of mine. Dave, Director of Development, School of Law, University of Virginia, was the first in his profession to have a University of Virginia Chair named in his honor. A former college football star, Dave, a Princeton graduate, is an articulate diplomat.

Dennis, Dave and I met on the football practice field for our combination work-out and symposium.

It was a time of great fellowship.

Early in his career, Dave had been an assistant football coach at Virginia and later announced the football games on the radio.

Naturally we discussed wide-ranging topics from poor officiating to disturbing world events.

We left no problem without a thoughtful solution.

It was refreshing to hear their opinions on psychiatric issues while I sallied forth on sports and the law. None of us ever acknowledged we were out of our field of expertise.

We enjoyed rubbing elbows with the coaches, all good men, all caring and responsible people.

How much these workouts meant to me I didn't realize until they ended. It was painful, to say the least.

I wanted to help

No man was more blessed than I was on that morning in May 2005.

The lush, aromatic Charlottesville spring was like an English country garden.

The visibility was so clear it seemed I could reach out and touch the distant mountains.

It reminded me of Edith Hamilton's book on Greece in which she explained that sculpture more than painting took root in ancient Greece largely because of its crystal clear atmosphere.

America was beginning its third year of 21st Century War in Iraq. We had bogged down in Afghanistan. The nation was anxious for an end to terror as well as the war.

The previously wordless cause of my restlessness now became articulate.

I wanted to help Soldiers fighting in 21st Century War.

Getting Hired

Without sharing my thoughts with my Dottie, my dear wife, I picked up the phone between patients and called an Active Duty Army

Post where I had previously served as Assistant Chief of Psychiatry during Operation Desert Storm and Desert Shield in 1991.

I was connected by phone to Dr. Eleanor Gagon, previously unknown to me but someone I soon came to respect and admire. Dr. Gagon was Chief of the Department of Behavioral Health.

"Do you need another psychiatrist?" I asked with an undeniable begging tone in my voice.

"We do need another psychiatrist, but we don't have a slot for one right now. I am the only psychiatrist here, along with Jason, a psychologist. We pretty much run the clinic and it is rapidly becoming nearly overwhelming."

Dr. Gagon reviewed my CV (Curriculum Vitae summarizing my education, training and experience). She set up an appointment for me to meet with her and LTC Kevin Smith, Deputy Commander for Clinical Services.

LTC Smith, a family physician, was a former military pilot. This young energetic bachelor was both a good doctor and a great administrator. He supported my application.

The hiring process took four months, but I was employed on 21 SEP 2005 as a staff psychiatrist. My patients would be active duty Soldiers directly involved in the Global War on Terror (GWOT), as it was called at that time.

Leaving my patients

It was not easy to terminate my relationships with my patients in Charlottesville, some of whom I had been treating for years.

Remarkably, without exception, all my patients understood my "calling" to help Soldiers whose lives had been transformed by the emotional horrors of terrorism.

Initially, I began my contract position with the Army on a part-time basis, three days weekly, leaving three days in Charlottesville for my patients.

Over the following several months, I found good psychiatrists in Charlottesville willing to take my patients. I also made myself available to my patients until the transfer of their care was complete.

In most cases, it was a mutually sad goodbye. Soon thereafter, I became a full-time psychiatrist for the Department of Defense.

My Beloved Wife, Dottie

The closing of my practice in Charlottesville may have been more difficult for Dottie than I had considered at the time. Dottie, as my former secretary, had developed a special relationship with my patients.

Dottie had been my secretary for many years. She knew my patients well.

After the office was closed, from time to time she would unexpectedly meet our former patients in a grocery store or on the mall. They would warmly exchange greetings and the news.

Later Dottie always conveyed to me the pleasure of these encounters with our former patients.

For years, Dottie had greeted my patients, taken their phone calls, and when called upon, she had given them words of encouragement at the end of their therapy session with me.

In addition, once I had taken up residence in a city distant from Charlottesville but close to the Army post, she prepared delicious and nutritious meals for each week. She packed my meals and I transported them back to the Army post in a cooler and a cardboard box.

I returned to Charlottesville each weekend for 48 hours at home.

Dottie, sensing protection from the three of our four children residing nearby, faithfully conducted the affairs of the household. She cared for Rosie, our spirited white West Highland Terrier, joined a book club, and, when possible, she joined me in my rented quarters away from home.

"Momma Brown"

It was a drive of several hours from Charlottesville to the Army post.

Soon Dottie was known by my Soldiers as "Momma Brown, the kind lady that makes and brings homemade vegetarian chili and velveteen cake," a treat after group therapy.

She is a very special person, always upbeat and cheerful, whose extraordinarily kind smile is contagious.

Now, 9 years after the decision to treat Soldiers was made, I asked Dottie how she felt about it.

"Looking back, it was a noble thing you wanted to do. You had been in the Army Reserve. You had a special feeling about it.

I never thought it was the wrong thing to do.

You had an affinity for the Army in the past.

It seemed like a natural transition.

You wanted to do something for the country.

It was never a question in my mind about changing your career. I knew you would be sensitive to your patients.

I always supported you. You have always provided for us."

How blessed I am to have a wife who loves me as I love her.

She rolled up her emotional sleeves, got into the trenches with me and the Soldiers, and from the first day, she became an irreplaceable team member.

Literally, I have no meal Dottie has not prepared. I wear no clothes Dottie has not washed or sent to the cleaners. I have no important encounter with a Soldier I do not share with her.

From the Soldiers to the hospital commander, Dottie's home-made vegetarian chili is tastily enjoyed and highly praised.

Each evening on the phone, we review our day. She is my counselor. Her wisdom helps get me out of tight spots of which there has been no scarcity.

I am soothed by Dottie's encouragement.

Last February, we celebrated our 60th wedding anniversary.

I look lovingly at a photograph of Dottie in her wedding gown. It was taken on the day of our marriage. It is readily visible from my desk just as she is readily visible to me in all that I do.

The best decision

As I reflect on the restlessness that led me to join the Civilian Army Medical Corps, I began to realize what it required of my wife, my family, and my patients. However, "there never was heard a discouraging word...." In real terms, it was overwhelmingly just the opposite. In Biblical terms, it was "as far as the east is from the west."

I was not the least discouraged by anyone.

I was mightily encouraged, thanked, supported, and esteemed far beyond that which anyone deserves who answers a call from one's heart.

Never, not for a second, have I considered my decision to join the Army's medical team was anything but the best. It was one of the most important decisions of my long life.

To the degree that it resulted in change and hardship for others, I am sincerely sorry.

Indeed, I am most thankful for their willing readiness to aid and support my action.

My close friend, John Sanderson, is a retired University of Virginia professor and long-standing Educational Consultant to the JAG (Judge Advocate General) School in Charlottesville.

John and Nancy, his good wife, are our favorite breakfast partners at the Boars Head Inn Porch.

John and Nancy is a couple we most admire.

Upon hearing of my determination to leave Charlottesville, John said to Nancy, "It's a shame Bob won't have much time now to enjoy his recently remodeled house, but he seems so happy."

Imagine the joy

Everything in our past prepares us for some great challenge, some great opportunity, some special calling and some rewarding fulfillment.

Most often, I believe, that preparation is to selflessly relieve the pain and suffering of others.

Our special preparation includes all our relationships, every moment of happiness, and every disappointment.

It is richly compelling when one is able to sense that special moment in time and to act upon it.

Validation of such a decision by others is unnecessary.

I imagine the joy is like the joy of inventors, explorers, and scientists when a goal is achieved. Certainly, it is not the end; difficulties lie ahead but a turning point is reached, a new direction is set and determination is as clearly focused as the vision of a blind person whose sight is restored by a skillful surgeon.

It was my very good fortune in the spring of 2005 to perceive a calling to provide medical care at an active duty post for Soldiers returning from combat in Iraq and Afghanistan.

No other experience in my career as a psychiatrist, forensic psychiatrist, psychologist, educator and an athlete has been more challenging.

No other experience has at the same time been more emotionally rewarding than entering into the suffering of Soldiers.

Today, our Soldiers deserve respect, yet seldom do they receive the appreciation they deserve.

In deepest humility I sense and I appreciate their acceptance. Mind to mind and soul to soul, I am honored to walk back with them into undaunted hopefulness of a flourishing life.

Recently, one of our good friends, quoting from a Catholic prayer written in 1905, explained my work with Soldiers in these enlightening, most tender, and accurate words: "Your heart has been pierced with the same sword of sorrow that has pierced the heart of our Soldiers."

At last, I know what this book is meant to be. This book is intended to help our nation learn to love our Soldiers as I have learned to love them by hearing their stories and sharing their suffering.

My story is intended to demonstrate how my heart was prepared to hear these precious stories and to guide the Soldiers to the real value of what they have selflessly sacrificed for our nation.

If I succeed, the reader's heart will also be pierced with the same sword of sorrow that has pierced the heart of our Soldiers. Pride and thanksgiving for our Soldiers will lessen the sorrow.

Purpose

In the words of one very brave Soldier, MSG (Master Sergeant) Keith L. Johnson, about whom more will be written: "War is easy; coming home is Hell." It is my intention, in the pages that follow, to prove the validity and reliability of his astonishing assertion.

My hope is to help enlighten the public about the life of the men and women, who volunteered to enlist in the US Army, were deployed to combat and struggle to return to a "normal life" after war.

We need to be reminded that our Soldiers serve wherever they are needed at whatever risk is required, and leave their families as often and for as long as the mission demands.

<u>Sacred Ground</u> is predominantly about the Soldiers I have come to know. It is about the persisting impact of their combat experience in Iraq and Afghanistan.

Their stories are told in their own words, either directly quoted or closely paraphrased.

A small number of US Marines were available and their stories are just as gripping, inspiring and informative as those of our Soldiers.

It is of interest that combat itself is often minimized in importance by our Soldiers. It is a contrast to the enormity of their challenge of adapting and acclimating to coming home from combat.

Too often our Soldiers are described by their family and friends as "changed persons," upon entering their home town doors.

Interestingly, these brave Soldiers rarely consciously acknowledge these subtle changes. Our combat Soldiers are forged and refined in the hottest furnaces, the furnaces of war.

Coming Home "Changed"

No one in combat is unaffected by its horror.

The inhumanity of terrorism is carefully designed to terrify its victims, eradicate its opponents and devalue and destroy all human life but its own.

Decent people are unprepared for what our Soldiers are expected to confront.

Our Soldiers, eye-witnesses of the devastation intended by terrorists to spread like an epidemic more toxic than the plague, come home schooled in a new appreciation of danger.

The skills acquired and exercised by Soldiers in combat become life-saving. In a word, these skills require constant threat-assessments and appropriate responses to their perceived danger.

Survival of Soldiers in combat against terrorists increases when they learn to expect the unexpected, a continual challenge often shared with a trusted battle buddy.

This survival skill, and others related to it, becomes as natural as sneezing.

Soldiers don't stop sneezing when they come home from combat.

Soldiers don't rid themselves of combat survival skills when they come home.

Persistence of the primary survival skills of combat forms the core symptoms of PTSD (Posttraumatic Stress Disorder).

"The song is ended but the melody lingers on," was a popular song in World War II. Of course, PTSD is nothing to sing about, until it is understood and conquered, but the old song conveys the message: "The deployment is ended but the danger lingers on."

How fitting to combat, yet how unfitting to redeployment (coming home) are all the thoughts and feelings of combat!

How dangerous it must feel to be alone in perceived danger without the protection of your battle buddy!

How anxious it must be to no longer have your weapon!

How naked, vulnerable and helpless Soldiers must feel at home where they still experience the presence of danger to their family and danger to themselves.

The Lost Self: What makes a person a person?

In <u>An Essay Concerning Human Understanding</u>, 1690, John Locke used the "Prince and Cobbler" to show the influence of experience.

"For should the soul of a prince, carrying with it the consciousness of the prince's past life, enter and inform the body of a cobbler, as soon as deserted by his own soul, everyone sees he would be the same person with the prince, accountable only for the prince's actions: but who would say it was the same man?"

Who would say the Soldier returning home from 21st Century War is the same man who left home 12-15 months earlier?

He or she may look the same, but will he or she be the same person?

Locke's notion may help explain the exchange of the Soldier's self before combat, with the self following combat.

The changes wrought by combat, to varying degrees, when perceived by the Soldier, are a sense of loss.

Some Soldiers refer to the change as a "loss of innocence," the sense that draws them to their youngest child, "the most innocent person I know and love."

Some Soldiers refer to the change as a "loss of my spirit."

Other Soldiers report the change as a "loss of part of myself."

Many Soldiers, unaware of the change, are surprised when told they are "different."

The application of Locke's insights sheds light on the question, what makes a person a person. "Consciousness is the awareness of one's thoughts and actions."

The simple truth of Locke's Prince and Cobbler story is that a person is the culmination and accumulation of one's experiences. The memory of one's experiences, churning every waking moment with the environment, influences one's sense of oneself and one's sense of others.

Emotional and sensory memories of combatting terrorists, in PTSD, trump all other memories. The soul of the combatant enters the soul of the redeployed.

The exchange of souls may occur instantaneously when it is caused by an unbearable trauma. More commonly, it occurs gradually. Like radiation, exposure to combat trauma has an accumulative effect.

Loss is often followed by grief, a painful emotion, one that Soldiers attempt to avoid, failing to know how to grieve.

When Soldiers lose the sense of themselves in combat, depression is difficult to escape.

Many Soldiers are grieving for the loss of who they were. Most are unaware of their state, only unhappy.

Some are stuck in the terrible, anger stage of grief.

Lost Time

"Who am I?" a Soldier asked the Tuesday Morning Post-Deployment Group.

"That's the question we are all asking about ourselves," was the sincere reply he received.

"When I was the First Sergeant, I went from point A to point B.

My job was to keep my company moving. I worked long hours, but I didn't mind. I took care of Soldiers. I gave orders and Soldiers followed my orders.

Now I'm home. I'm retiring. It is the toughest job in my life. I'm trying to hide my PTSD from my family.

When I was the First Sergeant, I knew who I was. Now I have nothing that tells me who I am.

I was driving my 16-year-old son to soccer practice. He spoke to me disrespectfully.

I stopped the car in the middle of the road. I told him he couldn't talk to me that way.

He could have said, 'Where were you when I was growing up? You can't come home and start acting like a dad.'

He could have said it. It is the truth. That's what I was thinking.

He said nothing.

It hurt.

It hurt real bad.

It hurt because he is a better kid than I am a father.

It hurt because all those 12-14 hour days I worked for all those years have no meaning now.

I am a stranger in my own home, resented and unappreciated.

Everybody hates me because I neglected everybody."

The group responded with silence.

Each Soldier in the group wondered to himself, "Have I neglected the people I love?"

The First Sergeant continued.

"I guess I've answered my own question.

Who am I?

I'm a stranger to my family.

I'm a stranger to myself."

"I don't know why I keep writing May 5th instead of August 5th."

It was a beautiful Monday morning in Charlottesville. The rain had stopped. The bright sun felt good.

I was waiting my turn in the Anesthesia lobby for blood tests at the University hospital. At least 30 or 40 patients, somber and anxious like me, were waiting to have their blood drawn, all facing surgery.

The staff treated everyone with kindness and respect.

In spite of continuous activity between patients, nurses, receptionists, in person and on the phone, there was a hush all about the large room filled with patients in chairs and on love seats.

"Mr. Brown," a thin, middle aged woman with bronze-framed eyeglasses and auburn-colored hair, called out.

Following her into the lab area, I took a seat in a grey plastic covered adjustable chair.

"Tell me your full name, all of it, and spell it for me, please, Mr. Brown. Good. Now tell me your date of birth."

I always add that I was born at 10 AM. Usually, I get a smile from the inquirer. It was not the case today.

She showed me the labels bearing more information about my identity than I am aware of. It was me, I agreed. The labels were attached to tubes with several different color rubber stoppers.

No motion was wasted. Speaking while working, almost incidentally or to herself, she said, "I don't know why I keep writing May 5th instead of August 5th."

"Do you have a special reason," I asked, "to have May 5th on your mind?"

The lab tech suddenly looked up at me. It was the first time our faces met. Curiosity and mild amazement described her eyes.

"That was my son's 25th birthday. Isn't that interesting that you would ask me about May?"

"What does your son do for a living?" I asked.

"My son is in the Army," she replied. Instead of the pride I expected her to express about her son's service to the country, she busily attended to her task and said no more.

"I think it is wonderful your son is a Soldier. Where is he stationed?"

"He's in Texas now, taking a class, but he is stationed in Hawaii. He is working in Intelligence."

Not wanting to distract her, but wishing to know about how the Soldier's life was going, I said, "Has your son been deployed?"

Before the lab tech replied, she carefully removed the needle from my left arm, inverted the purple top test tube several times, placed a bandage over the puncture site, appeared relieved and then said, "My son has that PT-something. I can't say the word right but you know what I mean.

People in this country are complaining about being spied on. We need to know what the enemy is planning. There is an attack on this country every day. We are just not told about it."

More animated now, she said her son had been sent to Afghanistan and has "horrible nightmares."

"He would get up in the middle of the night screaming, running through the house, not knowing what he was doing.

Then something strange happened.

He went to a pet shop to buy food for his pet rats.

There was a man with puppies to give away in front of the pet shop.

One of the puppies looked exactly like the dog my son had as child. He could hardly believe it, and it was free.

He took the dog home and takes care of it.

Do you know, Mr. Brown, since my son got the dog, he sleeps like a baby? The nightmares have gone away. Can you explain that?"

I explained my work, my dedication to Soldiers and my strongest wishes for the continual good health of her son. I confided having seen similar improvement in Soldiers with PTSD who care for a dog.

"Combat trauma can build walls that block out pleasant memories from the past," I said. "Your son's pet dog has opened a door to good memories from his childhood.

Good childhood memories can help weaken the grip of the painful memories of combat.

Even dogs can tell if they are liked. Your son loves his dog and his dog knows it.

Your son's dog loves your son. Your son feels valued, feels loved by his dog.

Sadly, many people know too little about the effects of combat on Soldiers. Lacking understanding, too many people feel uneasy around Soldiers with PTSD.

Combat may cause Soldiers to become sensitive to the feelings of others toward them.

Soldiers often try to avoid people. They do not want to be judged.

They don't want to be rejected.

It is upsetting when others are uneasy, indifferent or critical of them.

I know you will learn all you can about PTSD. Add that knowledge to the love you already have for your son, and he will continue to get better and better.

Thank you for sharing this wonderful story about your son.

I am glad you kept writing May 5th instead of August 5th."

"I don't believe in co-incidence," the Soldier's mother said.

"You were sent here to answer my questions. God bless you, Mr. Brown."

Longing for the past while dreading the future

In some important ways, our Soldiers become new, different, potentially even better persons.

Soldiers need help identifying their grief over their losses. Often, they have lost more than their sense of who they were before combating terrorism. This is a difficult but essential task.

As a nation, a superficial understanding of their sacrifices is not enough.

We need to more fully appreciate our military, remembering the sacrifices made by them and their families, day and night, to assure our safety and freedom.

One way to achieve these objectives is to share some of the experiences of these remarkable people.

The information about which I write is not easily obtained.

Soldiers are taciturn, reticent to disclose their inner thoughts and feelings.

Soldiers fear that expressing feelings is a "sign of weakness." They try to keep it all in. This common view too often deters Soldiers from accepting badly needed treatment.

The public, learning about Soldiers, also needs to know the story teller, his background, his biases, his experiences, and his deeply felt need to work with Soldiers who have deployed in combat.

Writing has not been easy. I often cried while reading passages to my wife, re-experiencing encounters with Soldiers I have come to admire and respect.

For the past nine years, I have resided in rental property of all types near the active duty military post where I am employed as a Staff Psychiatrist. My home is more than 100 miles away from my work.

The forty-eight hour weekends at home are spent with loving support from my wife, children, and grandchildren. If there were an exception, then it was from my five year old great granddaughter who appears to prefer Hershey's Kisses to my own.

If there is anything more deeply rewarding than combating terrorism's psychological effects on our Soldiers, and indirectly on the family of Soldiers, I have yet to learn about it.

Therefore, I frame the remarkable story of our heroic Soldiers in the context of remembering my own life. I feel strongly that I could have chosen no path more fitting than being a doctor to Soldiers.

I have embarked on no mission more important than telling their story to a nation needing to understand and to engage in the healing of our combat Soldiers.

Getting a Job Description

In 2005, I was asked to develop an evaluation and treatment program for Soldiers redeploying from combat with PTSD (Posttraumatic Stress Disorder).

I conducted diagnostic examinations and provided individual and group psychotherapy for these Soldiers. The individual and group psychotherapy I provide is based on CBT (Cognitive Behavioral Therapy).

CBT was developed by Dr. Aaron Beck who was a psychiatrist at the University of Pennsylvania before he retired to join his daughter, Dr. Judith Beck, a clinical psychologist, at the Beck Institute in Philadelphia.

Since 2005, I have conducted approximately 12,500 doctor-patient encounters with these Soldiers.

In many cases, in the presence of the Soldier, I have also interviewed the Soldier's spouse. This is an invaluable resource in probing the depths of suffering for which the words of the Soldier alone are inadequate.

Names and other identifying information about the Soldiers have been removed. Any similarity between the characters in the stories told here and actual people is wholly unintended.

Soldiers strongly believe that their trauma narratives are precious. Their trauma becomes the core of their new identity. Their combat trauma memories are tightly guarded.

Protecting the identity of Soldiers under my care is important. I respect them as people. I respect their right to privacy.

Several Soldiers edited the manuscript, looking for factual errors and for unintentional personal identification of individual Soldiers.

No significant errors of fact were found.

The reader will appreciate the thin line separating the need to inform the public and the need to protect the rights of Soldiers. No policy of the US Army, the institution for which the author has great respect, has been dishonored.

Method

Based upon my interactions with Soldiers and their spouses, this narrative is not intended to be academic, technical, perplexing, complicated, or a self-help book.

It includes no exhaustive review of the scientific literature.

The subject matter is the American Soldier subjected to the effects of terrorism in Iraq and Afghanistan during the first thirteen years or more of the 21st Century.

My enviable position as Staff Psychiatrist at a large Army Post, from 2005 to the present, provides a unique opportunity to have a long, intense, and emotionally rewarding experience with our Soldiers.

I have been permitted to know, admire, and respect our Soldiers, the most wonderful people in the world.

I learned to know them by permitting them to get to know me as a person whose behavior they could come to predict.

I intentionally satisfied their need to be treated consistently.

It may sound silly, but I stuck to their unspoken first rule of conduct: "no surprises."

I wear a navy blue blazer, shirt and tie, every day. I usually have a bottle of purified water and a cup of Twining's' Irish Breakfast Tea within easy reach on my desk.

I am attentive. Interruptions are minimized.

I often feel there is no place on earth I'd rather be than with our Soldiers.

Often, I made hand written verbatim notes. Sometimes I read back to the Soldier exactly what he or she had just said to me.

It let them know I was listening. It let them hear how they sounded.

For many Soldiers, it was the first time they heard their own thoughts out loud as I read them their script.

It was too often the first time their thoughts took on meaning and significance to someone who wanted to hear them.

Most important of all, it was the first time their thoughts about what they had endured in combat had ever found the courage to be uttered.

These are precious moments.

Tear-streaked faces often revealed the start of emotional cleansing.

It often led me to tell the Soldier that I feel I am on sacred ground while talking with him or her.

A long silence inevitably follows my revelation.

The Soldier stares into my eyes and through my eyes, into my soul.

It is the stare of recognition.

It is analogous to the "smile of recognition," in Object Relations Theory, in which the infant first recognizes the mothering person.

The smile of recognition launches the all-important stage of "Normal Symbiosis," a critical stage in the psychological birth of the child. It is evidence of the first human attachment.

It is also a critical stage in the Soldier's development of trust in me.

"Here is my professional card," I say in these special meetings of the mind.

"I am writing my cell phone number on the back of my card for you.

You put your life on the line for me. I want to put myself and my professional skills on the line for you.

Please call me between sessions or whenever you need me."

The psychological birth of a child begins with the "smile of recognition." It occurs when the infant, staring into the eyes of the mothering person, establishes its first attachment with another human being.

Through this attachment, the infant acquires love, nurture, trust, and the capacity to become a fully functioning, independent person. Its survival depends upon the attachment.

It is during this early stage that the infant acquires cognitive and emotional nourishment that contributes to later stability and sense of security.

This stage of psychological birth may be compared to fueling a rocket, preparing it for launching from its launching pad into interplanetary space.

The mothering person is fueling the infant with memories of warmth and security, preparing it for the final two phases, separation and individuation.

Consistency, sameness or invariance is essential for the successful completion of the normal, mutually beneficial early stage of development of the sense of self.

Every important relationship may begin with a "smile of recognition" or its equivalent.

The therapeutic relationship that I experience with Soldiers begins, I believe, with their visual response to my nurturing posture, consistency and non-judgmental stance.

My cell phone number becomes a transitional object, not unlike a child's teddy bear or other object that attaches us in a doctor-patient relationship.

Later in the therapy, I remain digitally attached to my patients through a series of DVDs and CDs in which I appear as their educator on matters of PTSD and its commonly related comorbidities.

Post-Deployment weekly group therapy sessions provide a smooth transition from the earliest stage of attachment between me and my patient.

The "separation" and the final or "individuation" stage of psychological rebirth of the Soldier is a slow process. The attachment between Soldiers in group therapy has a lasting quality.

Soldiers strengthened, first through attachment to the therapist and then to each other, are prepared to return to a flourishing life with meaningful relationships.

I have drawn from two complex psychoanalytic theories, "Object Relations" and "Attachment Theory." However, they are not the focus of this work, merely explanations that inform my approach to the care of traumatized Soldiers.

More may be said about this approach to combat-induced Posttraumatic Stress Disorder at a later point when DOD and VA-approved treatment methods are discussed.

One last, but maybe the most important, methodical fact is the function of my notes that are written during individual and group therapy sessions.

The notes are all written in the exact words of the Soldiers. On the average, I write at least 15-20 pages of verbatim notes each week, sometimes up to 50 pages.

The notes help me understand the suffering caused by PTSD. Notes read aloud help the Soldier understand him or herself. The ultimate goal is to tell the Soldiers' stories in their own words.

The words of Soldiers made me stop and listen.

The words of Soldiers will make the reader stop and want to understand.

The psychological cost of 21st Century War is seen in the faces of Soldiers and in the lives of their families.

When America understands the psychological cost of combat, it will have greater respect for our Soldiers. In a word, America will love them as much as I have come to love them.

The Army Chief of Staff

On October 23, 2012, General Raymond T. Odierno, in his Eisenhower Speech to the AUSA Conference, made these statements:

"Entering into our 12th consecutive year of war, approximately 1.5 million Soldiers have served in Iraq and Afghanistan, and a large majority of their leaders have served multiple times.

These young men and women have earned nearly 16,000 Medals of Valor to include 6 Medals of Honor, 26 Distinguished Service Crosses, and 660 Silver Stars, and these numbers continue to grow.

The Soldiers who have earned these medals for bravery, courage, and selfless service have told me, with striking humility that "they were just doing their job. They did what any Soldier would have done." That the medal they received represents and honors those who have served beside them. That is what our Army is all about. That is why I love to serve in this great Army of ours."

Small Feet Make a Large Difference

He sat quietly in a chair, near the door, surrounded in a semicircle by seven battle buddies in group therapy for PTSD (Posttraumatic Stress Disorder).

His back was to the wall.

His Army Combat Uniform pant legs were tucked tightly into his stained tan Army boots.

His pale face's grim expression recalled his recent Afghanistan deployment.

Up close he witnessed the death of two innocent Afghan children.

What struck me the most was just how small his feet are, at most size 6 or 7.

I wondered how those small feet walked around unclad in slippers in the dark of his cold bedroom this morning when he got up at 0400, put on his Army green socks and, as his last step in dressing for the day, slid his small feet into his boots.

If I could engage his boots in a meaningful discussion, then I would know exactly what he saw, smelled, touched, heard, and tasted in combat.

I would still not know what his mind perceived and what meaning he gave to all that his boot-clad small feet weathered in a "war" in which there are few victories and little to celebrate.

No war is painless or its memories uncostly.

In many ways, our 21st Century War has the most devastating effects on our Soldiers of all wars since the beginning of human conflict.

Now it is our job together to help him, this giant with small feet.

We need to help him rediscover the courage his tasks required, and how he repeatedly met and surpassed those requirements.

We need to help him believe, by understanding the effects of the complexity of combat trauma, that he can and he will become the hero of his own life.

Most important to the recovery of these Soldiers psychologically injured in action is an informed public.

We need to thoughtfully reflect on the protracted course of healing of these incomparably silent sufferers.

We must make them the heroes of our life.

They will heal, they will succeed, and they will find meaningfulness when they know that we, the American people in all our multiplicity, are one nation under God who is with them and for them.

3

WAR ON MOTHERS

The Brown Compound

I WAS BORN ON 11 JUL 1931 in the Norfolk General Hospital, Norfolk, Virginia, courtesy of the Department of Public Welfare. I was a typical "depression baby."

My mother, Johnny Louise Beale Brown, was born in Isle of Wight County, Virginia, 30 DEC 1898. My father, George Stanley Brown, was born in Norfolk, 10 JUL 1892. I was their sixth and last child.

I can't imagine that my arrival was a happy occasion. It was a muggy, hot day, well before air conditioning was within our imagination.

My father lacked the advantages of literacy. He worked when work was available on the construction of Foreman Field for the WPA. The WPA was a federally funded jobs program, unkindly denounced as "We Poke Along."

Additional demands on the limited rations around the Brown dinner table could not have been realistically welcomed. I was a college student before I learned that Campbell's Pork and Beans was not a thin soup with a few beans. Nonetheless, it still remains my preference to any other presentation of this, the most frequently enjoyed meal for supper during my early childhood.

Electric fans hummed away in vain attempts to cool down things in the homes of those who could afford the electric bill. I was a half-grown child before I saw an electric fan, an old black one, swirling stale air in the small house at 1231 West 47th Street, Norfolk, Virginia. This is where I resided for the first decade of my life.

I had a strong mother and a pipe smoking, intimidated father who was kind to me but emotionally unavailable. Randolph, an older brother ten years my senior, and Edith, a jitter bugging sister, 8 years my senior, also lived with us.

Christine, my oldest sister, lived next door with her husband Frank and their young son, Frankie, ten years my junior.

Frances, my second oldest sister, lived one street away with her husband Tommy and their infant son, Tommy, junior.

My two oldest sisters, Christine and Frances, had abusive husbands who often caused them to return to live in our household, along with their children.

George, Jr., the first of the Brown children, died of "pneumonia" in his infancy.

My Mother's Strength

Had it not been for the strength of my mother, my childhood and family life would, without a doubt, have been chaotic, hectic, and tumultuous. Principally, however, because of my mother, I felt loved, protected, encouraged, and safe, most of my childhood.

My mother's strength was evident in her will. She was a determined person. Her moral character was unblemished.

As a young child, I was permitted to select the switch from a wild cherry tree growing in our back yard. She used it like a lumber-jack on my legs and back to correct my misconduct. My tearful pleading for mercy was unacknowledged. Without exception, however, my post-switching conduct was impeccable for weeks. I always felt cleansed after a whipping.

My childhood offenses, wrongdoings, and transgressions increased, however, with my physical development.

I cannot recall the exact time in my young life when my privilege of choosing the instrument to be used for my correction was revoked. I vividly remember the dread, however, each time the leather belt, taken from its hanging place on the wall in the kitchen, left its red welts on my back.

My mother's strength of character was matched, even surpassed, by her physical strength.

I am told that the unafraid face the firing squad without a handkerchief. Imagine its extreme opposite in the case of my deportment facing my mother, leather belt in her right hand. To a flood of tears begging not to be beaten was added shrill, loud screaming with each blow to my body.

I remember that my father would quietly ask my mother to stop. I don't know that she counted the licks to match the crime, but the ritual went uninterrupted.

I hasten to inject, however, that my mother was as determined in loving as she was in punishing. I was never left in doubt about how she felt.

It is odd, looking back, that I cannot recall any of the reasons for which I was beaten with a belt. Vaguely I recall a whipping that followed my disobedience coupled with melting dry ice in a glass of water and drinking the sputtering concoction. Neither mother nor child knew its dangers, if any, but it frightened my mother.

Some of my discipline was remarkably like that Rousseau described for his son, Emile, in the 18th Century. I know of no access my mother could have had to his writings. In fact, I don't believe there were books of any kind in my home before the Bible.

Rousseau, for example, said in his chapter on the Spoiled Child, if Emile broke out the window above his bed it would remain unrepaired throughout the year. Emile would learn the natural consequences of his behavior.

Playing with Matches

I was caught playing with matches in the wood shed on 47th street. Fitting the punishment to the crime, endorsing Rousseau's natural consequences philosophy, I was tied with rope to the inside wall of the wood shed. Believe me, this I retained in my memory bank like a nightmare, never forgotten.

My hands were tied behind me and my feet were tied together.

I was bound in some ingenious way with my back to the wall.

My mother put newspapers under the brown shoes that covered my white socks.

Randomly, mother starting lighting matches all the while shouting, "This will teach you not to play with matches."

Soon the newspapers were on fire.

I screamed for help as loud as a 5-year-old frightened little boy in short, brown pants could yell, believing he was being burned at the stake.

My mother stomped out the burning newspaper. She untied me. I never played with matches again.

When traumatized, you may ask, do children get PTSD. "Dr. Brown, did you get PTSD as a child from the punishment you received for playing with matches?"

I did not get PTSD from the punishment my mother meted out to me, and here is why: the meaning I gave to the experience determined its effect upon me. I had a secure attachment to my mother. I trusted her. I never doubted that my mother wanted the best for me. She was the master sculptor of the most formative years of my life. When my punishment ended, I did not feel abused. I felt relieved. I did not have nightmares. I felt corrected. I learned about the danger of playing thoughtlessly with matches.

Even ghosts obeyed her commands

My mother convinced me in my childhood that she communicated with "spirits," also referred to as "ghosts." She could command their presence, calling them into a room to which they entered through a keyhole.

Happily, I never saw the ghosts, but I realistically felt their presence and feared them. One of her brothers, she certified, had seen a ghost while locked in a closet for "his own good." It was said by my mother to be a pedagogically sound way to learn.

If her pedagogic theory was correct, it may have accounted for knowledge I could have acquired nowhere other than in the dark, claustrophobic, locked closet under the stairway.

Thankfully, I recall only the merest details.

The most accurate comparison that comes to mind, all these years later, is the emotional equivalent of "waterboarding." It was done with a sound purpose in mind. It was done by a person who believed in its effectiveness. It was acceptable at the time it was used.

I feel twinges of betrayal of my mother as I make these entries in the record of my life. No intention could be further from my mind. She was a bold, creative, inventive, and loving mother. Her love and discipline made me the person I became.

Tension in the Family

Tension between dad and my brother Randolph and between mom and my sister Edith was cyclical, but fell into insignificance in comparison to other more wrenching events, both within the family and in the world around us.

I discovered a hiding place in my mind, a station short of tranquility, but one that I counted on frequently and reliably: lying flat on my back on the floor of 1231 West 47th Street, I stared at the ceiling. It was, I imagined, as calm as a restful sea, undisturbed by conflict, clutter, anger, concern, or even furniture. There I tuned out the chaotic times, but I was still present to all that was happening on the floor.

Randolph did not meet my dad's expectations. Randolph became the object of what I now would call emotional abuse.

Upon Randolph alone, dad inflicted harsh and perhaps mostly undeserved criticism.

For example, Randolph did not bring in the stove coal in a timely manner each night before dark. The coal bin, a wooden enclosure built adjacent to the "wood shed," was located in the back yard, no more than 15 yards from the house.

Two buckets of coal were required to heat the house at night and to bank the fire in a pot-bellied black coal-burning stove. It was our form of central heat because it sat in the center of the house. In the winter months, it was cold in the adjacent but infrequently occupied rooms with their doors closed.

Houses in Lamberts Point were not insulated.

My sister, Edith

Edith, dark hair, dark eyes, shapely, outgoing personality, independent, and almost as strong-willed as my mother, loved to dance and she was good at it.

"You are beautiful," my mother would say to Edith, "I wish people could come to a window and see your beauty." In an uncanny way, people did come to a window and behold Edith's beauty when she later worked in a glass enclosure as a cashier at the Roxy Theatre on Granby Street, near its intersection with City Hall Avenue.

"But beauty is as beauty does," my mother often reminded Edith, "and sometimes your behavior is ugly."

Before I was 10 years of age, late one dark summer night, one of Edith's male admirers climbed up and onto our front porch roof and crawled through the window of the bedroom I shared with Edith.

The presence of the amorous young man, Ernest, was soon detected by my mother, who, screaming angrily, beat him down the steps and out the front door with a wildly swinging, potentially lethal weapon, an old black high-heeled shoe whose pointed heel repeatedly found its target, the back of Ernest's hard and risk-taking head.

I don't believe Ernest ever returned to our house, by day or by night, by a second floor window, by the front door, or by any door.

My Mother's Chair

I took many weekly baths in the kitchen behind the stove where it was warmest, using a pan of water heated on the top of the gas stove, a bar of red, disinfectant-smelling Life Buoy soap, an old wash rag, and towel.

Steam rose from the pan of water as it boiled on the top of the gas stove, humidifying the kitchen windows, providing unintended privacy.

Interior design architects today, looking back at my home on 47th Street in the decade between 1931 and 1941, would identify the coal stove as the central organizing feature of the entire 2-level house for which the monthly rent was $12.50.

My mother's chair, an undistinguished appearing old wooden rocking chair, was used by no one but her. The rocking chair was occupied only after the dishes were washed in the kitchen sink and dried with a dish cloth. Her chair rocked slowly, standing a few feet away from the front of the pot-belly stove.

In the poorly lit kitchen, seated upright in her wooden rocking chair, my mother slowly read the Norfolk Ledger Dispatch newspaper, from the back to the front. She strained her eyes to overcome both the inadequate lighting and the early onset of glaucoma. I don't recall that we discussed what she read in the newspaper, but it was an inviolate ritual. Quiet conditions favorable to reading in an otherwise noisy house were assured.

Family Sculpting

Many years later, during a group therapy workshop at Virginia Beach, I volunteered to make a living sculpture of my family by selecting people from the audience to represent each member of my family.

Literally, figuratively, and emotionally, I became immersed in the exercise, transported in time back to the way I experienced my childhood family.

I first selected a middle aged woman with auburn colored hair, freckled faced, fair skin, and erect posture to be my mother. Her similarity to my mother was striking. I quickly seated her in my mother's chair.

From the audience, I positioned a man with graying thin hair, six feet tall, on his back on the floor to represent my father. My "mother's" left foot rested on his chest.

A younger man, representing Randolph, was also placed on the floor. My "father's" foot held down my brother Randolph in this family-sculpting exercise led by Peggy Papp whose husband, Joseph Papp, directed "Shakespeare in the Park," in New York.

Each of my two older sisters' representatives stood on either side of my mother. Along with my mother, my sisters' hands were raised lifting me upward. I stood behind my mother, more as an observer than a member.

Each family member representative, still in my family sculpture, stated how awkward it felt to be in their particular positions. All were obedient to their assigned roles, but no one felt comfortable.

Interestingly, I left out my sister, Edith, and was unaware of it until the family sculpting exercise ended.

It was a strange but mysteriously uplifting experience for me. Perhaps it was the first time, then in my forties, that I conceptualized how I had perceived and experienced my family during the most formative years of my life.

I could hardly wait to drive back to Charlottesville to share with Dottie my newly discovered view of my family.

Lawyer Jett

Randolph's assumed negligent passivity infuriated my dad whose fault-finding seemed endless. Dad's disapproval went beyond my ability to understand it at that time in my life. Maybe, I cannot say for sure, but most likely, it was my mother who came up with the resolution to this conflict between father and son.

Randolph, then 17, young appearing, face inflamed with acne, and inexperienced for his age, would enlist in the Navy.

The plan met with difficulty. The poor economy, said to be the worst and longest economic depression in the history of the United States, made the US Navy an even more financially appealing organization to a lot of young men. This meant the Navy could be very choosy in recruiting Sailors.

None of us had ever noticed it before the Navy, but Randolph's enlistment was declined because his face was said to be asymmetrical. The Navy maintained that one side of Randolph's face was noticeably flatter than the opposite side. Weeks turned into months while the barriers to his enlistment continued.

"Lawyer Jett" was a term I heard several times during my childhood. I did not know its exact meaning, but I knew it meant something important was about to be undertaken.

Only my mother used the term "Lawyer Jett." She seldom invoked it, but it nearly always meant she was going to solve a conflict that meant additional sacrifice.

Years later at Maury High School I met "Lawyer Jett's" son, an attractive, successful member of our high school tennis team.

On December 7, 1939, exactly two years before the Japanese attack on Pearl Harbor, "Lawyer Jett" had loosened the Navy's grip on Randolph's enlistment barrier.

As I recall, the process of getting Randolph enlisted in the Navy was further delayed because my father then refused to sign, literally to mark his "X", on the second signature block after my mother's name.

"Randolph was sworn in"

My mother prevailed and Randolph was sworn in the U. S. Navy. After weeks of boot camp at the Norfolk Naval Operating Base, we visited him.

I had never before or since seen such large, bulging red blisters on Randolph's feet or anyone's feet in my 7 years of life. Close order drill or marching caused the blisters. Randolph's blistered feet were a major source of worry because a member of the Royal Family in England had died from blood poisoning.

We all shared the wide spread dread, common in the pre-antibiotic days of medicine, of an infection of Randolph's feet.

Randolph sent home a monthly allotment check in the amount of $18.00 from the beginning of his enlistment in the Navy. Today, $18.00 does not sound like much money, but in 1939 it paid our monthly rent and a week's grocery bill. Ironically, some of it even helped pay the monthly coal bill.

Randolph wrote my mother a letter every week. He was stationed on the USS Craven, a Navy destroyer, whose home port was Pearl Harbor, Hawaii.

When at sea, the USS Craven traversed a route from Pearl Harbor to Sydney, Australia, and back. Later in the War, Randolph served on the U.S. Reno, a cruiser, and much later on a battle ship whose name, sadly, I do not remember.

Altogether, during World War II, Randolph was in 14 major battles in the Pacific and went "over the side" when his ship was torpedoed. His ship was expected to sink, did not sink, but limped like a crippled, bedraggled person to a shipyard for repairs in the Charleston, South Carolina port.

Randolph sent gifts to us from Hawaii. I received a pair of pearl handled cap pistols, a good gift for a 9 year old boy. The pistols worked perfectly, advancing a roll of caps that fired with a loud flash with each pull on the trigger. The pistols fit nicely with their holsters. I wore the pistols as part of my Army suit, the one for which I always wished every Christmas.

Later, Randolph sent me a silk short sleeved pale yellow shirt from Hawaii. A multicolored image was sewn on the left pocket. It was a stylish shirt, commanded a lot of compliments, maybe some envy, and remained my favorite shirt until I wore it out or I out grew it.

I don't recall the gifts other family members received from Hawaii.

Pearl Harbor became a real, very personal place for the Brown family.

Staying in my own back yard

For the most of my childhood, I had been confined to one side of 47th Street because my mother did not want me to "play in the street and get run over by a car," although few cars were driven on our dirt street.

I did not have free rein to leave our fenced in the front yard to mingle with certain "foul mouthed, riff-raff children" who resided across the street.

The rules lessened somewhat as I approached 10 years of age, but crossing Hampton Boulevard, the busiest street within miles of my home, a street that led directly to the Norfolk Naval Base, street-car tracks in its center, cars readily whizzing past, was by no means permitted to me without an adult "crossing" me over it.

Thus Edith held my hand and we walked to Gray's Pharmacy with a purpose.

I spent a lot of time during the first decade of my life, I remember, peering through the tiny spaces between the wooden plank-fence. I've heard others refer to being reared on an island of one city block in a large city.

In my case, I was reared in a space defined by a front and back wooden plank-fence. I was further restricted by a narrow alley between our house and the residence of my oldest sister, Christine, who was a second mother to me.

The second story of the house on the left was rented by the Johnsons. The Johnsons were a family of Norwegian ancestry. Mrs. Johnson was a very kind and generous mother who often threw home-made cookies, wrapped in waxed paper, down to me from her second-story window.

Mr. Johnson was a busy father who rode a street car from the corner of 46th Street and Hampton Boulevard early each morning to a destination unknown to me.

Munroe, their mean son, often delighted in tormenting me on those rare occasions when I was permitted outside my yard but not out of view of my front porch.

Mary Elizabeth, their friendly daughter, one might say was perhaps my first girl friend, if that title is appropriate for a female two years my senior when I was about five years of age.

Occasionally, Juan DeVala, about a year my senior, who lived across the street, a member of a Puerto Rican family, was permitted to come into my yard to play.

For the most part, my world was experienced through the visual perceptions that reached my retinae as I strained to see the world through the narrow spaces separating the boards that formed our fence.

Vividly painfully, eight decades later, I still remember my loneliness, piteously pleading with passers-by children to come into my yard and play with me. However, they were assertively indifferent to me.

I saw children from both sides of the street playing together in what appeared to me to be perfected bliss. I saw the same children later engaged in vicious name-calling and fisticuffs.

I heard the special ring of the ice cream man who slowly peddled a bicycle-like vehicle in which dry ice preserved special treats. I heard the wagon wheels drumming over the rough dirt road in front of our house, the unique signal that the sweet aroma of baked trumpets, cream-puffs, doughnuts, and raisin buns were verbally marketed by the resonant voice of a kind man dressed in a white coat and dark pants.

My love of art, I conjecture, may have its origin in the visual orientation of the world required of me by a loving, firm and protective mother. For my love of ice cream and bakery goods, however, I hold no one more responsible than yours truly.

Gray's Pharmacy

On Sunday afternoon, 7 DEC 1941, my sister Edith held my hand as we cautiously walked across Hampton Boulevard, on our way to Gray's Pharmacy, from our home, 1231 West 47th Street, Norfolk, Virginia where winter weather was ordinarily not severe.

It was a cold, overcast day.

Dr. Gray, the pharmacist and owner of Gray's Pharmacy, was a thin middle aged man with thick eye glasses and even thicker eye brows. His was a stern, no nonsense demeanor. This serious, tall man with graying tips of his full head of hair was acknowledged by my mother as a vital resource of medical information, a person whose opinion was sought when she reached the limit of her natural healing knowledge, and before Dr. West, Norfolk Department of Public Health, was contacted.

We had no telephone in the house at that time. Messages were delivered in person. My mother's handwriting was barely legible, another reason that messengers were employed.

Gray's Pharmacy was not a large store in 1941. It was located on the east side of Hampton Boulevard at the corner of 48th Street. Next door to Gray's Pharmacy was Butler's Barber Shop. "Save the sideburns," my mother always demanded, to my embarrassment, before the barber was permitted to tonsorially address my "best feature," my brown curly hair.

Dr. Gray stood behind a glass-encased counter, the main attribute of the store. If he had other employees, it was never more than a middle aged plain woman and a teenage delivery boy.

I do not remember that the store was ever crowded with customers or obviously a busy place of business. The exception was Sunday afternoon, December 7th 1941. President Franklin Delano Roosevelt, a man much loved, admired, and respected by my family and by everyone known to me, was speaking on the radio.

The volume of the radio, turned up by Dr. Gray, filled the store's one large room, about 25 feet wide and 15 feet deep. A small, quiet crowd, appearing more like they were attending a funeral service, had gathered in the store on this dreary Sunday afternoon to hear the news.

Some of President Roosevelt's words had no meaning to me, but when he announced that the Japanese had attacked Pearl Harbor I was suddenly gripped by fear. I knew that my brother Randolph was stationed in Pearl Harbor.

Randolph had mailed our gifts from Pearl Harbor. We had deep blue end-table cloths with exotic designs of Hawaii, and a large brightly colored tray gaily displaying a map of Pearl Harbor. Its place was on top of an old mahogany dresser. My pearl handled cap pistols were sent to me by Randolph from Pearl Harbor.

Edith, without uttering a word, grasped my hand and left Gray's Pharmacy with uncommon speed.

"What's wrong," I begged.

"We are going home to tell mother about the news."

"Our Father in Heaven, Protect Randolph"

We had a radio at home, an Emerson, often repaired by my dad, a man with incredible manual skills. The radio was only played in the evening, to conserve electrical expenses. Several nights a week, as a family we enjoyed our favorite programs: "Jack Benny," "Fibber McGee and Molly," "The Shadow," "The District Attorney," "The Eddie Cantor Show," and "Jack Armstrong, the All American Boy."

Edith and I ran to our modest, two-story, rented house on 47th Street, probably without crossing Hampton Boulevard cautiously, taking less than two minutes from Gray's Pharmacy.

"Mother," Edith, then 17 years old, and, like me, out of breath, shouted upon opening the front door, "The Japs have bombed Pearl Harbor!" Edith's voice was piercing, loud, and ominous.

Mother, as usual, was in the kitchen, donning a white apron. The kitchen was a fairly small room at the end of a narrow hallway from the front door, the opposite side of an adjacent middle room.

My mother screamed in fear, "Our Father in Heaven, Protect Randolph."

We all cried. We knew nothing of Randolph's status and we were not to find out for weeks.

My oldest sister Christine, married to Frank, lived next door. My next older sister Frances, who by this time was married to Roy, a Navy Chief Petty Officer, out to Sea, lived with us. My unemployed but never unoccupied father was in the back yard working at his work bench.

In seconds, all six of us crouched around the radio, crying, praying, and listening to the worst news of my lifetime. The news of the war was incomplete but bad. It was the worst attack on the US Navy in all its history.

As a ten year old I imagined the Pacific Ocean ruby red with the blood of our Sailors stationed at Pearl Harbor, possibly including the blood of my only brother, Randolph.

My mother's plea to "Our Father in Heaven, Protect Randolph," was screamed from the seriousness of a mother's boundless love for her son.

Her sincere prayer did not spring from a rich, regular, ritualistic religious education, training, or experience.

My mother's prayer was answered.

There may have never been a more urgent or a more plaintive prayer. I never heard my mother utter the same prayer again, but I am confident it remained in her heart throughout the war for Randolph and for those who served in the war.

My Mother, a Prayer Warrior

My mother, kneeling for a different reason but for a reason also directly associated with World War II, later in the same decade of her answered prayer for my brother, Randolph, became a prayer warrior.

My mother's dramatic transformation into a prayer warrior led her to pray for many souls, including my own. Her prayers helped many of us navigate through troubled waters. These pages will provide the essential details of this miracle, one deserving prominence and gratitude.

My family was neither spiritual nor religious until I was well into my teens. A greater integrity than one might expect from my minimally educated and often welfare-supported family, however, was demanded by my mother. I was taught the value of hard work, the painful consequences of failing to keep my word, of lying, cheating or stealing.

Edith reminds me today, "We were proud but poor."

Even though it was alien to my nature to do so, I was reared to fight for myself. "If you don't fight for yourself I will beat you when you come home," I was told in solemnity not unlike Moses reading the Ten Commandments. I saw it as a "lose-lose" situation. We are talking here about physical fighting, a common activity in my neighborhood, something I came to dread and did my consummate best to avoid.

In fact, Edith's shepherding me around to nearby churches as a small child, was the only religious practice in the Brown family at that time other than being "tucked in bed" each night of my life reciting for my mother the well-known child's prayer, "Now I lay me down to sleep; I pray Thee Lord my soul to keep. If I should die before I wake, I pray thee Lord my soul to take. Amen." It was our unbroken ritual.

World War II spread through our neighborhood like an epidemic, touching everything and everybody known to me.

I wanted to fight in the war. I always wanted to be a Soldier. Why could not a ten year old help defend his country?

I loved the American flag. As a child, the present I most often begged my mother to acquire for me was a small American flag. A Soldier suit, designed like those worn by American Soldiers in World War I, is all I ever wanted as a child for Christmas.

Somehow, despite marked financial restrictions, I had several small lead Soldiers. Realistically painted Army brown, these little six-inch figures, my most cherished toys, were to me as alive as the men who served in the military.

Earlier in my childhood, nearly daily I played with my Soldiers, strategically placing them in critical locations within the protective dirt walls that defined my fort. Small amounts of water mixed into the dirt made the walls, I imagined, impenetrable. The soft, black soil, slightly below which was sand, typical of Tidewater Virginia, comfortably accommodated my material needs for the construction of an Army fort. The best location for the readily available valuable resource was in the mostly shady, darkened alley between my house and my sister Christine's house.

I spent untold hours in this solitary endeavor between age five to eight.

With ever so slowly increasing physical growth and even more ever so slowly increasing latitude from my mother to occasionally leave my yard, I spent less time with toy Soldiers and more time with real, living Soldier substitutes: peers about my age whom I trained in close order drill, skilled use and maintenance of weapons, read sticks, in realistic warfare.

Edith recalls this period in my life as "the times you were dressed in little more than rags and used sticks as rifles as you marched children around the neighborhood like Soldiers."

The Beale Name

My mother's maiden name was Beale. She was proud of her name, her family, and no one could reflect discredit upon her name or her family and fail to face the consequences.

My grandfather, a quiet and humble man, despite his every instinct opposing it, was forced to borrow money from a relative in order to set up housekeeping in Norfolk for his wife and children. When he was unable to repay the loan, my grandfather's relative took all of my grandfather's furniture that was permitted by law to be taken for unpaid debt.

One of the few pieces of furniture retained by my grandfather, 100 years ago, was a small, drop-leaf walnut dining room table.

The table came to me by a very circuitous route. I use it daily in my home as our kitchen table, a cherished connecting link with my grandfather. I hardly knew my grandfather as a child because he lived in the Norfolk City Tuberculosis Sanatorium most of my childhood.

My Grandfather, John Wesley Beale

My grandfather, John Wesley Beale, came to Norfolk in 1912 by boat and returned by hearse in 1945 to the cemetery in Chuckatuck where members of the Beale family have been interred since 1824.

He and my grandmother brought their 3 sons and 5 daughters to Norfolk from Isle of Wight County by boat on the Nansemond River in the midst of financial misery.

I don't think he ever knew the meaning of financial security. He was known as a good family man, a man of his word, a hard worker, even under harsh conditions and a man of impeccable character. He was a quiet man in demeanor and speech who lived a long, virtuous life and was never known to be of severe or violent temperament. He endured hardship like a Soldier.

I knew more about my grandfather from stories my mother told me about him than I heard from him directly. Sadly, I recall that he talked to me only on rare occasions.

He faithfully loved my grandmother, I am told, and at her request, as she lay dying in bed at home in early middle age, with her weeping children gathered respectfully around her bed, my grandfather sang her favorite hymn, "Till We Meet Again."

Here, I imagine, is a shy and grief-stricken man, a man of few words, mastering all the emotions that engulfed him, rendering an audible tune to his dying wife that she may depart from her human mantle in the peace, comfort, and security of the inspiring promise that they will, and of course by now they will have already met "on that beautiful shore."

My grandfather and one of his three sons, John Addison Beale, affectionately known in the family as "John A," at one time worked for the City of Norfolk in positions that required the use of trucks. Their truck was struck by another vehicle and both my grandfather and my uncle John A. were injured.

My grandfather suffered a punctured lung and John A. was even more seriously injured. After days of suffering in the Norfolk General Hospital, both gentlemen appeared to be improving; however, John A.'s left arm injury became infected with gangrene.

During the dark night of one of the summer's worst electrical storms, the decision to amputate John A.'s left arm above the elbow had to be made, according to the physicians, by my grandfather. A more sad and grave dilemma is difficult to picture for my grandfather who had already buried his 12 year old daughter, and whose twin infants had barely lived a year.

Poll Tax

To complete the profile of my mother's father, the person who most significantly influenced her childhood development and her deeply held beliefs, I repeat here one final story.

It is about the quiet, humble pride that most typically described my grandfather's character. It may well have been his nonassertive style of communication that contributed to my mother's quick temper and assertion, and when necessary, her tendency to resort to aggression in the service of aiding and abetting her children in the cause of justice.

Several years after my grandmother's death, my grandfather remarried. The vignette that follows may not be entirely unbiased because my grandfather's five daughters opposed the marriage. These daughters were all grown into adulthood when this union took place. Nonetheless, fault finding gained momentum among the daughters, my aunts. I am told that the most egregious of their step-mother's faults occurred as follows.

My grandfather, like all the Beale men before him, was a staunch Virginia Democrat, read "conservative" in today's political terminology. He took to voting like ducks take to water. He voted in every election, big and small, and was well known by his neighbors and friends who manned the polls during elections.

Poll taxes were in full force during my grandfather's day. To his great embarrassment, however, when he lined up to cast his vote in the first election after his remarriage, he was told he could not vote.

In utter embarrassment and humiliation, he was told that his poll tax had not been paid. It was said that he had been assured by his new wife that she, the manager of all his finances, had paid the poll tax in a timely manner.

His head lowered, he painfully looked for the exit. Silently and slowly walking with a purpose, he left the polling station never to return again. Not long after, and in a similarly silent and slow, speechless manner, he walked out of his new wife's residence never to return again.

Christmas Day 1945

The Brown household was particularly happy with life on Christmas Day 1945.

World War II was over. Peace seemed world-wide and everlasting.

A log fire was lit in the fireplace built earlier by my mother's brother, Henderson Beale, called "Brother." The wonderful sights, smells, and happy mood almost unique to Christmas morning filled the house. The wonderfully matchless aroma of nutmeg sprinkled on top of mugs of hot eggnog enriched the kitchen.

The special eggnog was made from a treasured recipe passed down from several generations. It is still maintained in a special place in the Brown household, christened the earliest part of the day. Christmas carols playing on the radio further lightened our mood.

Dad was slicing the Smithfield ham, the traditional Christmas culinary treat, at the kitchen table and mother was busy with last minute tidying before the rest of the family was scheduled to arrive.

I loved the Army dress officer uniform of that period and I wore a pair of new pants of similar color to "Army pinks," and a dark brown, long sleeve shirt that replicated the essential features of the Army dress uniform of WW II.

The phone, 38636 (no area codes in those days), remembered from many years ago, was located in the middle room, a room sometimes used as a dining room, but it was most often unheated and unused. The phone rang. I ran to it and said, "Merry Christmas, the Brown residence."

The caller identified herself as a "Nurse from the Norfolk City Hospital. Is Mrs. Brown there? I'm afraid I have some bad news for her."

Even today, all these decades later, I cannot acceptably explain what I did, or rather what I failed to do. There must be hundreds of reasons; I just don't know. At age 14 years I knew or should have known the right thing to do. My mother was so happy. WW II was over. God had answered her prayer; Randolph was protected. It was Christmas morning.

"Mom," I said, "it's for you." I omitted the crucial preparatory words…"It's the nurse from the Sanatorium where Papa lives…its bad news." It may have been one of the cruelest things I ever did. As I plead for mercy from the judge in my mind, I say that I intended no harm, but what I saw and heard does little to justify mercy.

"Is it for me?" my mother happily inquired. "Who is it?"

We had no long phone extension cords or mobile phones in 1945. I did not answer her question, uttered as she walked quickly towards me. Robbed of speech, like a coward, I just passed her the phone.

"Merry Christmas," my mother happily spoke into the phone. "Yes, this is Mrs. Brown."

The few seconds that followed abruptly ended with ceaseless, loud, shrill screaming.

"My father is dead...my father is dead...he died alone...he died alone...Oh No...I don't believe it...we have to go to him now...George. George, drive me to Water Works Road," the name she used to partially disguise the shame of one's father in a city sanatorium for TB.

In some ways my mother's crying never completely stopped. That Christmas morning her tears were like a heavy rain fall in a thunder storm, interrupted only the lightning of her piercing, high-pitched screaming.

She had visited her father only the day before his death, Christmas Eve, and took his and her favorite food, Smithfield ham, but she was guilt-laden that she had skimped and had been ungenerous, in her harsh, judgmental mind, in the amount of Smithfield ham she shared with him.

I never saw my mother sadder. Nothing I observed ever came close to the painful grief she endured that Christmas Season and beyond.

I never told her how bad I felt for failing to prepare her for the "bad news." It would have been less shocking. I wonder if it would also somehow have lessened the pain of her intolerable, unbearable grief.

Years later, I would observe the same, but seldom expressed traumatic grief in the Soldiers about whom I am writing for our nation.

The next few days were consumed by my grandfather's funeral service at the Derry Funeral Home on Colley Avenue, in Norfolk. He was buried at Oakland Christian Church in Chuckatuck, Isle of Wight County. A crowd of loving family members and friends attended his services. No one cried as painfully as my mother. It created vivid and lasting memories in the mind of his 14-year-old grandson.

My Sister, Christine

Christine, my oldest sister, at least 20 years my senior, was the most serious-minded and most responsible and intelligent of my five siblings. Christine and her eccentric and abusive husband, Frank, lived next door to us for the first 10 years of my life, making her readily accessible when needed.

It was to her house that I ran when my mother terrified me, now seemingly playfully, by calling up spirits through key holes in the sliding wooden doors separating our two front rooms, telling me that her brother John A. once saw a ghost in our closet, the one formed under the stairway leading upstairs, the one in which I was sometimes locked in the dark when I misbehaved, or convincing me that our house was haunted.

In the warm arms of my over-weight sister, I found solace and safety; not infrequently, I was invited to stay for supper.

I enjoyed supper with Christine most when her husband Frank was not there. This was frequently the case because Frank, at the end of his work day as a City of Norfolk Street Sweeper Operator, drove his dilapidated, old wooden-sided dump truck nightly to his farm at Bird Neck Point, Virginia Beach.

Frank's unsightly truck was filled nightly with garbage collected from several downtown restaurants. He used it as slop to feed his squealing hogs.

Unpleasant olfactory and visual memories remain in my mind from the many times I joined Frank in his silent sojourns to his grateful hogs, oblivious to their squalid, stinking state or to their destiny, some weighing hundreds of pounds, clamoring unkindly over each other, squealing so loudly that I tried to cover my ears as well as my nose when slop over-filled their troughs. When his pigs reached the desired weight, Frank drove his proud progeny to market in Richmond.

Frank's truck, a sentinel memory, transported him to work each day, to his hogs each evening, and to his favorite country store on old Virginia Beach Boulevard. Stopping, sometimes for hours, at the country store was an inevitable part of his unbroken circuit. I sat on one of its wooden barrels countless times.

Frank's conversations with the middle-aged couple who owned the store were largely devoid of words. Finally, Frank drove the truck to his home at night, but not before 9:30 PM.

It was Frank's truck that moved my family to 1321 West 39th Street, the Lambert's Point section of Norfolk, shortly after the beginning of WW II. Frank's truck bed must have been cleaned before it became our moving van, but its odor, weakened by the air its motion circulated, attracted the attention of those we passed.

Embarrassed, I lowered my head closer to the floor of the truck as we neared our destination, fearing that I would be recognized, and teased by classmates at James Madison School. I was already a familiar target for their scorn. I feared there would be an increase in their personal attacks, now rearmed with explosive ammunition.

In at least two important ways, my family was like the majority of people around whom I was reared during the second decade of my life. We had a family member in the military service during WW II, and the economic status decidedly improved as a result of WW II.

My father was employed as a painter at the Colonna Ship Yard where Liberty Ships were reconditioned.

My parents purchased, for $1300, the first house of their life-time, a mansion in their long view, one that required the sweat and impatience of my father whose every driven nail was supervised by my mother. Today, this type of unrepaired domicile would have been posted with "Uninhabitable and Unsafe" and other equally uncomplimentary signs.

A more exacting master than my mother could not be found. I can see my father's sweat drenched face, frustration in every wrinkle, too numerous to count, peering helplessly through his eye-glasses with his one good eye, the other blinded accidently with battery acid while working on a tug boat in the Elizabeth River at age 12.

He pled unsuccessfully with her, "Pig," his term of affection for my mother, "it can't be done…you just can't build two separate entrances after you come through the front door." Never raising her voice, she replied willfully and with the confidence of a credentialed New York architect, although she had no formal education beyond the fourth grade, "George, it can be done and you will do it. Let me walk it off for you."

It was done.

Undeniably, there is something universally appealing about an unambivalent person who knows what she or he wants, takes no compromising position, and has the strength of will and character to achieve almost unimaginable goals.

Having no building inspectors to contend with, the renovation became a reality with every sawed board and every disputed decision. In the end, my parents together created two second floor apartments, each with a kitchen and bedroom, and a rented room on the first floor with a separated entrance.

For mom, dad, Edith, and me, they formed two bedrooms, a large eat in kitchen, a dining room, and a living room with the cherished fire place built by my uncle, Brother.

Except for the fire place, all the manual labor was done by my father.

Green canvas awnings adorned the front porch where on many evenings I sat in my mother's loving lap, even until I was twelve years of age, with dad sometimes seated next to us in the freshly painted glider. Those evenings were peaceful. The pride of mother, her dream come true through their combined efforts, was palpable.

Mr. and Mrs. Riley

Housing in Norfolk was in great demand during WW II. Mr. and Mrs. Riley, a middle aged couple from Brooklyn, New York, rented the rear apartment upstairs. His degree of friendliness depended upon his degree of inebriation. He frequented Robins Confectionary, a popular meeting place on the corner of 38th Street and Bowden's Ferry Road, across from James Madison School, where he was known for glib extraversion and a feat that went awry.

I was not present when the event occurred, but I observed its lingering, unfortunate consequences. He was fond of spraying a mouthful of an inflammable liquid and blowing it out between his pursed lips onto a lighted match or cigarette lighter, producing a homemade flame thrower. It often drew a crowd because real flamethrowers were a popular American weapon during WW II.

On the occasion referred to here, however, the stunt backfired, burning Mr. Riley's face severely. I believed it ended the carnival-like part of Mr. Riley's entertaining personality despite ongoing requests from his previously entertained audiences. In my childhood, I thought of Mr. Riley as a good person, an intelligent, hard-working person whose overly serious side, I now rationalize, was unlocked and set free with libation.

Mrs. Riley, a devout Catholic, unlike her husband, did not smoke or drink. She baked the most pleasant smelling aromatic and gustatorially delightful date-containing cookies. She was generous by nature. A plate of freshly baked cookies awaited my arrival at the top of the stairs. Too often, I consumed Mrs. Riley's cookies with the zeal that today easily meets the diagnostic criteria of an eating disorder.

Not unlike Mr. Riley, I too did not know my limits. Eating and drinking habits start early in life and too often are lasting. I pray that Mr. Riley was more successful in conquering the habit of ingesting ethanol to excess than yours truly in breaking his cookie weakness.

Christine and Frank

I have no recollection of how it happened, but Christine and Frank had already moved to 39th Street into a dark brown shingled house directly across the street from us before our move was completed.

Christine had dropped out of public school early, but was astute with finances and I suspect she had something to do with the purchase of my parents' property, perhaps co-signing a bank loan. Next-door to Christine and Frank's house was an unoccupied dwelling in a maximum state of disrepair; in its side yard stood a large, prolifically productive pear tree and a space sufficient for Frank to park his unsavory smelling truck each night.

"That's Frank," we all habitually said each night as we listened for the loud, distinctive clunking sound made by his truck tires climbing over the curb late each night to curl up in its parking space only to awaken not many hours hence, taking Frank back to work in the lightless morning hours.

The neighborhood was spared the ugly view of the abandoned house by gangly green hedges that grew at least 15 or 20 feet high, the result of neglected trimming for scores of years by some long forgotten home owner whose horticultural views intended an attractive little hedge row, not the obstructing canopy it grew to become.

One dark night the anticipated clunking sound of Frank's truck went unheard.

Christine's youthful love for Frank had not faded; it had been abused into oblivion. His nocturnal neglect of her and Frankie, their 10 year old son, matched, if not surpassed, his silent hateful, nearly daily abuses of Christine; and so on both sides of West 39th Street the Brown family slept undisturbed through Frank's failure to return home.

Frank was discovered unconscious the following morning trapped under a large tree he was attempting to clear from his Bird Neck farm with a borrowed bulldozer. His broken neck, treated with 3 Crutchfield Tongs bored deep into his skull, and his concussion, led to confusing delusions, persistent pain, and protracted immobility.

Frank's medical condition gradually stabilized. While he remained weeks more in the Norfolk General Hospital, Christine and Frankie disappeared and were not heard from by anyone for many years.

I remember Frank, encumbered by a large metallic brace encompassing his head, neck, and back. Emaciated, and walking robotically, barely surviving alone across the street from us and barely cognitively processing what happened to his wife and son, never really understanding that he drove them away.

His eyes depicted the melancholy of his existence, but he complained only of not understanding what happened to his family. He defiantly assumed a dependent role, begging my mother, "Lou, where did Christine go? Why did she leave? I never dreamed it would come to this. Please tell her to come back and bring my son to me."

He was not easily convinced that no one, not even my mother, knew where Christine had fled. All but Frank knew why she left him, but no one in our family knew where she went. It was a terrible devastation to all of us at that time. There were no safe houses for abused women in those long ago days.

Examples of Frank's cruel treatment and equally cruel neglect of Christine do not come to mind easily. He towered over Christine by at least a foot, but I have no recollection of any physical abuse inflicted by Frank.

His was an unusual form of meanness. He would not be engaged in conversations, seldom responded to questions of even the most innocent and polite. He was not a grumpy or complaining person; even that would have been preferable to his painful periods of long silence.

Frank liked to gather eggs each morning from his small flock of laying hens he raised in their back yard on 39th Street. When he learned that Christine had gathered the eggs earlier one day, perhaps to be used in baking a cake for her husband and son, he became enraged and imploded.

Standing threateningly over Christine, because she had breached one of his unspoken rules, robbing him of the pleasure of gathering his eggs himself, Frank forced Christine moments after his discovery to scramble a dozen eggs from his supply in the refrigerator and to eat the entire dozen eggs while he loudly cursed and belittled her, harshly teaching her a lesson.

One can only imagine the indelibility of countless emotional scars left by Frank on Christine's soul.

Alone in his dark brown-stained shingled house, 1322 West 39th Street, Frank slowly recovered from his broken neck, but he never recovered from the loss of Christine and Frankie.

He unsuccessfully attempted to fill his empty life with ethanol. I am not certain he ever returned to work. He came across the street to visit us fairly frequently initially, and then he was seen less and less.

One episode occurring during Frank's self-imposed isolation and chronic quandary over the inexplicable loss of his family stands out vividly in my memory.

Frank, foaming at the mouth, tied to a gurney, was carefully lifted by several men into the rear of an ambulance, parked in front of his house, and thus in front of our house as well, its engine still running, its unpleasant smelling exhaust creating a thin fog, a ghost-like scene.

I was told that Frank was having a grand mal seizure, a diagnostic term having little meaning to me at that time, but I was not too young to appreciate the gravity of his condition and its likely connection to the excessive ingestion of ethanol.

The years passed slowly. Christine and Frankie were gone. And then one day they returned as suddenly and unexpectedly as they departed. Frankie left as a little boy, but he returned as a tall, lanky adolescent. Frankie had changed, matured physically but emotionally scarred.

I could see the enduring pain in his eyes. He avoided my questions about his long journey, the decision to return, the emotional costs of being on the run, the persistent stress of avoiding detection.

Already, as an early teenager, his eyes had the "one-thousand mile stare" that I have come to recognize in Soldiers returning from combat. I can't explain the nearly overwhelming melancholy feeling and thoughts of Frankie's return trip to Norfolk from California that still possesses me when I happen to hear Dvorak's, Symphony No. 9, From the New World, Largo, "Going Home."

Frankie and I walked into the field behind our 39th Street house and shot a few baskets of basketball. It was like meeting someone for the first time. We both felt awkward. Earlier Frankie had been like a little brother to me.

I walked several feet in front of Frankie back to the house. Frankie was closing the back gate, his back to me. I gasped in surprise when I looked toward our house and saw, standing quietly by my father's work bench, Frank. We both stared at Frankie's back; he was still trying to fasten the back yard gate.

If birds had been singing that clear early spring mid-afternoon in Tidewater Virginia, no chirping or any other sound was audible.

Frankie, as if in slow motion, turned, gazing at his father for the first time in years, nearly drowning in confusion and uncertainty.

I sensed that Frankie's initial response was to run out the back gate, propelled by fear and alarm.

"It's all right, Frankie," I shouted.

I looked back at Frank. With huge tears raining down his cheeks from his large, unbelieving eyes, Frank ran towards his long absent son.

Frankie froze. The love of the father about which we are told in the Bible when his prodigal son returned could not have been greater in those precious moments of reunion.

Frank, no longer moving robotically, no longer the man with a broken neck, fell to his knees weeping, hugging and kissing Frankie.

All of Frank's past haughty pride, irrational anger, and meanness dissolved in his unashamed tears and was cleansed away in a flash in front of my witnessing eyes.

Over the following years until Frank's death, father and son rebuilt a lasting relationship.

Christine remarried, but I never observed her as care-free, fun-loving, or really happy. Nonetheless, Christine remained a steadfast, stable, responsible person, readily available to help meet the needs of family and church until her death in the seventh year of her lonely widowhood.

4

WAR ON SOLDIERS AS PEOPLE

Combat Death: the Loss of Attachment

SURVIVAL IN COMBAT depends upon strong, secure attachments between Soldiers.

The attachment between Soldiers in combat is the most intense of all human relationships. The loss of a Soldier with whom one has a strong, secure, intense attachment is unspeakably shattering.

Is death ever painlessly accepted?

Is watching death traumatic?

Is witnessing shocking injury ever free of pain and regret?

The burden of serious injury and death of fellow Soldiers in combat is worsened by attempting to avoid thoughts and feelings about the loss.

The loss is irreplaceable.

The void it leaves is enormous.

The void, the awareness of emptiness, will be faced when the Soldier is finally able to grieve.

If there is a theme or underlying connection between the stories told by Soldiers in <u>Sacred Ground</u>, it is the suffering of emptiness when meaningful attachments are lost.

Each injured Soldier is honored, admired, and respected. Each loss must be mourned by battle buddies in unique and individually meaningful ways

Soldiers who discover how to accept the truth of the meaning of their combat traumas are often released from overpowering suffering and irrational guilt. When Soldiers learn how to grieve and how to bear its suffering, they will remember their losses with less pain.

Quincy's Loss

Daniel Quincy, a 30-year-old married Soldier, recently returned home from his fourth combat deployment to Afghanistan. The tall, stocky, soft-spoken, somber man was tense, agitated, and uncertain about his first session with a psychiatrist.

He said nothing during our long walk together down the hallway to my office. He sat down quickly, visually scanned my office, and stared at the door.

The SFC (Sergeant First Class) spoke. "I hold everything inside. I've had 4 deployments, only this time…" he paused for a long time, looking as if he wanted to say something, but he just couldn't say it. I imagined it was something too difficult to say out loud, too emotional to disclose.

His pause continued. I said nothing.

"I'm scared all the time…just like I was down range. When I get scared I get real angry. It's like I want something to happen… something bad. When it does happen, I will give it all I've got like I did down range.

Does this make sense?"

"Yes," I replied.

"Good. I was afraid I was losing it."

I observed the first, although very brief, sense of relief.

"Before this last deployment, I was afraid of nothing! All that's changed now.

I'm even afraid to ride my motorcycle at home. I am afraid a bomb might be under the road and it will blow me up.

The tattoo on my back says, 'God is Love.' The only thing that got me home is God.

The last deployment proved to be more than I could manage.

What is the only emotion I feel? Is this the day I will die? I'm scared all the time…and angry.

I'm broke to the point I question my own ability.

I learned my mortality. I realize how close I came to die.

I keep my mind shut."

"What was special about your last deployment that made it different?" I asked.

"I gave him everything…everything I knew…I taught him.

He was my gunner.

He was very young…didn't even have a driver's license…but he had heart…I kept him because he had heart.

I gave him a combat nick-name…'Cheddar Bob.'

The Senior Platoon SGT took him out of my vehicle the night of the mission. My Soldier asked me why…I told him the Senior Platoon SGT wanted it.

We were in an 8 vehicle convoy…almost 9 months ago to the very day…in Afghanistan. His vehicle took a direct hit. The Senior Platoon SGT ordered everyone to help with the rescue.

We thought the gunner and TC (truck commander) had been captured by the enemy…the door of their vehicle was half-open.

We searched the wood-line and along the river.

We didn't know what happened to them; we didn't know until the vehicle stopped burning."

Another long, important pause helped Quincy keep his thoughts clear, his cheeks dry.

"They had burned to death.

We didn't hear them screaming because the attack made an incredibly loud noise."

"What is that black bracelet you are wearing on your right wrist?" I asked.

He removed it and quickly passed it to me.

The thin metallic band was about an inch wide. Pressed into the black band were the dead Soldier's full name, his combat nick-name, the identification of his unit, and the date of his death.

I quickly returned it to the patient's outstretched hand, complying with his unspoken request.

"Did you attend the memorial service for your Soldier?" I asked.

"I hate remembering," he shouted.

"I hate remembering! You re-live it. You feel it in every part of your body. You even feel it in your skin. You get upset."

His voice continued to rise. "Rather than cry, I get upset and angry…and disappointed."

I said nothing, silently accepting him and his mistrusted self. You could hear a pin drop. The silence seemed endless before he spoke again.

"I cried that day…the day he died. I cried at dinner. I cried that night when I was alone.

I just don't want to be scared any more…I want to be able to calm down from being very upset. I want to be able to sleep again. I want to keep my mind from moving so fast.

It makes me feel weak to cry…and ashamed."

"Have you attempted to reach his family?" I asked.

Staring at the floor, not speaking, he slowly shook his head, indicating the negative.

"You taught him everything he knew, SFC Daniel Quincy. What did 'Cheddar Bob' teach you?"

My question caught SFC Daniel Quincy off guard.

"I never thought of that, Sir," he replied. His puzzled look sprung up quickly. In an uncanny way, his gaze appeared hopeful to me.

"Your tears tell me that 'Cheddar Bob' taught you how to become attached to a young Soldier who had 'heart.'

Your bracelet bearing his name tells me how he taught you to stay attached to him even after his death.

Is it really a sign of weakness to weep for 'Cheddar Bob'? Is it shameful to cry for a brave young man who gave his life for his country?"

SFC Daniel Quincy, without weakness or shame, wept.

"What could you say if you phoned 'Cheddar Bob's' parents?" I asked.

The SFC had often thought about contacting his Soldier's parents. He said he knew it was important but "I never found the right time...the right thing to say...until now."

Wiping away tears, seated as erect as a Soldier standing at attention, Daniel Quincy spoke without hesitation.

"This is SFC Daniel Quincy. I was your son's Platoon SGT in Afghanistan. I was with him when he died in combat. He had heart. He was the bravest Soldier in my unit. He taught me important things. I can't tell you how much I miss him. He will always be in my heart."

Soldiers

"Soldiers are the proudest people in the world," said SFC Albert North, a plucky Soldier in the Monday Afternoon Post-Deployment Group Therapy session. His fellow group therapy members smiled, nodding in agreement.

Soldiers are also very sensitive people. It is the sensitive nature of Soldiers that led many of them into the military in their youth... like a higher calling. Sensitive people who can be inspired find the military gratifying. Enlistment peaked, for example, following the terrorist attacks on the US in 2001.

Soldiers are idealistic. They are led by their heart to serve their country. If necessary, Soldiers will not hesitate to die for their country.

In so far as it can be proven, sensitive young men, and more recently, sensitive young women, have always answered the call of their country for Soldiers.

Their numbers have not dwindled as the weapons of warfare become more terrible and the chances of death and horrible injury more likely. The near certainty of losing a cherished fellow Soldier, closer than a brother, inhumanely and helplessly before their eyes, has not weakened their strong sense of duty to serve their country.

Appreciation of Soldiers

How could any citizen fail to appreciate and to honor the men and women in our military services?

Being appreciated and respected is vital to our Soldier's sense of worth.

Many Soldiers return home from combat perplexed by their estranged sense of self. Their newly emerging self, the post-traumatic self, needs to be understood and valued by others to lessen the turmoil of their change

How could any citizen fail to appreciate the weight of the burden that Soldiers bear for our safety?

There are two important answers to these questions that are crucial to the understanding and restoration of our Soldiers returning home from combating terrorists.

Simply, first of all, the public knows little about the suffering our Soldiers endure in antiterrorism combat in two countries for the past decade and even less about their stress in coming home.

Equally importantly, our Soldiers are highly reluctant to disclose the nature and the extent of suffering caused by terrorists and their ever evolving, sophisticated weaponry. Recently, for example, during his first encounter in my office, a Soldier politely refused to tell me his trauma narrative. He said, "I don't know you that way yet."

The vast painful, nightmarish, unrelenting nature of the terrorism, ushered in by the brutal, unprovoked attacks of "9/11," is locked tightly in the souls of our sensitive Soldiers.

Our Soldiers' reluctance to divulge the details of their combat trauma is strongly influenced by their deeply held belief about the trauma itself. I was surprised by this belief until I found it to be nearly universal and deeply meaningful to combat Soldiers.

Soldiers regard their combat traumas as "precious."

SFC Tommy Kennedy, a 40-year-old thrice married man of medium height and build, with short black hair and black penetrating eyes, spoke solemnly. "It is a cherished part of me. To a significant degree, my combat trauma memories define who I am."

SFC Kennedy's combat trauma has harmfully shaped the course of his life. Speaking with the seriousness of a person on his death bed, he said, "The man who sleeps with my wife would be better off than the man who steals my combat trauma."

SFC Kennedy's strong sentiment arose from the misconduct of an unscrupulous Soldier who heard SFC Kennedy's combat story in one group and then retold it as his own combat experience in a different group. Fortunately, this highly infrequent, unacceptable behavior was identified immediately and corrected. "Trauma theft," another form of "Identity theft," is even more disturbing.

Why is the public's knowledge of the human cost of our current armed conflicts so unacceptably limited? It's plainly clear that the public has no idea of the psychological cost of our current armed conflicts.

"They don't know what I went through in combat," is a common theme among our redeployed Soldiers. "They don't know the good we did…the good things we did over there like building schools, caring for the sick, providing food for starving children."

"They get the most news about the few bad things our Soldiers did over there."

"They don't know what it means to free a country from a hateful dictator."

"We get the feeling that our country does not care about the war any more."

The Maine Troop Greeters

There are exceptions. The Soldiers tell me, for example, they are "treated like heroes...the people really show they care about us. It seems like the whole town turns out to greet us. They open their hearts to us," when they land at the airport in the state of Maine.

According to the Bangor Daily News, 10 DEC 2011, the "Maine Troop Greeters meet at the Bangor International Airport, a transfer stop for some military flights, whenever they hear of an inbound troop flight. As Soldiers leave their plane for a brief layover at the airport, greeters line up to shake their hands and welcome them to US soil."

The "Troop Greeters" have faithfully carried out their mission since 2003. "It's our pleasure to welcome them and to make their stay here as comfortable and as friendly as possible...," quoting greeter, Clayton Dodge. "The group operates a lounge where troops can use prepaid cell phones to make calls to family and friends."

"It means a lot that people are supporting us. It shows that we're doing something right, that somebody cares," said SPC (Specialist) Stasha McDonald.

If the "Troop Greeters" from Maine skim this page of my book, let them be told that countless Soldiers have lasting, pleasant, and thankful memories about what you did for them... that you cared for them in a very special, unselfish, exceptional and touching way.

Our nation is indebted to you. If your model of showing Soldiers that you care for them could become more widespread, all-embracing and lasting, then our Soldiers would experience unsurpassed healing.

"Troop Greeters" of Maine, we need to follow your warm hospitality throughout our returning Soldier's days, weeks and months into the future.

Perceptive Soldiers

Our sensitive Soldiers perceive immediately when they are liked, cared for, or treated indifferently.

It is not necessary for the public to know the details of the horror our sensitive Soldiers endured, both natural, such as blinding sand storms, and unnatural ones concocted in the shameless minds of terrorists.

However, this much is essential: as a nation let us never neglect our duty to treat our Soldiers with kindness, dignity, and respect. Sales clerks must not be rude. Drivers must not hog the passing lane. Family members must not be impatient or unduly inquisitive. Children must not ask, "Did you kill anybody?"

Remember how much we are in their debt. In a word, we owe our Soldiers our lives.

But let me hasten to say that our Soldiers are not asking to be treated with kid gloves. They need to know that you know what they did for you and for you to act accordingly.

Combating terrorists in Iraq and Afghanistan has made our perceptive Soldiers even more sensitive, more vigilant, more aware of unexpected dangers and more conscious of internal turmoil.

Our fine Soldiers are keenly responsive to perceived injustices, indifference, and rejection by anyone and by everyone encountered.

We are indebted to a host of complex defensive measures devoted to the protection of our nation for which we are thankful. However, our Soldiers are the embodiment of our greatest national defense.

It is not my purpose to educate the public about the sickening details of war, only to ask for patience and understanding in dealing with our military whose behavior, at times, may appear less desirable than is expected.

Please observe, however, with increasing admiration and deepening respect, that our Soldiers, even at home, are just as conscious of our need for safety and protection as they were in combat.

In particular, our Soldiers are burdened for the safety and protection of their families.

Our Soldiers are trained to be conscious of danger wherever they are, and remain competently skilled to appropriately respond to it.

Every symptom of PTSD (Posttraumatic Stress Disorder), for example, is little more than highly efficient combat readiness. In fact, many Soldiers returning from Iraq and Afghanistan will tell you they expect and therefore stay alert for more terrorist attacks in America.

Caring Too Much in Combat

Soldiers fight again and again when called upon in 21st Century War. These Soldiers develop behavioral health disorders to a degree yet to be understood. It does not seem to vary with the number of combat deployments.

I wonder if some of our combat-induced behavioral health problems come from our Soldiers "caring too much." The following story may help make this observation more understandable.

SGM (Sergeant Major) Sheldon McInnis recently retired from the Army. The SGM, a blond haired, blue eyed 41 year old, twice married Irishman wore a Ranger patch, indicating a Soldier with extraordinary military skills.

He accepted a managerial position with a large corporation near our military MTF (Medical Treatment Facility). He requested the night shift in order to continue to attend his weekly Post-Deployment Group Psychotherapy sessions.

"I can't give up my group. It is the highlight of my week." A brighter light, unfortunately, one he too often switched on, was his fondness for alcohol.

He was paid an excellent salary, treated respectfully by his employer, and he enjoyed his work. However, after only three weeks of employment, he quit abruptly, angrily and impulsively.

His employer encouraged him not to quit. "Take off the rest of the shift...go home...get some rest...take off tomorrow, but don't quit."

Nonetheless, the Soldier could not be dissuaded. He left indignantly.

He explained his action to his Post-Deployment Psychotherapy Group.

"It was like commanding a company of Soldiers who never had basic training, never had advanced individual training, never been trained on the range how to fire a weapon...and I was expected to take them to war.

The first week, I was in charge of 50 associates.

By the third week the number of associates was up to 150.

No matter how much I explained their job to them, they did not seem to get it."

A wise, recently retired NCO listened intently. He then said, in a matter of fact manner,

"You cared too much...those associates or whatever you called those civilians could not have cared less...they didn't give a shit.

The problem is we care. Sheldon walked out in anger because he cared. His associates didn't care.

Most people don't care and there are more of them than us. From zeroes to heroes, they get the same pay whether they care or not."

How likely is it that combat PTSD, the most common health impairment of our Soldiers from GWOT (Global War on Terror), has its fundamental and primary etiology as caring too much?

How many of the symptoms of combat-induced PTSD emerge from creative, inventive ways to ward off or disguise excessive caring?

The abundance of the evidence suggests that PTSD cannot develop in a context of indifference or of ambivalence. It requires sensitivity to suffering, and most often it arises out of the emotional pain of witnessing the suffering of others.

Witnessed suffering imprints itself in the memory of the combat Soldier as permanently as a brand burned into the hide of bovines. Try as one may, memories of witnessed suffering revisit awareness relentlessly.

To dampen the burning and painful memories of witnessed suffering, Soldiers try to stay very busy, try not to think about it. Too often Soldiers distract themselves with alcohol.

Most often and most costly emotionally, Soldiers seek solace in emotional numbness.

Emotional numbness robs the Soldiers of significant and important dimensions of existence.

Often the only feeling preserved in the emotionally numb Soldier is anger.

Imagine the quality of existence of living with the capacity to feel and express anger, but little or no capacity to feel or express other important feelings such as tenderness, love, or sadness or the ability to grieve losses, frozen in the numbness of emotional detachment.

Mercifully, many of our Soldiers, robbed of their healthy emotions, are often unaware of their deficits. MSG (Master Sergeant) Yoder's story may add clarity to this difficult and challenging predicament.

MSG Yoder's Story

MSG Michael Yoder, a 35-year-old, fair skinned, soft spoken, articulate, humble, intelligent man, a member of Combat Team B, was flown by helicopter with his team in Iraq to relieve Combat Team A.

"Chopper 909, your LZ (Landing Zone) is Cherry Hot. Repeat. Cherry Hot (Danger All Around)."

The Helicopter pilot informed the crew chief there were no moments to spare during the landing operation. He would have preferred to have heard the LZ was "Ice," without apparent danger, giving him more time to land and take off.

"This is Chopper 909. Reading LZ is Cherry Hot."

The operational plan required the rapid exit of Team B from the helicopter. Immediately following the exit of Team B, Team A would enter the helicopter and fly out of harm's way.

Something happened that day that changed MSG Yoder's life.

On the ground near the helicopter landing site, MSG Yoder spotted his best friend. His friend, a member of Team A, was seriously injured.

Instinctively, MSG Yoder scooped up his friend in his arms and carried him onto the helicopter.

He held his friend in his lap and prayed for a miracle that did not come as the helicopter speedily took off to return to headquarters.

His friend stared into MSG Yoder's eyes and died.

MSG Yoder did not and could not cry. His only thought, "I let my best friend die," haunted him.

His guilt was irrational. His grief, blocked by his guilt, seemed interminable.

On his worse days, for years after it occurred, MSG Yoder sensed and even saw images of his best friend.

He was terrified by these experiences and shared them with no one until he joined the Tuesday Morning Post-Deployment Psychotherapy Group.

MSG Yoder had "good days and bad days" but he was mentally imprisoned by the suffering memories of the death of his friend in his arms.

The years pass slowly.

MSG Yoder retired from the Army.

Still a young man in his early forties, MSG Yoder never went to work. He had no vitality.

Recently, MSG Yoder experienced another significant loss.

MSG Yoder's nephew died of cancer. His nephew was like a brother. Only a year separated them by age.

MSG Yoder attended his first group session following the death.

"I want to tell you," he said to the group with confidence, "I had a breakthrough.

I was with my nephew when he died.

I broke down and wept.

I wept for all those years I had blocked out my feelings.

A feeling of calm came over me. I felt relieved. I feel so much better.

I can't say I understand it.

The only time I expressed emotion before my nephew died was in this group or in dreams or nightmares."

The group sat silently. The group felt good, real good for MSG Yoder and they told him how pleased they were for him.

I looked carefully at the group. I saw facial expressions of authentic doubt. I can only imagine their thoughts: is it really good to have an emotional breakdown? Can an emotional breakdown really be a breakthrough? I have been thinking that expressing emotion was a sign of weakness. Does it really bring a calm feeling? Suppose I started to cry and lost control? What would people think of me then?

"The night sky is so beautiful in Iraq"

The Wednesday Morning Post-Deployment Psychotherapy Group was asked to consider the "caring too much" model of PTSD, an observation made the day before in the Tuesday Morning Group.

The seven members of the Wednesday Morning Group discussed the merits of the "caring too much" model of PTSD, suggested there may be some truth to the model but concluded it may be too simplistic.

For example, MSG Ken Compton, a mortuary affairs Soldier said, "I have feelings of all types. I am confused by my feelings…by my mixture of feelings…and how they change every few minutes."

MSG (Master Sergeant) Keith L. Johnson said, "I have no sexual feelings at all…I have a fear of loving…of getting rejected. I feel all alone…deserted. I feel I want to be home (down range).

It doesn't help me feel better any more to restore my antique cars (a previous source of pleasure)…I just stand and look at my cars and look at my tools but it doesn't excite me any more.

I have my serene moments.

The night sky is so beautiful in Iraq. It feels so close…nearby… it's like a beautiful blue sea and the moon is just amazing…I would stare at the moon and wonder what my family was doing on the other side of the moon…the feeling is hard to describe."

Fellow group members nodded their heads in agreement and in amazement that a long-forgotten pleasant memory, the beautiful night sky in Iraq, returned with this imagery.

Suddenly, as if a new but related feeling came into his awareness,

MSG Johnson said, "I feel like a stranger in my own house. My girlfriend wants a reaction from me, but I am as numb as a mouth full of Novocain."

The Spiritual Domain

Gunnery SGT Frank Martinez, a tall, muscular, quiet, US Marine, attending the Wednesday Afternoon Post-Deployment Spiritual Domain Psychotherapy Group, said, "I made it back from Iraq but not all of me came back. I left my spirit over there. I just imagine my spirit is roaming around over there and I want my spirit back, but I believe I can never get it back.

Without my spirit, I feel incomplete. I don't feel the same. I feel hollow from the inside…like an alien…like somebody that does not belong here any more. I don't want to die. I want to live, but I can't fully live without my spirit.

I visited my grandmother in Mexico. An old girlfriend was there.

She said, 'You don't seem happy.' She could see it in my eyes.

I can laugh, but there is no pleasure in it. It is different. I used to laugh with pleasure.

I feel like a machine. I do things, but it is like second nature. I feel like a robot walking down the road in a uniform."

MSG Barry Walker, a tall, large 38-year-old, twice married, talkative, insightful, caring man with soft blue eyes spoke in response to Gunnery SGT Martinez's statement that he left his spirit in Iraq.

"When I came back from Iraq I felt evil. In Iraq, you see the worst of what human beings can do to other human beings.

Terrorism affects the soul. Terrorism affects and scars your spirit. I felt lost. I could not rediscover myself. It is like being born again.

In some remarkable ways, I felt like a child again. I had a pretty rough childhood. I had to take care of myself. It was remarkable to me, but I have many of the same feelings I had as a child. I felt abandoned. I could not trust. It was like these feelings had been imprinted on my mind from childhood and it was being repeated again coming back from Iraq.

I asked one of the providers in the WTU (Warrior Transition Unit) to help me understand it. She told me that neglect or abuse in childhood increased the risk of a Soldier getting PTSD in combat."

I concurred. Childhood abuse and/or childhood neglect may cause permanent changes in the brain. A history of abuse or neglect in childhood increases a Soldier's risk of developing PTSD from combat.

A history of childhood abuse and/or neglect in Soldiers with combat-induced PTSD may also contribute to resistance to treatment. Imagine what childhood abuse and/or neglect does to the fragile, developing sense of basic trust.

The injury of childhood abuse and/or neglect in combination with combat-induced PTSD wears down the capacity to trust. The ability to trust is necessary to form attachment bonds. Without strong attachment bonds there is no enduring healing of PTSD.

Trauma

<u>Sacred Ground</u> is about the effects of a unique, special, and horrible form of trauma, the trauma of terrorism encountered by our Soldiers primarily in Iraq and Afghanistan during the first decade of the 21st Century and beyond.

Trauma, a French word meaning "wound," has become a household term, popularized by the increasingly widening acts of terrorists to inflict havoc, typically in shocking and phenomenally dramatic ways.

Posttraumatic Stress Disorder (PTSD) was first officially recognized as a mental disorder and included in the <u>Diagnostic and Statistical Manual of the American Psychiatric Association</u> in 1980. The Vietnam Veterans Association and the Women's Movement combined their efforts to make this happen. The details of PTSD, as induced by combat, and its closely associated diagnosis, mild Traumatic Brain Injury (mTBI), will be told by Soldiers, mainly in their own words, throughout this manuscript.

Death and Terrorism

"I need to accept death," SFC Gene Rivera, a Puerto Rican depressed man, told the Monday Afternoon Post-Deployment Group.

"Since Iraq, I am not the same person I appear to be on the outside. My wife says I am a cold person. I don't express my emotions to others...but when I am alone I have lots of feelings and my emotions come out.

If I hear of a death, for example, even if I don't know the person, I get very hurt inside. It is so emotionally draining internally. It is hard to explain."

"What has been your experience with death?" I asked.

"I had lots of loss to death in the war. I am so far out in rehab. I don't know why I am still feeling this way. Maybe it's because I pushed so much into the background.

In combat, we had to keep moving. If there was a death, I tried not to deal with it then. Now when I hear of a death in my neighborhood, my emotions leak out and it makes me feel so heavy-hearted...just hurting."

Tragically, there was a house fire in SFC Rivera's neighborhood in which a Soldier and his child died from smoke inhalation.

"Life is precious," he said. "I think of what the family will have to go through...the funeral...and all. It was just five houses down from mine. Christmas lights were up. I have children."

He stared at the floor vacantly.

Terrorism

The word "terror," coming from the combination of both French and a Latin word, means "great fear."

Numerous attempts have been made to satisfactorily define "terrorism," a subject with a long history, but I am informed by the literature that no single definition of terrorism is universally accepted. Nonetheless, the ultimate fear by which terrorism inflicts its most deadly objective is the fear of death.

Soldiers who have successfully fought in our 21st Century War tell me they functioned "beyond the fear of death."

These Soldiers, inundated with courage overflowing, accomplish feats of unimaginable achievement during the pitch of battle. Not uncommonly, however, once the mission is accomplished, psychological and physical exhaustion take their toll.

Death anxiety is an important subject to which we will return again and again as we try to understand the emotional impact of Soldiers combating terrorism.

The following example meaningfully describes how some Soldiers approach death. Here are the words of a former combat medic addressing the Wednesday Morning Post-Deployment Group.

LT Mike Bloom, 74 inches tall, physique of a weight-lifter, fair skin, and light brown eyes, may sit through a 90-minute group session declining to speak. On other days, he may be difficult to interrupt. Today, a talkative day, he said, "I was a combat medic in Afghanistan several years ago as an NCO (Noncommissioned Officer). Since then I have gone to Officer Candidate School and I am now a commissioned officer...but in my heart I am still an NCO.

The other day, my 8-year-old son, my friend, and I took our German Shepherds for a walk.

We came upon a house with a large dog chained inside a yard. Somehow the dog got unchained and tore into my friend's dog.

He badly injured my friend's dog.

Immediately, I ran to my truck, got my medic's bag, put the dog in the back of my truck, and I sutured up all his wounds. It was almost automatic. I was completely calm. I knew my friend could not afford a vet's bill.

I checked on the injured dog the next day and he was doing fine.

I was not going to tell anybody what happened, but my son told his mother, his teacher, and his friends. To me it was nothing. I just did what I did. I have not spoken to my son about it yet…so I don't know how he feels about what he saw.

This is what I do not understand," continuing to address the group, "shortly after it was over I saw blood on the front of my truck. The dog was never near the front of my truck.

When I went home, I saw my children lying on the floor covered with blood. I knew it could not be real, but it seemed very real to me at the time.

Can somebody help me understand what was going on? I was perfectly fine during the crisis. Everybody was running around screaming. The dogs were growling and fighting. I was perfectly calm. I had inner peace…even a feeling of power during the crisis.

It was only afterwards that I started to feel strange…even weak. What happened to me?"

MSG Walker, described above, a mature Soldier with PTSD, said "PTSD is all about triggers, and the triggers can sneak up on you.

The blood of the injured dog, the one whose life you saved, was your trigger. The blood of the injured dog triggered a delayed flashback. It transported you back into a real combat situation.

The dog's blood was a delayed trigger because your training as a combat medic kicked in. You felt powerful saving the dog's life. After the crisis was over, you felt weak. The trigger kicked in when you felt weak. The flashback followed.

The blood you saw on the front of your truck and on your children were components of your flashback, a scary, miserable feeling. Man, I know. I've been there. Everyone in this group has been there.

Fortunately, your flashback did not last very long. Like the rest of us in this group, you were caught off guard by your trigger.

You are new in our group. We are pleased you are here because we have a lot to teach you. We are all in the same boat. You also have a lot to teach us.

Your finely perfected combat medic skills enabled you to function like a combat medic to save the dog's life. Your adrenalin provided the confidence you needed for the task. But when the mission was over, just like in combat, the adrenalin wore off...your guard was down...the fear that often surrounds combat missions became real again."

MSG Walker continued speaking.

"I had a trigger sneak up on me so bad yesterday that I could not sleep a wink last night.

I was in my car with a friend going to Virginia Commonwealth University to see a professor. My friend was giving me directions. The area was crowded. I drove into an area that confused me. I cursed out my friend. I exploded on her.

I couldn't understand what upset me so terribly. I was surprised at my outbursts.

Later, I realized that the whole area looked like a traffic circle in Iraq where two VBIDs (Vehicle Borne Improvised Explosive Devices) detonated, causing mass casualties. I had a sense of panic. In Iraq there was a grassy median and a round-about circle.

I didn't understand why I panicked in Richmond at VCU (Virginia Commonwealth University).

Later I processed it in my mind. I was so upset I couldn't sleep. I was enraged. I was angered by the things in my head from Iraq. I was high-strung. I was paranoid. I had to check the door all night. While I was coming down, I felt stupid that I let those things sneak up on me. The trigger kicked in when I took that turn and saw a military set-up.

In Iraq it was in Section 11. It had a traffic round-about…lots of traffic…a market place.

I had always felt comfortable coming through there. It took 7-10 minutes to get through it.

VBIDs are very destructive.

We turned around.

The Team Leader said, 'What the fuck was that?'

We said, 'It's a fucking VBID.'

Let's go back!"

The Leader shouted 'No, when there is one VBID there is always a second one.'

We watched the second one go off.

It was awful. It was mass confusion.

An Iraqi Policeman was carrying a detached arm…a perfectly good arm.

There was screaming, wailing.

I felt detached from my body.

I was motionless and emotionless.

It was like I was lifted out of my body and watching it.

A child was crying all the time and a mother was also crying.

I felt helpless."

An overpowering silence of understanding filled the group room.

It was written on each Soldier's face.

Yes, that's the way it happens.

Yes, our triggers catch us off guard.

Yes, our triggers are painful because they cause us involuntarily to re-experience the worst parts of our combat memories.

Each Soldier stared at the floor and then slowly looked at me.

"Is this the way I am going to spend the rest of my life, Dr. Brown," they wordlessly shouted at me.

'This is not a prison sentence, gentlemen," I said with confidence.

"You are going to be free, released from the power of your triggers. Try to be patient.

Let time and understanding do their work.

MSG Walker talked LT Bloom precisely through each step of his flashback. Knowledge based on truth is powerful.

MSG Walker, however, was not able to sleep last night. He could not talk himself through his own flashback. It was too fresh. He needed time to understand it. He'll sleep tonight.

You had the courage to fight terrorism in combat. No one can take that from you.

It will take the same kind of courage to recover, to become the fully functioning hero of your own life.

Every one of you is a hero to me!

You are a hero to everyone who knows you.

Commit yourself to therapy.

Together, as Soldiers we can win this battle. Believe it. Believe it 100%!"

Is the feeling of helplessness a form of the fear of death?

Is the fear of the loss of control another special form of the fear of death?

In how many forms, configurations, and appearances do our brave Soldiers in 21st Century War experience and encounter the fear of death?

Our courageous Soldiers will answer these crucial questions in their own voices and describe how they continue to master their fear of death.

Roll Call

The war makes SGT Underwood appear 40 years of age, although he is 10 years younger. He spoke as if he had a mouth full of mashed potatoes. He is inarticulate but unsurpassed in sincerity and authenticity.

He spoke with conviction and determination to his Monday Afternoon Post-Deployment Psychotherapy Group.

"I will never go to another memorial service again."

His supervisor ordered him to attend a memorial service last week. He told the supervisor, "Sir, I can't go. I just can't handle it."

SGT Underwood's supervisor replied angrily, "You will go or you will face the consequences."

The soldier told the following account.

"We had a memorial service on the post last Friday. One of the soldiers in Iraq was home on leave and died. We didn't know it was going to be a memorial service until the last minute.

I can't stand those services because they are so upsetting. They had a roll call at the service. I could not bear it.

Just as soon as the service was over, I left the chapel and got in my car.

I drove no more than 25 miles per hour for several hours. That's the fastest I could travel safely while crying.

I cried my eyes out. I didn't feel any better afterwards."

I asked the group to explain to me the meaning of a "roll call."

They all chimed in almost at the same time with the same disdain.

Eight men, all combat veterans, said they dreaded roll calls.

One of them went to the blackboard. He drew a diagram of a fallen soldier's boots with the rifle bayonet extended, stuck in the ground, and his Kevlar, or armor and helmet on top of his rifle. Beside the Soldier's boots lay his dog tags and awards.

The members of the fallen soldier's squad are called to attention.

The name of each member of the unit is called alphabetically.

It goes something like this:

"Private Johnson?"

"Here, Sir;"

"Private Jones?"

"Here, Sir;"

"Private Larson?"

Silence.

"Private Larson?"

Silence.

"Private Larson?"

Silence.

The fallen Soldier does not answer.

The fallen Soldier has been killed in action.

The silence is ear-piercing.

In the distance, not a very far distance, a 21 gun salute is fired. The bugle sorrowfully bleats out Taps.

With each Soldier's lamentable death, part of every Soldier in his unit dies with him.

Little else is more disturbing to a Soldier than the loss of a battle buddy. The attachment between Soldiers whose very survival depends upon their close working relationship is emotionally costly.

Acute traumatic grief in combat challenges one's sanity. Its devastating memories endure.

Jules Masserman identified the "Ur-defenses" as a set of "three fundamental beliefs essential for psychological integrity of the individual. They are 1. A delusion of invulnerability and immortality, 2. Faith in a celestial order, and 3. A wishful fantasy that fellow human beings are potential friends available for mutual service."

Our Soldiers, in the midst of the loss of a fellow Soldier, closer than a brother, have body armor for protection of their body. Sadly, however, there is no protection for their overwhelming feelings of unexpressed grief. They are robbed of their "Ur-defenses."

They must "move on." They must "stay on task." Scouring for the enemy, their tasks are ceaseless.

All soldiers come to dread roll call.

Inevitably, each Soldier must think there might come a time when their own name will be called three times, but they will not answer.

I am told by the soldiers that the roll call and a memorial service must be conducted within 24 hours of the death of the soldier. A memorial service sometimes associated with the roll call must be brief. Fellow soldiers, especially leaders, make a few comments about the fallen soldier.

There is a "communication blackout" following the death of a Soldier in combat. No one is permitted to contact the outside world until the Soldier's family is personally delivered the sad news by a Casualty Assistance Officer and team. The grief and other feelings experienced by the dead Soldier's family are unimaginable.

I asked the group if they thought I should write a letter excusing SGT Underwood from attending memorial services in the future because he has such difficulty coping with it.

Surprising to me, they all said no.

The members of SGT Underwood's Post-Deployment Group Therapy thought he must somehow find the courage to face roll calls and memorial services.

I reminded them that it was difficult for Soldiers with PTSD to have the additional stress of dealing with grief following deployment.

They reminded me they already know about the stress of memorial services and roll calls because they suffer from PTSD as well. Furthermore, even SGT Underwood himself said he did not want an excuse from me to miss the next roll call or memorial services.

Witnessing

Our Soldiers are required to be warriors. Our Soldiers are also required to be witnesses. Soldiers must report or testify to every detail of combat that can be recalled, ideally as soon as possible after the engagement with the enemy ended.

Their report may be vital to the operations to follow, to planning, and to future combat training.

Soldiers may perceive, however, that what is reported may reflect unfavorably upon their actions and upon them personally as Soldiers, unintentionally influencing their performance in combat and, grievously, their flawed memory in the years to follow.

Witnessing the Serious Injury of a Fellow Soldier in Combat

CPT Thomas, a tall, handsome, dark-skinned, physically fit officer, was self-confident in the past. He served a total of 30 months in combat, from 2006-2010.

CPT Thomas, however, is no longer fit or confident. He is very depressed.

This 28-year-old married man, father of two small children, is deeply sad appearing. He continues to be burdened by the indescribable agony of guilt.

Thus far, all treatment has failed to help the CPT.

Initially, CPT Thomas resorted to doctoring himself with alcohol. Even large amounts of alcohol, for long periods of time, did not bring relief.

Finally, several months ago, he was sent to Behavioral Health. Following two lengthy psychiatric hospitalizations, he came to Post-Deployment Traumatic Grief Psychotherapy Group.

Reluctantly, CPT Thomas told his fellow group therapy members his trauma narrative.

"We were under pressure to get our numbers up...to look good on paper.

The battalion commander wanted us to have more soldiers qualified on the rifle range.

We were in Iraq. The nearest range was an hour and a half away by convoy.

Convoys are always dangerous.

The MAJ was putting pressure on me because the battalion commander was putting pressure on him to get more Soldiers to the range.

PVT Billy King, a small farm boy from Indiana, was only 17-years-old. He was fresh out of AIT (Advanced Individual Training), immediately following Basic Training.

He had only been with us for two days.

I ordered him to go to the range in a convoy. It was against my better judgment. It was an unnecessary risk.

PVT King did not complain.

His convoy got to the range safely, but on the way back they were hit by explosive weapons.

The PVT was in a vehicle with one other soldier.

Their vehicle was hit. The other Soldier was killed. The PVT was seriously injured.

I heard the whole thing on the radio. They did not call out names, but they called out numbers that we identified as our Soldiers.

I looked up the numbers and found the PVT's name on the list.

I went to the CASH (Combat Army Support Hospital) to check on his condition.

He was not there. He'd been flown to Baghdad.

I got to Baghdad in a helicopter and found him.

He was incapacitated by narcotic medication. He could not speak to me.

He went from Baghdad to Landstuhl and then to Walter Reed.

I never heard what happened to him.

I just think about him all the time.

I feel like it was senseless to order him to the range. He was too young to be severely wounded."

I asked CPT Thomas what he would say if he could speak to PVT King today.

He did not know exactly what he would say.

"I would be asking for forgiveness," he whispered.

CPT Thomas has not been able to grieve for PVT King's traumatic injuries nor for the Soldier who was killed.

CPT Thomas had nothing to do with ordering the other soldier to the range, a decision made by someone else. However, he felt responsible for the serious, life-altering injury to PVT Billy King because he directly ordered him to the range.

CPT Thomas was not blamed by his chain of command, there was no investigation of the incident, and no one knew that CPT Thomas held himself personally and directly responsible for PVT King's injury.

There are at least two important lessons to be learned from CPT Thomas' witnessing a serious combat injury.

First, the "witnessing" of the injury took place by hearing a real-time radio description of the attack that caused the severe injury of one Soldier and the death of another soldier in combat.

Listening to the trauma instead of seeing it or being personally present did not lessen its powerful shock upon CPT Thomas.

Secondly, the next lesson to be learned from CPT Thomas' case is the degree of guilt which, as in many combat cases, is extreme. By its very nature, CPT Thomas' excessive guilt persistently interferes with the normal grieving process.

CPT Thomas suffered to such an extent, primarily over his misperception of causing the injury, that he required multiple psychiatric hospitalizations in the previous seven months.

CPT Thomas acknowledges that he has not been able to grieve. He acknowledges that he does not have closure. He would likely benefit from meeting with PVT King and having a heart-to-heart discussion about what happened.

This much is clear: CPT Thomas perceived that the convoy trip to the range was unnecessary, the risk outweighed the benefit, and no alternative options were considered.

CPT Thomas saw the situation as "a type of fraud, one in which I willingly and regrettably participated, a costly one, one for which the price was paid with PVT King's health and wellbeing."

"It is what it is," mistakenly thought CPT Thomas.

It is never what it is, dear CPT, dear Soldiers, and dear readers. It is always the meaning we give to it.

The meaning we give to every experience significantly influences its effects upon us. It behooves us one and all, therefore, to make an accuracy check of the meanings we assign to our experiences.

For example, as a new Soldier assigned to a combat unit, PVT King's skills with a weapon likely needed honing. In order to most suitably assign PVT King to a team position, his trip to the range was critical.

The life of the Soldier to his right and the Soldier to his left depended upon PVT King as a rifleman. PVT King's life and the lives of the members of his unit depended upon his ability as a Soldier with a rifle.

Another Kind of Witness

"We don't understand."

The Appeals Board in Washington was questioning the "witness" for SFC Albert North exercising his right to appeal the decision of his MEB (Medical Evaluation Board) rating.

The MEB process is a complex procedure in which a Soldier is financially compensated for all "in line of duty" injuries rendering him or her unfit for duty.

"How could you rate SFC North "excellent" on most of his NCOER (Noncommissioned Officer Evaluation Report) bullets? At the very same time, his psychiatric diagnoses included PTSD, TBI, and Cognitive Disorder.

Can you explain this apparent contradiction to this PEB (Physical Examination Board), 1SG O'Malley?

You were his 1SG for two years.

No one knows a Soldier better than their 1SG.

Your days with SFC North began at 0430 and ended at 2230, or even later, depending on the circumstances.

For the sake of SFC North and for the sake of this board, help us address this challenging question.

How is it possible that a Soldier said to be burdened with PTSD and TBI deserves superior marks on his NCOER?"

SFC Albert North's former 1SG, now a MSG stationed at another, distant military post, responded articulately on a speaker phone for all to hear at the Washington, DC, Appeal's Board hearing.

"At first, I did not notice it, but the longer he worked for me the more I could see that he was different.

He was an AIT (Advanced Individual Training) Platoon SGT.

He graduated two classes of 100 AIT students in the first six months of the two years of his assignment with me.

It was difficult for him, but he stuck with each class from the beginning to the end.

He had to write down everything I told him, entering it methodically into his cell phone.

I noticed he walked with a limp.

He requested no Profiles (medical excuse from duty).

He always answered my questions, but he never requested special consideration or claimed to have consequences from his combat deployments.

I made him my Senior Platoon SGT over 5 or 6 other Platoon SGTs."

When his former 1SG made her next statement, SFC North, seated in front of the panel of judges, cried. Tears streamed down his saddened face. He considered it an unmanly act, especially in the presence of other men of superior rank.

The Soldier, humiliated by his spontaneous tears, quickly turned his face away from his attorney and the 3-member panel of military judges.

"I arranged his assignments around his Behavioral Health appointments," she said, "because on his worst days he tried harder than all the other Platoon SGTs on their best days."

After a long silence, the panel's senior officer, bursting with tears successfully trapped securely inside his own sternum, quelling, proud chest, without emotion said, "Thank you, MSG O'Malley. We will need to speak to no more witnesses." SFC North's MEB disability ratings were increased significantly.

My Soldier Died in My Arms. "Te amo Papa"

CSM (Command Sergeant Major) Eric York was referred for Post-Deployment Group Therapy. I evaluated him as an appropriate patient for Group Psychotherapy. He chose to join the Dream Interpretation Group.

Small in stature, solemn in demeanor and facial expression, articulate in speech, mild in manner, he was physically exhausted from protracted insomnia. He was significantly depressed.

He had a business-like manner, a person, I deduced, unlikely to share his emotions or to value psychological phenomena.

Without visible emotion, he said, "One of my Soldiers died in my arms.

Five of us were walking side-by-side. We had just left the mess hall. It was dark.

An explosion...out of nowhere...seriously injured two of the five of us. We ran for the bunker, but I had to reach out and pull Suzy back into the bunker.

She slumped forward in pain. I yelled for help and started CPR, but I could hear gurgling in her chest. I felt totally helpless.

A woman, not a Soldier but a civilian contractor, opened Suzy's blouse. Blood was pouring out of the left side of her chest.

In Spanish, Suzy said "Tell my Papa I love him." Suzy was one of my Soldiers...only 20 years old.

It should have been me.

If only I had walked in the front it would have been me.

It should have been me."

"Where is it written that the injury and death should have been yours?" I asked.

"I just feel strongly it should have been me.

It happened at the beginning of the war in Iraq, a long time ago, but it keeps coming back into my mind like a fresh memory.

We redeployed to Fort Lewis, Washington.

I went to see her father in Arizona some time later. I needed to do that for closure.

Suzy's father is not American. He spoke very little English. I was able to tell him in Spanish what his daughter said before she died.

Her last words were for you, "Te amo Papa."

Her father fell to the ground. It broke him apart. He could not stop crying.

The word Suzy used for daddy was the most intimate word in Spanish for father.

Her high school honored her memory. The students built a 50 foot American flag design garden with flowers showing the red, white, and blue of our flag...in her honor.

I just can't get over feeling completely helpless as she died in my arms..."

"Are you thinking you should have saved her life?" I asked.

"Yes, I think that is what I have been thinking all these years. I think that is why I felt so helpless."

"Could you have been there with Suzy for some other reason?" I inquired.

"Like what...what other reason could there be?"

"You tell me if another reason comes to mind," I said.

His eyes filled with tears. "Do you mean was I there to take her message back to her father?"

"He will never forget you," I said.

The Soldier wept.

"It took courage, energy, and time to go find Suzy's father," I said with confidence.

"It was not easy, I am certain.

What you did makes me see you as a Soldier of old, charging with the flag, ahead of the troops, on a mission of great importance, nothing deterring you.

You obeyed your heart. Taking her dying words to her father was the most precious gift of his life."

"Thank you," he said gratefully. "What you said is a big help.

I have seen many counselors and no one ever said that to me. It really helps.

I have been so depressed that I have considered suicide with a sense of joy, the sense that, if necessary, I could stop my despair by suicide, but I have tried to argue against that thought.

My individual therapist, Dr. Michael Regal, has been really helpful, reminding me of all the good reasons I have to live."

Based on thousands of conversations with Soldiers, witnessing the death of a fellow Soldier, one with a close emotional attachment, is more traumatic, more enduring, and more painful than the Soldier's fear of the loss of his or her own life.

Most of us are spared the horror and sadness of the sudden, senseless, traumatic destruction of the human body of someone to whom we are closely attached.

Many of us may find it incomprehensible, even unimaginable, to fathom what our Soldiers experience in 21st Century War.

Our Soldiers, however, are not removed in time or place from the dreaded catastrophic, intended destruction of the ingenious terrorists whose immoral financial and political sponsors remain largely unidentified.

Our Soldiers defend us with their selfless courage in Iraq and Afghanistan, or wherever they are needed. They sacrifice their life to keep us from more home-grown terrorists' attacks.

In our 21st Century War, our Soldiers live on volcanoes, known to erupt at any unpredictable moment.

God, we have to love our Soldiers.

Our Soldiers have seen in one day, depending upon the stage of our 21st Century War, more traumatic injury and death than a thousand of our citizens collectively witness in a life time.

Memories of Combat Death

Many soldiers tell me their unpleasant memories of combat trauma seem real and "fresh," as if they had just happened, despite the fact that many years have passed since the trauma occurred.

It is as if combat memories, particularly those associated with witnessing the death of a fellow soldier in combat, are stored in a part of the mind in which the passage of time is not relevant.

"Will I be like this the rest of my life, Sir?"

Of course, there are no guarantees in the field of medicine or in life itself.

However, over time and with an appropriate therapist with whom the Soldier becomes attached and trusting, these memories will be recalled with less pain.

With effective treatment, Soldiers will discover a perspective through which to meaningfully interpret and understand their memories. In this way, the irrational components of the memory will be corrected.

The Soldier will experience relief.

Fortunately, unnecessary emotional, self-induced suffering is remarkably lessened when the truth of the meaning of trauma is discovered and accepted, free of all misrepresentation.

Death is accepted with appropriate sadness when the attachment is understood.

Witnessing serious injury and death of a fellow Soldier in combat is never free of deep pain and regret. It is part of the price paid for caring.

5

Little Bobby Brown

Coming of Age ...Too Soon

Frances, my second oldest sister, eighteen years my senior, was physically frail most of her life. She spent much time seeking medical care; however, like the other women in my family, she lacked no assertive skills.

As a young married woman, Frances was modest appearing: brown-blonde short hair, brown eyes, medium height, thin, weak and anxious.

Frances was the designee or volunteer to take me to the emergency room at the Norfolk General Hospital whenever it became necessary. Fortunately, it was infrequent.

I was never adept or manually skillful, barely passing Wood Shop at James Madison School in the seventh grade. The wooden tie rack or corner what-not shelf I made was unrecognizable by all but those who loved me.

I recall "building" a go-cart and accidentally dropping a heavy metal wheel from which protruded a large nail for an axle. It fell like a WW II bomb landed precisely on top of my right foot.

I don't remember the pain, but I sustained a large bruise and a through-and-through penetrating injury. Frances took me by bus to the emergency room. The strong odor of ether in the emergency still lingers in my mind.

Frances was most often kind and caring, never one to talk or act hatefully, although she was my second sister to tolerate an abusive marriage. Tommy, her husband, was an attractive, likable, athletically talented man who was a good prize fighter.

For reasons never shared with me, Tommy ultimately was a state penitentiary inmate. He made friends easily, often randomly. He laughed readily and heartily, but most at the misery and suffering of others.

Tommy's full head of dark hair, sharpening the deep blueness of his eyes, often fell down over his face. He pushed it back with his hand or uniquely shook it back into position by an odd movement of his head.

Frances and Tommy lived in a second story apartment on 46th Street, within easy walking distance from my parents, but on the opposite side of Hampton Boulevard.

Strategically and geographically, their apartment and their life were less susceptible to my mother's direct observation and scrutiny.

"Pretty is as pretty does," my mother often reminded all of us. Tommy had an ugly side, hidden from most of my family.

"Half-laughing and half-scolding…"

The following incident, never previously disclosed, happened when I was not more than five or six, during one of my frequent visits to Frances and Tommy's apartment. Of course I could have never gone there on my own because the dangers of "crossing" Hampton Boulevard prevented it.

Tommy may have been drinking. He was in a playfully sadistic mood.

He wore boxer shorts and had been on the bed with Frances who wore a pale white night gown. He was not through with whatever he had been doing with Frances on the bed.

He forced her to sit on the floor at the foot of the bed, pulled up her night gown, and pried her legs apart.

Half-laughing and half-scolding, Tommy made Frances expose her most intimate female anatomy to me.

I stood back only to be pulled up close by Tommy to examine the forbidden scene.

Using crude terms intermingled with terms familiar to a child, like "pee-pee," Tommy slowly and painstakingly repeatedly touched each anatomical feature and described its physiological function, instructing me of their great pleasure.

In retrospect, it was not intended as a first lesson on the facts of life for a five or six year old boy.

It was solely a memorable humiliation, mortification, embarrassment, and shameful degradation of Frances for the gloating, cruel, heartless, callous, nasty, appalling pleasure of Tommy, even crueler than the physical beatings he habitually inflicted upon her.

The incident was never discussed.

It did not lessen my love for my sister.

I am aware of no grudge I held against Tommy, a man I had admired.

Psychoanalytically, it happened to me during Freud's celebrated "Oedipal Period."

If the incident happened to a six year old boy today, it would unhesitatingly be reported as child abuse.

Child protective services investigators would classify it as "founded."

Today, the perpetrator would be appropriately punished. The child victim would be subjected to a vast variety of alternatives such as possible removal from the home, individual play therapy, and family therapy may also be likely.

None of the alternatives sounds appealing to me now all these years later. No criticism of our current child protective services is intended.

It was not the only time in my childhood that I was exposed to inappropriate sexual conduct by adults.

"Do You Want a Ride Home?"

Two other instances, neither previously disclosed, come quickly to mind. I will briefly describe them, not for their sensationalism, but for their lack of conscious meaningfulness to me or apparent influence on my life that I can determine.

I share these incidents, and other childhood experiences, to show that I am no stranger to early trauma.

As I honestly reflect on my own life, withholding none of its ugliness, thankfully only a small amount compared to its beauty and the love I received, two ideas emerge into my awareness.

First, "what's good for the goose is good for the gander." If I want the Soldiers I treat to be honest in fully disclosing their combat trauma and re-entry trauma of coming home to a new life, can they expect less honesty from me? I think not. The Soldiers who read <u>Sacred Ground</u> will discover a facet of the life of their therapist that has been shared with them in no other way.

In making this comparison, dear reader, please permit me to assure you that I do not equate the tiny traumas of my life with the massive, multiple traumas of the sacrifices made by our Soldiers in combat.

Second, even unacceptable, hideous early childhood sexual abuse need not mar a person's life indefinitely, without therapy then or a later time.

The next instance to which I refer occurred when I was ten, walking from Colley Avenue on 47th Street to my home. Ninety percent of my transportation during the bulk of my childhood consisted of walking or riding my Western Flyer bicycle.

A car slowed down. The driver was a middle-aged over-weight man, with a reddish face. I later saw him in public meetings where his presence was noted to be important. He was dressed in a business suit, and he asked if I wanted a ride home.

I preferred walking, but I got into his car, not wishing to disappoint him.

Making small talk, he placed his hand on my left knee, and then on my genitals.

A white handkerchief partially obscured his penis from which small amounts of semen leaked out as he moved his right hand rhythmically.

"You need a girlfriend," I said forthrightly.

He was too engaged in this self-stimulating act to reply, but then he moved my hand to his penis and his to mine.

Strangely, I was unafraid.

Fifteen minutes passed. He stopped the car, cautioned me to keep his secret, and signaled me to leave.

At the time, as I distinctly recall, it was not sexually stimulating. It was more of a non-event for me.

I realized it was wrong. Of course, I told no one.

Forty Whole Minutes

"Forty whole minutes," captures the third instance of sexual conduct with an adult during my childhood.

Rudy is a close first cousin, two years my senior and one foot taller. He and I were on a bus from Lamberts Point to the Trail Way Bus Station in downtown Norfolk.

We were going to take an early evening trip to Chuckatuck, Isle of Wight County, in which was located the modest residence of the Beale family. We were seated on the rear of the bus when approached by a man who said he would like to please us sexually.

I believe I was 14. The man was physically unattractive, effeminate, but pressingly insistent.

We declined his offer, saying we had a bus to catch. Nonetheless, he accompanied us to the bus station and read the bus schedule sign.

"You have forty whole minutes," he said, grabbing my arm. I told him that Rudy was older, inferring his sexual maturity was more advanced.

Neither Rudy nor I had any interest in the man's proposal, but under pressure Rudy fell prey, went with him to a nearby darkened set of steps and in an instant was relieved of his sexual arousal by the man's perfected oral sex.

"What happened," I asked Rudy after we boarded the bus.

"Nothing," Rudy said, hiding his embarrassment.

It was never discussed again. I am unaware that the encounter ever affected either of us.

Witnessing Abuse

As a child, I witnessed some of the physical abuse Frances undeservedly and too often received from Tommy's fists.

I was never privy to all its reasons, but Frances left Tommy and returned home with her young son, Tommy, Jr. He was not more than five or six when they came to live with us on 47th Street.

Frances' divorce from Tommy was unassociated with the incident disclosed above in which I was precociously introduced to the anatomy and physiology of adult female sexuality.

That secret was locked in a safe whose combination remained undiscoverable until now, and the secret had left no vivid, lingering memories because it was enveloped in dense mental fog. The fog that comes to mind is the bewilderment for which flashing yellow lights caution drivers approaching the ridge of Afton Mountain in the nearby Blue Ridge. As Dickens wrote in Great Expectations, "...it left a stain that faded with time but never completely disappeared."

Amazingly, "big Tommy," as we called him after "little Tommy's" birth, remained in the good graces of our family, always warmly greeted by my mother, and stayed in contact with us throughout his prison sentence, shortened by volunteering as a human subject for medical research in the penitentiary, until his death several years later.

Before we moved to 39th Street, immediately after the very beginning of WW II, Edith married Johnny Loftin. The marriage is noted principally for its unromantic brevity.

She later married Coker.

Christine, my oldest sister, lived nearby during the most formative years of my childhood, was like my second mother, chronically overweight, divorced Frank and married Jimmie (after WW II).

Frances divorced Tommy and married Roy.

Interestingly, at one point in my life I had three sisters and six brothers-in-law. Fortunately, basically all parties eventually showed mutual respect for each other, likely out of respect for my mother.

My Mother's Relationship with My Father

My mother was staunchly loyal, a person who loved her five surviving children beyond the telling of it.

In a painful contrast to my mother's love for her children, I never observed my mother showing the least amount of affection or even tenderness towards my father. He was not indifferent to feelings of affection. She was often openly critical of him, suggesting she lacked respect for him for reasons that to this day remain unknown to me.

He was not a dashing figure and cannot be blamed for his natural physical traits. My dad was 6 feet tall, slim, never athletic, and during his waking hours, from his lips hung an unlit pipe.

My mother must have compiled a mental list of my dad's worst traits. No list of his least appreciated traits was ever written. I record the list posthumously from her repetitious statements about him that reside in my memory. My dad's unacceptable traits were important to my mother. Objectivity is claimed for the list, permitting no feelings even akin to pity. It would be accurate, and it would be heart breaking to all those who read it except for my mother.

The list in my mother's voice (without profanity, but she made up for its absence):

(1) "He is round-shouldered. A man should stand erect (she always did, and she always reminded us to square our shoulders, to stand up straight);

(2) He starts talking before he enters a room, leaving us dumbfounded about the topic he is delivering;

(3) He has no common sense;

(4) He lies on his back on that sofa (pointing to a day-bed in the kitchen) all day long whenever it rains (as a house painter, most of his work was out of doors, dictated by the weather);

(5) He runs his mouth too much and that's what gets him into trouble;

(6) He has always been half deaf;

(7) He would not sign the consent form to get my hernia operation (her long-standing feelings about this unrepaired perceived physical flaw were very strong);

(8) I am embarrassed by his tremor (familial hand tremor that sometimes contributed to a tremor in his voice);

(9) Getting blinded in his right eye at 12 years of age on a tug boat in the Elizabeth River was his own fault; he should have been in school; and

(10) He follows me around the house like a puppy, and I don't like it, and I don't like him."

Still to this day, forty years after her death, I was never told why my mother did not love my father.

Sad Rainy Days

Rainy days meant my father, a house painter, was often home asleep on the cot in the kitchen. It rains frequently in Tidewater, Virginia.

My mother was intolerant of my father's confinement to the house when it rained.

Rainy days upset my mother terribly. Often she openly belittled my father. Awake on the cot with his eyes closed, my father heard her shouting to me, "Don't end up on your back like him; get an education."

The curse of the rainy days in Norfolk was visited upon my family primarily prior to WW II or in its most early phase when dad worked for my mother's brother-in-law, Cress Richardson.

In a painful recollection, dad punched Cress with all his might in the middle of Cress' protuberant abdomen.

It happened in our kitchen during a much heated debate over dad's perception of Cress' failure to fairly pay for the work he had done for him as a house painter that week.

Cress' wife, Aunt Daisy, the eldest of the Beale children, was ordinarily quiet, controlling, judgmental, and intelligent.

My mother often spoke for and supported my dad in situations where his passivity was deemed inappropriate.

Aunt Daisy and my mother participated loudly in the dispute in question. Soon both women started screaming with horror, terrifyingly attempting to break up the fist fight between their respective husbands.

I was about 10 years old. Failing to comprehend the severity of the situation, I had Tommy Fentress, my 2 year old nephew, in my arms as I lay on the infamous kitchen cot.

I was playing a modified game of peek-a-boo, raising and lowering Tommy up into the air. I was even mimicking the pre-pugilistic language of the disputants, never imagining it would become a real fist-fight in the small confines of our kitchen.

I was repeating over and over such, to me meaningless, words as "cheating me," "not working like you say," "I have the hours in writing," and "I do all the work while you stand around or are not even there."

I sprang to my feet when the fighting began, approached the four adults in confusion, not knowing what to do. It seemed to end as quickly as the fist-fight started. The Richardsons exited, dad was fired, and the physical and psychological injuries hardly ever healed.

Ocean View Amusement Park

My mother equally loved her parents and siblings, and invented situations that brought family members together. I remember summer picnics at Ocean View Amusement Park where my cousins, aunts, uncles, and parents really enjoyed playing on the beach. Lettuce, tomato, and bologna sandwiches with Pepsi Colas were followed by ice-cold watermelon.

My favorite ride was the Bumping Cars. I collected refundable soft-drink bottles and cashed them in for stashes of pennies to pay for my Bumping Car rides.

It was at one of these summer family days at Ocean View that I first learned about a mean ugliness.

Junior, perhaps my closest friend at age 10, the Filipino son of a U.S. Navy Chief Petty Officer, joined us at Ocean View. I proudly placed twenty pennies on the counter of the ticket booth and requested two tickets, my treat.

The middle aged woman selling the tickets gave me one ticket and returned ten of my pennies. When I complained she pointed to a sign, "Whites Only," and said, "Your friend is not white."

Junior and I were close. I never knew he was "not white," and I never cared that he was "not white."

"You don't understand," I pleaded, "Junior is my friend."

"I don't make the rules," devoid of emotion, she announced.

If a ten year old boy can be enraged, then I was enraged and hurt and helpless.

I felt upset for Junior and for myself. I wanted to show my friend the great fun of bumping multicolored metallic bumping cars with rods from their rears poking up to the ceiling where an electric circuit powered the cars.

I can see Junior's face now in my mind, hiding his feelings of rejection; lips pursed tightly in unexpressed anger, a single tear fallen to his cheek.

"No, it's okay. You go ahead. Really… it's okay," he kept repeating, all along gently pushing me to the entrance of the Bumping Cars gate.

We both felt hurt. It was my first witness to this unkind senselessness and the pain it provoked.

I am ashamed to confess that I rode while Junior stood at the fence and watched. It was a ride without joy, a meaningless repetitive circling of the floor. It was no fun to bump into cars driven by strangers. I recall merely riding haplessly.

The real bump, the crash that day, stupidly repeated in many forms, crushed my ignorance of the fallacy of generalization of devaluing any human life for any reason. Small-mindedness today is no less disturbing than it was 7 decades ago.

Junior lived with his parents in a small second story apartment not far from my house on 47th Street. I remember his mother as small, shapely, and quiet and his father as stocky, stern, and unfriendly.

I sensed that Junior's parents were not doing well with each other, confirmed by the disgusting aging of foods stored in their refrigerator. I knew the prices of the foods that were limited to us because of the great depression. Ground beef, 29 cents a pound, was a luxury, but I watched it turn green in Junior's ice box, unattended, unimportant to a couple soon to separate.

Not long after the Bumping Cars disappointment, my good friend Junior, and his mother, moved away, never again encountered except in the rich memory of our youthful friendship. It was one of the earliest important losses in my life.

Religious Influence

Family Christmas parties were another of my mother's favorite traditions. Family, friends and neighbors came to our house to celebrate. Santa Claus, a job I was assigned during my teens, was dressed in a realistic Santa suit of red velvet and white fur. We exchanged gifts, enjoyed the delicious, abundant food my mother prepared and sang Christmas carols.

These were stress-free, happy events.

Windows were decorated. Standing in a most pleasant contrast to the blue Christmas tree lights, the tree was covered with long, thin strands of tinsel. As I remember the family Christmas parties, they did not come off as very religious. They were more like the memorial of an undoubted historical fact.

The origins of religious influence in my family cannot be traced with certainty. Someday, MapQuest may sketch out the direction of one's religious beliefs and practices. It would require sophisticated technological refinement. Even in combination with the most expensive GPS, MapQuest would suggest another approach. Here is how my working memory recollects the beginning of religious influence in my life.

First, my sister Edith comes to mind. She not only held my hand crossing Hampton Boulevard to Gray's Pharmacy, but she held my hand walking several blocks along Hampton Boulevard to a Christian Church on some Sunday mornings.

I was too young to absorb any theology, too naive to understand the stern faces of its congregation, but amply suited for its red and green boxes of hard Christmas candy that it generously made available to the children.

Uncle Earl

When I was almost ten years of age, Edith took me to a meeting held in a large tent, its dirt floor covered with sawdust, on the east side of 47th Street "to watch the Holy Rollers." She said it was like a carnival. We stood in the dark, outside the tent on a warm summer night.

I was not amused and I begged Edith to take me home. It frightened me.

"Wait a few minutes," Edith said, "it will get better."

People, fervently praying and shouting, ran up and down the aisles formed by spaces left between the wooden benches. Some performed forward rolls in the sawdust. More frightened, pulling at Edith's hand, I beseeched her to leave.

"Look," she said, surprise in her voice and pointing to the makeshift altar at the front of the tent, "there's Uncle Earl. We can't leave now. I think he is going to say something we need to hear."

Taking my hand, Edith accompanied me to an unoccupied bench on the right side of the tent, near the front.

For some inexplicable reason, I suddenly felt comforted.

Uncle Earl was my mother's youngest brother. I suspect he was also her favorite brother. Uncle Earl is someone I am often told by others in adulthood I most "favor," having similar facial features.

Uncle Earl was a quiet, soft-spoken, judicious and kind if not passive, junior accountant for Texaco. My mother loved and respected him and he often came to visit us on 47th Street and later on 39th Street.

Uncle Earl spoke from his heart, battling tears, to the thirty or forty people gathered in that tent. His wife, Teeny, slovenly attired, large dark eyes peering confusedly if not disoriented, stood next to him.

Now crying without shame, Uncle Earl said, "My wife has not spoken for one year. No one knows what is causing her failure to speak. I have taken my wife to the best doctors and to the best hospitals, even to Johns Hopkins Hospital in Baltimore, but nothing has helped her.

I bring her here tonight, to be anointed with oil and prayed for that God may heal her.

If God heals Teeny tonight, I will give my life to Him and serve him all the days of my life."

Everyone in the tent, including me and Edith, tears running down our cheeks, prayed.

Many people shouted their prayers loudly to God. The evangelist asked Teeny to bow to her knees, placed oil on her forehead and prayed earnestly, sincerely, confidently, faithfully.

A spirit of oneness filled the tent. "God," we all prayed, "please heal Teeny."

I can't tell you how long the healing service lasted, but no one wanted to leave.

When the evangelist announced the Amen to conclude the prayer for healing, Teeny stood up, staring lovingly out of her newly sparkling eyes.

A supernatural noiselessness silenced the tent.

Teeny spoke her first audible, articulate words in three-hundred-sixty-five days and nights.

"Earl," she uttered.

Joy filled the heart of every soul in that tent with its sawdust covered floor. The "carnival" to which we came seeking entertainment had been transformed into nothing less than a miracle.

The celebration of thanksgiving, if it were possible, was even more sincere, genuine, honest, heartfelt, and authentic than the prayer for Teeny's healing.

Teeny lived another half-century, free of her debilitating malady.

Uncle Earl kept his promise. Ultimately he became a pastor, taking God's message to countless people including most of my family, about which more will be said later.

Burrows Memorial Baptist Church

From my earliest memories, when I went to bed, as I said earlier, I was "tucked in" by my mother. It was a special, gentle and loving time as my mother heard my prayer.

Some nights, my mother sang to me: "Two eyes that shine so bright. Two lips that kiss good night. Two arms that hold so tight...the little boy of mine. Nobody knows just what his coming has meant. He's like an angel that Heaven has sent. He's all this world to me. He climbs upon my knee. To me he'll always be that little boy of mine."

Mother pulled the covers up to my chin, kissed me good night and I slept soundly.

Burrows Memorial Baptist Church, the Norfolk Public Schools, and the Norfolk Department of Recreation's James Madison Community Center were the three institutions that most influenced the first two decades of my life.

They were all located within walking distance of my home in Lamberts Point.

To each of these firmly established institutions, I can trace, with the strongest sense of gratitude, most of the moral and intellectual virtues I value, the desirable goals and objectives of my life, and my earnest wish for strong citizenship, acceptable scholarship, and to be worthy of friendship.

In addition, of course, my mother, siblings, my father, and my very good friends completed the formation of my character.

Burrows Memorial Baptist Church stood on the corner of West 38th Street and Blue Stone Avenue, the heart of Lamberts Point in Norfolk, Virginia. It was the social center of my life as an adolescent.

"Bible drills" taught me the basic truths of the Old and New Testaments.

BTU (Baptist Training Union) taught me public speaking.

Singing in the choir taught me to appreciate a category of music with which I had little familiarity.

My three best friends, Bobby Clyburn, Baxter van Pelt, and George Munden were all active members of Burrows. In every activity we joined boisterously more often than religiously, but always together.

If Burrows Church won architectural awards for its construction, I never heard of it. The brick structure, however, was a tribute to the hard-working blue collar neighbors who joined in raising the funds for its creation and maintenance for over a century.

The sanctuary, furnished with a dark red carpet and handsomely assembled deep brown wooden pews forming a wide semi-circle, looked up at large, beautiful stained glass windows.

When the conditions of light and life were just right, the Biblical characters portrayed in the stained glass appeared powerfully real.

Until Rev. George Euting, one of Burrow's spirited former pastors, pointed it out in one of his inspiring sermons, I was unaware that several small window panes on the side of the church were long overdue for repair.

On more than one occasion, I recall walking up to the church, loving what I saw, and almost magically drawn to envelope or absorb it, to take it in to my being. I wanted a mental image of all that Burrows Church meant to me, to carry with me. In several important ways those valuable images remain very real in my mind today, thank God.

The Heart of Lamberts Point

Street car tracks ran down the center of 38th Street, directly in front of Burrows Church.

"Pulling the trolley" was considered by some to be great fun, by others to be sheer meanness. In Lamberts Point it was considered a manly act to "pull the trolley."

"Pulling the trolley" meant yanking down the metal rod extending from the end of the street car to the electric wires suspended above. Pulling the trolley disconnected the street car from its power source.

The street car came to a sudden stop, all the lights went out, and the street car conductor, tired and impatient, angrily climbed down from his seat and, in the dark, tried to reposition the trolley to restore its electrical power.

Of course it was dangerous, thus adding excitement to the trick, because it was executed in the dark of night, and required running down the tracks unseen. Stories were told of amputees who had sacrificed a limb in the line of duty to stop a street car by "pulling the trolley."

In several identical ways, "pulling the trolley" was not unlike "hopping" a Norfolk and Western Coal Car as the trains lumbered down the railroad tracks, slowly gaining speed. The rail road tracks paralleled West 38th Street, to and from the Lamberts Point Coal Pier at the very west end of 38th Street.

Cargo ships from around the world, nudged safely into the Lamberts Point Coal Piers by red tug boats on the Elizabeth River, waited to be filled with coal mined in Virginia and West Virginia.

When the trains were sufficiently slow, one could easily "hop" on the rear of a coal car at Bluebird Park and soon jump off, unless too much speed had been achieved, on Granby Street, conveniently located near City Park. Alternatively, after a relatively short walk, one arrived in downtown Norfolk.

Boone's Corner was the second street car stop after Burrows Church on West 38th Street. "Boone's" was a tavern frequented by international merchant marines whose ships came to carry coal from the Lamberts Point Coal Pier to their home countries to warm their domiciles.

The merchant marines, rarely able to understand spoken English, came to Boone's Tavern to carry beer back to their ships in the warmth of their lifeblood.

At one time, long ago, blood was spilled at Bone's Corner Tavern as often as beer, but with greater passion because Norfolk native men loved their neighbors but not the foreign merchant marine intruders.

I am told, on the other hand, that Norfolk native women who found conviviality at Boone's had enough love for both their neighbors and foreign merchant marines.

The love of life became secondary to the pride of personhood when the wives of Norfolk native men, searching for their unfaithful husbands at Boone's, discovered more evidence for their jealousy than they anticipated.

Saturday night specials were fired, knives larger and sharper than those found in the US were savagely wielded, and too often the Police arrived too late.

I was never permitted by my mother to go near Boone's corner. A bar of an all too different type, however, opened on the corner of 38th Street and Hampton Boulevard, a quiet, genteel place where men sat at a counter or at small tables and calmly drank their beer.

Several times, Callas, our renter, took me to this place whose name escapes me, where I enjoyed a Pepsi Cola. I could not understand my mother's degree of anger, perhaps rage, upon learning of my visits to this bar with Callas.

As a twelve year old, I was puzzled by her severe reaction because the patrons seemed so harmlessly friendly, always asking me questions about myself, and welcoming me in the most friendly, warm ways.

My mother was not a religious person at this time in her life, but she knew right from wrong and in her judgment I was wrong to go in the first place and must never, ever return to the place or any place like it. I am hazy about the punishment I received.

38th Street

Except for several places mentioned above, and several more to be mentioned later, 38th Street should have no special meaning for me, but it does. In reality, it was my main thoroughfare by bike or perambulation from my home on 39th Street to James Madison Grammar School, to the James Madison Community Center, to Burrows Church, to Blair Junior High School, to Maury High School and to just about everywhere else I traveled from age ten until I entered college.

38th Street was the very center of Lamberts Point, the lowest socioeconomic and perhaps one of the most detested sections of Norfolk. It was infamous for its crime, poverty, and indifference to ambition.

Lamberts Point was paralyzed by the Great Depression. It was the blight between Larchmont and Ghent, the upwardly mobile and picturesque neighborhoods. There of course were the exceptions in Lamberts Point, the strong families, cleanly kept homes, and loving, protective parents.

Fortunately, as time churned onward, crime and poverty became the exception and that change was significantly happening as I entered my early teenage years. Although I left Lamberts Point for college and medical school, I often returned to it. Recently, the Honorable Alfred W. Whitehurst, Circuit Court Judge, my former neighbor in Lamberts Point and former Sunday School Teacher, took my wife and me for a tour, a real sentimental journey, to witness phenomenal changes in Lamberts Point, not all to our liking.

George Munden and Baxter Van Pelt, two of my very best friends during the second decade of my life, and I formed a trio, inspired by the music of the Ink Spots. We sang "Paper Doll" with more passion than imaginable.

Together we played football, baseball, and basketball in the Norfolk Community League, sang in Burrows Church choir, and hung out at Robbins Confectionary on 38th Street.

We ran long distances at night on the asphalt-covered streets throughout Lamberts Point.

We ate ice cream cones at High's on Hampton Boulevard. In a word, we were inseparable. Nearly all day was spent at Burrows Church on Sundays. We attended Sunday school, sang in the church choir, and went to the Baptist Training Union on Sunday evenings before the Sunday night church service.

Bobby Clyburn was a high school football team mate, and a friend from our days together at James Madison Elementary School. His family also attended Burrows Church. His parents were church leaders.

Mr. Clyburn was a deacon and Mrs. Clyburn was Director of the Junior Department Sunday School Teachers. I had been attending church inconsistently; however, at Easter, during a church revival at Burrows, when I was twelve years old, I responded to pastor Kenneth E. Burke's invitation to make a public profession of my faith.

Two Baptisms

I distinctly recall the experience of joining the church. It happened in an evening service during a revival.

I was sitting near the front, near Bobby Clyburn, on the left side of the church, the old brick building with some of its window panes missing. The dark wooden pews, worn maroon carpet, and pulpit were circa early twentieth Century.

Less than adequate electric lighting at night in the aging building created a subdued setting. My young heart was stirred and my mind was determined to become a Christian, but it was not easy to leave my seat, walk down the aisle to the front of the church, and take the pastor's hand.

The church was full. It must have been a successful revival service. Mr. Noble was playing the organ flawlessly. The choir, up in the loft behind the pastor, was led by Mrs. Burke, the pastor's assertive wife. This stern woman was known for calling me and other boys like me, a "scamp."

Angelically, the choir sang, "Just as I am with one dark spot...I come, I come to Thee."

I had a "now or never feeling" as I burst out of my seat and nervously walked to the front of the church and took the pastor's hand. I said nothing.

"Bobby," Rev. Burke inquired, "do you wish to make a profession of faith in Jesus Christ, to be baptized, and join this church?"

"Yes," I said, nodding my head as well.

"Welcome," he said. "Have a seat on the front row, and one of the deacons will take your information after the service is concluded."

On the Thursday night before Easter 1943, in the very midst of WW II, wearing a white choir robe, I was baptized by Rev. Kenneth E. Burke in front of the congregation of Burrows Memorial Baptist Church, 38th Street, Lamberts Point, Norfolk, Virginia.

A special visitor, next to whom I sat before I was baptized, my mother, came to observe the ceremony. I believe it was her first and her last visit to my church.

Several years later, however, she was "baptized in the Holy Spirit" in our home on 39th Street, nestled less than a city block from Burrows. It was the major life-changing experience for my mother and led to her faithful membership in the small Church of God where her youngest brother, Earl Beale, became her pastor.

Rev. Burke, standing up to his waist in a pool of water, submerged behind the pulpit, removed for the occasion, took my hand as I descended several steps into the pool. With both hands clinging on Rev. Burke's left arm crossing his abdomen, his right hand covering my nose, he eased me backward, immersing me in the water with these unforgettable words, "Bobby Brown, I baptize you in the name of the Father, the Son, and the Holy Ghost. Amen."

As if in one complete motion, I was immediately pulled upright out of the baptismal water by Rev. Burke.

The peace that I felt at that moment, I later learned, is best described in the Bible as "the peace that surpasses all understanding."

If I could have kept the pure heart and the clean mind with which I ascended those few steps out of the baptismal pool that spring night until this mid-winter night nearly seven decades later, my regrets, I believe, would have been minimal and my faith extraordinary.

A rare incident occurred in my family shortly after my baptism, something I learned many years after it transpired. It was a long kept secret. Its significance may have remained untold.

The white choir robe in which I had been baptized had to be washed and ironed and returned to Burrows Memorial Baptist Church several days after the baptismal service.

During the second decade of my life, my mother spent most of her day in the kitchen, probably at the sink. Her kitchen was like her sanctuary. Here stood her old rocking chair in front of the coal-burning stove in our renovated house on 39th Street.

After I had fallen into a deep, serene sleep following my baptism, my mother, in the presence of no one but God Himself, baptized herself with the baptismal water she managed to squeeze with her work-hardened hands from the white robe in which I had been baptized.

My mother held the white choir robe over her bowed head. She whispered to God, "I baptize myself, Johnny Louise Beale Brown, in the name of the Father, the Son, and the Holy Ghost." I suspect her tears of repentance were more plentiful than the residual water she pressed from my baptismal robe.

A Prayer for Dad's Healing

Uncle Earl kept his promise. He made the promise years earlier in the tent meeting the night his wife Teeny was healed. As mentioned earlier, I was in the tent meeting with my sister Edith the night Uncle Earl promised God to devote his life to Christian work if God healed Teeny. It was the night Edith took me to be entertained by a carnival, the night I first witnessed the miraculous.

Uncle Earl kept his day job with Texaco. He also became an ordained minister in the Church of God, a Pentecostal denomination, and opened his own small church on 26th Street near its intersection with Granby Street, Norfolk, Virginia.

Uncle Earl was busy but never too busy to come to one's home to pray. No one met Uncle Earl without receiving his warm handshake and his even warmer welcome to attend his church.

My dad's first lucrative employment, made possible by WW II, was painting Liberty Ships at the Colonna Shipyard in Norfolk. The shipyard operated twenty-four hours daily during the worst part of the war.

Long hours, physically challenging labor, and rotating shifts were not easy for a fifty-one year old man. I believe my dad also lacked the social skills required to work effectively with a diverse group of men under pressure.

One day he came home from work with a painful black eye. It was embarrassing, painful, and medically dangerous for a man with vision in only one eye. We were never told what happened.

Not long after the black eye, my dad "fell" forty feet into the hold of a ship under repair at the shipyard. It was said that he may have been pushed, but this was never investigated.

No matter what its cause, my dad sustained life-threatening injuries. He was hospitalized for a long period of time. He endured several major surgical procedures. He remained partially disabled the rest of his life. I vividly remember the painful suffering he experienced and the loss of some of the functional capacity of his arm.

My mother called two people for help: Lawyer Jett and Uncle Earl. I was never informed about the success of the efforts of Lawyer Jett, but I witnessed the results of the phone call to Uncle Earl. I also remember that our phone was always listed in Edith's name because of our past bankruptcy.

The details of the healing service for my dad at our home on 39th Street were not shared with me, then thirteen or fourteen years old.

Brother Hunter, a tall, strong, strapping deacon in Uncle Earl's church, accompanied Uncle Earl and Teeny to my house. Literally following the Bible, Uncle Earl anointed my dad's forehead with oil. Those who were able, including my mother, got on their knees. Their thoughts and their words went up. No doubts remained below. With unsurpassed sincerity, their prayers flowed and flowed.

It was a bright, clear, warm spring day. I was walking home from school when I heard loud shouting coming from the direction of my house. I was embarrassed. I hoped this disturbing shouting was coming from another house, not from my home. Until I heard the noise, the prayer meeting was unknown to me.

I made an excuse and ran ahead of my friends. I entered the back door. Uncle Earl, Teeny, Brother Hunter, and my mother were crying and laughing joyously. Hands raised high in the air, these blessed people were running in and out of the several rooms of our house, praising God.

My dad was still lying on his sick bed trying to silently manage his pain.

The healing service for my dad had an unintended outcome.

Dad remained unhealed, but my mother had been "saved...baptized by the Holy Spirit...and had spoken in tongues." Truthfully, dad and I were the only ones present in that kitchen on that bright spring afternoon that were not speaking in tongues and shouting praises to God. The rest is history.

Dad was later saved in the same way, as well as all three of my sisters and my brother, Randolph. Ultimately, they all joined Uncle Earl's church, tithed faithfully, and nothing ever became more precious to them than their love for Jesus.

Uncle Earl's church thrived and moved to a larger facility to become the Ballantine Church of God. I remained a member of Burrows Church, the only family member not to join the Church of God, but I respected the integrity of their faith and their complete dedication to God.

During the infrequent occasions I fell ill during my adolescence, Uncle Earl was called to my bedside for prayer. Inevitably, his prayers were answered.

The Prayer Warrior

My mother became a prayer warrior.

More often than I knew, I was the subject of her prayers. However, no special occasion passed without my mother saying, "Let's get on our knees and pray, Bobby."

She prayed for God's protection whenever I left home to travel. She prayed for every aspect of my life. She knew my heart.

After a disappointing first year in medical school and a decade that followed, my mother prayed and requested prayer for me.

Her prayer requests for me, by my name, made me "familiar" to her congregation. By my mother requesting prayer for me so often in her church, I became known to nearly every member of her church.

During one of my occasional visits to my mother's church, I was warmly greeted with kind words saying, "Bobby, we know you through your mother's prayer requests."

If there is anything more powerful than prayer, it is the love that leads one to pray.

Despite frequent hospitalizations for coronary artery disease, my mother lived a full but all too brief life. She suffered her first heart attack at age 62. Her second heart attack at age 72 took her life in 1971.

The circumstances of my mother's death are decidedly miraculous. Dottie and I, separately because one of us necessarily remained in our car with our children, visited my mother in the hospital several weeks before she died. I told her that I loved her and that she had been a good mother, not knowing it was the last time I would see her alive.

The decision was made that I would open my practice as a psychiatrist in Charlottesville. Dottie worked selflessly to make my office-opening a very special occasion. We perceived it as the end of the rainbow where there is happiness. Together, we had searched for it over a long, difficult journey.

We mailed formal office-opening celebration cards in Charlottesville to our family and friends. My mother received my card in the Norfolk General Hospital on the same day it was mailed from Charlottesville, an unheard of US Postal Service achievement. In 1971, it ordinarily took 2 or 3 days for mail to reach Norfolk from Charlottesville.

According to my sisters, Christine and Frances, only a few hours after reading the announcement of the opening of my medical practice, my mother died on 27 June 1971.

Her prayers for me had been answered.

Love at First Sighting

The choir loft of Burrows Baptist Church was elevated about ten feet behind and above the pulpit. It provided a perfect crow's nest to keep watch over the troubled waters of the congregation below.

Mrs. Burke, our choir director, with inexplicable regularity and rigidity sat on the front row of the choir, nearest to the organist.

Her gaze was fixed on some imaginary spot forty-five degrees from the back of the congregation at the level of her eyes. She avoided even the slightest glance of the congregation.

Mrs. Burke's self-discipline, though greatly desired, was never achieved by the basses, tenors, altos, and sopranos in the choir.

The incredible wide-screen view of the entire congregation was far too tempting to be ignored. Seated in the choir between George Munden and Baxter Van Pelt, I sometimes would whisper to my friends to check out a beauty spotted below. Most of the time, we were also appropriately attuned to the sermon.

It was done in light-hearted fun. It became a contest, however, to determine who could first spot the most attractive young woman in the congregation below.

During a Sunday sermon that my mother would have described as "dry" or "dead," I got tripped up by my own game by the most sparkling smile that my eyes had ever beheld.

The wonderful smile was matched by golden blonde hair and clear blue eyes.

The game ended with abrupt suddenness.

I fell in love in an instant.

"Who is that," I whispered to George.

"I'm not certain," George replied, "but I think her grandmother lives on 27th Street."

Baxter had no intelligence on the matter.

The sermon seemed endless. I could not wait to meet her.

Rather than hanging up my choir robe, I just snatched it off, stuffed it in the closet, and ran down the steps.

I caught her as she was coming out of the church with her parents and grandmother.

"I'm Bobby Brown," I said just short of a stutter.

"We know who you are, Bobby. We saw you singing in the Center Theatre last summer. I am Kathleen Hinkle. This is my mother, Mamie Heath, my husband, Hinkie, and my daughter, Dorothy Ann."

Dottie smiled. I was smitten!

Never before and never since that moment have I ever romantically loved another person.

Recently, we celebrated our sixtieth wedding anniversary.

I can remember its painful beginning.

At times it was like a severe case of influenza. I was in love's grip.

It engrossed my sixteen-year-old mind like nothing before it.

We saw each other at neighborhood parties, on church hayrides, and, of course, in Burrows Church.

Will you be My Girlfriend for 1947?

On New Year's Eve, I walked Dottie home from the Burrows "Watch Night Service."

We stood on her grandmother's 27th Street front porch.

I could not have felt more awkward.

Looking back, I felt very much like when I left my seat to be baptized. Instead of a profession of faith, it was a profession of endless love.

I had the same sense of urgency; "it is now or never."

Fortunately, it was during the dark of midnight. The level of stress must have contorted my face.

Somehow I managed to form the words and to enunciate them pleadingly, "Will you be my girlfriend for 1947?"

She said, "Yes."

I kissed her quickly and ran off her grandmother's front porch. I continued running the 3 city blocks to my house...and haven't stopped running since.

I don't believe I have ever been more excited in such a very special way.

I was a very jealous boyfriend. I learned more than I wanted to know from my informants, George and Baxter. I was a counselor at Camp Greenbrier every summer for the five years. From early 1950, I was in Charlottesville attending the University of Virginia, leaving little time for the attention our relationship deserved.

On the other hand, Dottie was attentive and thoughtfully caring when I was available.

Toll House cookies made by Dottie were delivered to me by her younger brother, Buddy.

We kept our love alive and thriving through the US Postal Service.

Perry Como's fifteen minute Chesterfield Supper Club radio show was listened to every night at 27th Street and 39th Street, respectively.

Supposing I could sing like Perry Como, I called Dottie on the phone after each radio show and sang to her lovingly, if not quite like our idol, the same songs we had just heard on the radio.

Perry Como's music and his soothing voice inspired our love for each other, taking us to a special place.

Sadly, it remained an unfulfilled dream to meet Perry Como in person. Many years ago, the opportunity unexpectedly came while we were at the Williamsburg Inn where Perry was filming his annual Christmas television show.

We missed meeting him but, interestingly, we met and talked with John Wayne, Perry's guest for his Christmas show. We most enjoyed John Wayne's robust laughter, an incredible man who knew then his diagnosis of terminal stomach cancer which took his life not long after the Perry Como Christmas Special.

Dottie came to Mid-winters and Easter's at the University. We danced to the music of Tommy Dorsey in Charlottesville.

Dottie was an honor graduate from Granby High School, Norfolk, Virginia. Several years earlier, I graduated from Maury High School, known less for good grades than for athletics.

She sang in her school choir, had the lead in her senior class play, Romeo and Juliet, and was voted the most talented in her senior class. I sang in the Maury Fifth Bell Chorus, played football, had the lead role in the senior class play, and was also voted the most talented in the senior class. However, with honor I must admit that I graduated in January in a much smaller class than Dottie's, with far less competition.

What is more, Dottie was an Honor Graduate with a GPA of 93.5. For me it was an honor to graduate, having the good sense never to inquire about my GPA.

Will you be My Wife?

On Christmas Eve, during the semester break of my first year in medical school, I asked Dottie to be my wife.

I got on my knee in her living room.

Her parents were in the kitchen. Only the murmur of their talking could be heard; however, her father was hard of hearing from his many years of working around and in the noise of the Norfolk Naval Ship Yard.

Dottie was seated on the sofa. Her father's chair was immediately to her right. On the chair was an invisible sign saying "Keep out of this chair. It is reserved for the man of the house. Do not disturb when he is scrutinizing the Friday night fights or dissecting the Sunday afternoon Washington Redskins games."

In some ways I felt I was proposing to her father, dreading his reply.

Dottie and I kissed and my tearful proposal of marriage was accepted.

Hand in hand we walked from the living room, through the foyer, into the kitchen.

Dottie's father was best described as a private person. He was ill-at-ease outside the presence of his wife. He was very self-conscious of his worsening deafness.

I had to repeat myself when I asked, "Mr. Hinkle, may I speak with you?"

Looking somewhat perplexed, her father slowly nodded his head. He and I walked back to the living room.

"I love Dottie, Mr. Hinkle. I want to marry her." I spoke uncomfortably loudly, leaving no chance to be misunderstood.

Immediately, he said, "I have no problem with that. What does Dottie say?"

"She accepted my proposal a few minutes ago," I replied with confidence.

Passing me his hand to shake, her father said, "Then it's fine with me and her mother…I think…let's go ask her mother."

In the kitchen, Dottie and her mother were sharing tears of happiness. The deal was sealed on that memorable Christmas Eve. No couple in all of history could have been more in love.

I had come home to Norfolk as a single man for the Christmas break from my first year in medical school. I returned to Charlottesville as a very happily engaged man.

The classmates who drove me back to school were happy for me and soon the whole medical school class of 1957 was cheerfully joking with me about marriage, particularly teasing me about the intimacy and the familiarity of marriage.

A medical student in love, separated from the woman he is in love with, as in my case, finds little appealing in the study of Biochemistry or Physiology.

I think now in looking back, the biochemistry and physiology of love itself may have become too overpowering.

We could not wait for a June wedding. We moved the wedding date up four months sooner.

Misty-eyed, we found ourselves standing up for our wedding vows in Burrows Church in front of friends and family.

Bobby Clyburn was my Best Man.

Will We Ever Have a Honeymoon?

We drove back to Charlottesville that Saturday afternoon immediately after the wedding ceremony. We took the ferry from Norfolk to New Port News. The ferry is now replaced by two tunnels.

We had removed the tin cans tied to the back of the car and erased all the "just married signs" scribbled on the car windows in order to have no obstructed view from the car.

I was very puzzled, therefore, by the ferry-ticket salesman who said, "Congratulations on your marriage."

Thinking he must have been an unrecognized wedding guest, I asked, "How did you know we were just married, Sir?"

Without hesitation, passing me my change from the purchase of the ferry ticket, he said, unsmiling, "There is rice in your hair."

Our wedding night was spent in a small two story brick home I had just rented from Mrs. Berlin Eye on Jefferson Park Avenue, a mile from the School of Medicine.

Unbounded passion and enchantment reigned, filling the small bedroom with light brighter than the sun that woke us early the next morning, accompanied by a knock on the front-door by Ed Weise, a medical school class mate, anatomy lab partner, and now a life-long friend and Pediatrician in Jacksonville, Florida.

I covered up my infuriation, thinking how anyone could intrude on the first morning of my honeymoon, finding Ed's early morning unwelcomed visit incredible.

In reconsidering Ed's disrupting early morning visit, I remember he was returning from church that Sunday morning. He knew that I had missed several days of class.

Ed had heard I was being married in Norfolk. He had not been invited to the wedding (only because I did not want him to miss class).

He genuinely wondered how I was doing.

Our friendship began four years earlier when we lived in the Baptist Student Center located next to the University Baptist Church. We were laboratory assistants in Biology. We both admired Dr. D. Runk, Biology Professor and Director of the Biology Labs. We studied together as pre-medical students and we sang in a quartet about which I will say more.

Ed Weise was the younger brother of Reinold.

Reinold was a flamboyant person in whose shadow Ed quietly restored most of what "Reynolds," as he was fondly called, and later to become a general surgeon, tended to shake up or dismantle.

It is in Ed's nature to care for others, making him a faithful friend, husband, parent, and physician. He is and has been a treasured friend for more than sixty years. I can't count the times I have relied upon his authentic friendship.

Ed knew Dottie from her earlier visits to Charlottesville. He congratulated us with unsurpassed warmth. He never knew how much I disliked his unwelcomed visit. Dottie was her usual friendly, kind, and hospitable self.

It was the first day after our wedding. I was meaninglessly bothered by an incident I misunderstood, perceiving it as intrusive. Dottie was loving, friendly, supportive, patient, understanding, caring and gentle. Little did I realize then, as I do now, that this would become the precedent of our lasting relationship.

Six decades and a half later, I still flourish in her respect. Her love is like an endlessly glowing warm and bright light. How could anyone ask for anything more?

6

WAR ON MEMORY

"A glimpse into the suffering…"

WHO CAN HEAL our Soldiers injured with Posttraumatic Stress Disorder? Who can replace their idealism and hope? Who can restore their soul? Who can cleanse their memories?

The task is too great, too important, and too precious to be left only to physicians and other behavioral health specialists.

Is the task of healing these most deserving men and women too big for our nation?

In my professional opinion, based on thousands of privileged encounters with these, our nation's best, only our nation itself, not its government, not its politics, but its people can and must be trusted with this honorable challenge.

The nation's first step is to dedicate itself to understanding the extent and the intensity of suffering that our Soldiers have experienced in 21st Century War. This can be accomplished without having to know the gory, sickening details.

The second step for our nation in the healing process is to understand and accept the painful fact that redeployment or coming home from 21st Century War, for many of our Soldiers, is as difficult as facing the enemy in combat.

This chapter provides only a glimpse into the misery of suffering from PTSD.

The following section is graphically told by a Soldier just as it happened.

"I Never Saw So Much Blood"

"I am not doing well, Sir.

I have no energy.

I jump in my sleep.

I have lost all interest in sex."

MSG Keith L. Johnson (Soldier's real name and rank, used at his request) is a physically strong man in his mid-forties. This intelligent Soldier is a "Soldier's Soldier," a compassionate, natural leader.

He is the first patient I saw after the Christmas break in 2012.

I have known, admired, and respected him since he came under my care in 2007.

His usual self-confidence was replaced today by despairing bleakness. He had nearly given up.

"I jump with any noise.

I'm stressed out at work...

I don't know, Dr. Brown...

I don't think the Lexapro (antidepressant medication) is working any more.

I see my country doctor for check-ups. I trust him."

MSG Johnson was on Testosterone patches for three years, but they were recently stopped.

Its discontinuation may be one of several likely causes of his low energy level and decreased libido.

The most likely cause of his present terrible mental state, however, is told below.

"My legs move 58 times an hour in my sleep. That's what the sleep study showed.

They wanted me on medication for Restless Legs Syndrome, but I read up on it. I don't like the side effects. I refused to take it."

From his description, his whole body "jumps," when he sleeps, not just his legs.

On 21 DEC 2012, MSG Johnson was emotionally distraught.

It was the eighth anniversary of the suicide bombing of the chow hall in Mosul, Iraq, 2004.

He remembers this combat trauma every day.

However, he re-lives the unbearable experience on its anniversary. No detail of the carnage is forgotten. His memories of the trauma suddenly mutate into reality.

His memories become a living daytime and nighttime nightmare from which he cannot fully awaken.

"That chapter won't close...l don't know why...it really upsets me."

"What keeps the chapter open?" I asked.

He replied, "So many people got fucked up...it was hit everywhere...

The blast tore up some shit...

Utensils became shrapnel...!

I never saw so much blood...

The floor was so cold the blood clotted like pudding...

Four of my men were killed."

MSG Johnson, unlike others, did not run for cover.

Out of dedication, more than duty, he said, he stayed in the wrecked building and saved lives.

He stuffed a plastic trash can liner into a gaping hole in a woman's chest. Until he acted, she was painfully, unsuccessfully gasping for breath.

The American woman Soldier was able to breathe again because MSG Johnson acted speedily. He intuitively relied on his training.

"She looked young. I don't know, maybe in her early twenties. She may have been Hispanic. I don't know, Dr. Brown, her black eyes were wide with fear.

She couldn't make a sound until I closed the hole in her chest. Then she breathed and thanked me. She was med-evacuated. I heard later she was okay.

Soldiers everywhere were crying …some were screaming.

Everywhere you looked, somebody was crying…

Tables were all blown apart.

When it was over, I just went to my hooch (temporary military housing).

I sat on the stoop and smoked one cigarette after another…just staring…

My body was there but my mind was gone…!

I just lost it…

My SGM (Sergeant Major) came to talk to me…

I have no idea what he said.

They burned our uniforms because there was blood all over them…

The SGM came back 3 days later.

He said I had to go back into the chow hall…

I did not want to go back inside the chow hall…

The CID (Criminal Investigation Division), FBI, everybody was there.

They were drawing chalk marks where the bodies were found…

They took us in 10 at a time…

The evidence table was in full view…

A combat boot with half a leg sticking out…

The smell was there…

Blood…

A giant hole was in the ceiling…

They tried to say we were hit by a rocket…

With a loud, angry voice, I said, 'No, it was a suicide bomber.'"

Tears, initially undetectable, now flowed unashamedly down his chiseled face.

No suitable words came to my mind.

Perhaps, sometimes just being silently present for our friends who grieve may be the best we can do.

MSG Johnson slowly shook his head from side to side.

He was recalling the unbelievable. No, he was re-living it, each vivid sight, sound, smell.

He was conducting a personal memorial service in the theatre of his mind.

The memorial service, affecting his every thought, starts every December. Never completely ending, it recedes with the common distractions of life.

Like a burglar hiding in a closet, it pounces on its victim with full force, making December the most dreaded month of the year for MSG Keith Lamont Johnson.

Unhurriedly, I offered reassurance. We both knew that words now had little value.

We quietly sat together. Our silence seemed soothing.

Later, I suggested we try augmenting Lexapro with Buspar, an antianxiety medication.

He declined.

He is helped most, he said, by group therapy.

"Only guys who have been through combat understand it, Dr. Brown."

"You Can't Take Away Memories"

Memories are biologically and chemically stored in the brain. They contribute to our sense of who we are and make it possible to function adequately in our environment.

To be devoid of memory is a pitiful state.

Of the many types of memory, combat trauma memories are often the most disturbing and the most relentless.

Too often, combat trauma memories are notoriously inaccurate. The trauma itself causes nearly every part of the mind to focus on survival.

Survival reflexes trump rational, cognitive elements of the experience, blocking out detailed aspects of the trauma of which later reflection may lessen self-incrimination.

Often an acceptable truthful explanation of the meaning of the Soldier's conduct during and immediately following combat trauma is only discovered and recalled under special, precise conditions afforded in treatment.

The "worst combat memories" produce psychologically incriminating emotions such as guilt, regret, remorse and helplessness. These self-condemning emotions impair other memory functions - often at the expense of accuracy, blocking recovery.

This chapter focuses on combat trauma memories reported by Soldiers being treated for PTSD at an Active Duty Army Post. It emphasizes two powerful principles.

First, to be understood is to be immediately comforted.

Second, errors in combat trauma memories cause unnecessary suffering and too often delay healing. It is imperative, therefore, that the errors in thinking are identified and corrected as soon as it is feasible.

In their own words, Soldiers with crippling combat trauma memories must repeatedly tell their combat narratives in order to identify and correct their cognitive or thinking mistakes.

Combat trauma memories shared with a trusted person who wants to understand the Soldier and is willing to enter into the Soldier's suffering is an essential first step towards recuperation.

"Sacred" is the best word describing this healing relationship.

Attachment

"Attachment" is a psychological term describing one's capacity to meaningfully and consistently relate to others. Too often in combat-induced PTSD, attachment is superseded by detachment, emotionally and physically, avoiding, withdrawing and severing connections with others.

One way to conceptualize combat-induced PTSD is to imagine the Soldier as detached from most if not all significant attachments. The few residual attachments are insecure, anxious or ambivalent. The required emotional nutrition ordinarily supplied by meaningful others is thus rendered unavailable.

Secure attachment is essential to a sense of safety and protection.

For Soldiers with PTSD, secure attachment is all but forgotten. Secure attachment is often eradicated by combat trauma.

Secure attachment gradually returns, albeit slowly, as the sacred relationship between Soldier and doctor strengthens.

It begins with individual therapy and it blossoms, in my opinion, in post-deployment cognitive group therapy with fellow Soldiers with the same or similar combat exposure and remarkably comparable combat trauma memories.

Healing takes time and commitment. "How poor are they that have not patience. What wound did ever heal but by degrees." Shakespeare.

Dissociation

SGT Roberts arrived at 0815, 15 minutes late for group therapy. He apologized for being late.

He sat down in his favorite chair in the center of the semi-circle formed by his 8 fellow Soldiers. SGT Roberts has occupied the same seat each week for the past 7 years.

SGT Roberts is a tall man who covers his dark, shining bald head with a deep blue baseball cap. The brim of his baseball cap is always pulled down, concealing the top half of his face, covering his wire-rimmed eye glasses.

Occasionally, SGT Roberts momentarily lifts his cap from his head and face. When he lifts his cap, it reveals the pleasant, caring, kindhearted expression of a man appearing younger than his 46 years.

On this particular day, SGT Roberts looked subdued. He was attentive, but he did not speak for the first 15 or 20 minutes after he arrived for the group session. He then came out of his silence.

"I remember every smell of combat." It was an appropriate statement for SGT Roberts to make because the group was discussing olfaction. However, it was made like an announcement, catching the group off guard.

A soldier sitting immediately to SGT Robert's left described the smell of human remains on his hands. Difficult to describe, he said, "It is a sweet, sickening, unique smell.

I didn't know why the smell returned," the Soldier said.

"It came back the other day. It's been a year since I worked with human remains."

He described how he had been unable to remove the odor with repeated washing of his hands with strong soap.

"The last human remains I processed were those of a young American Soldier who committed suicide in Afghanistan," the Mortuary Affairs Soldier reminisced.

"Dr. Brown helped me figure out why it came back at this time. Tomorrow is the one year anniversary of the last human remains I touched with my hands."

The details with which the Soldier spoke about the smell of his hands could be described as disturbing to Soldiers unfamiliar with the work of Mortuary Affairs.

I saw SGT Robert's left leg moving up and down rapidly. This commonly observed PTSD symptom I have come to call RLM (Rapid Leg Movement).

SGT Roberts was staring into space. He was peering straight ahead but seeing nothing.

He looked like a person in a trance.

SGT Roberts did not answer when I checked on his emotional status by calling his name.

The group, kind and understanding, called his name out loud several times.

Receiving no reply, the group then carried on, discussing other topics.

I calmly asked the group not to touch SGT Roberts. Touching may have been misunderstood as a threat by this partially conscious

Soldier. The same principle applies to Soldiers in the midst of the terror of a nightmare.

After 4-5 minutes that seemed to pass very slowly, SGT Roberts raised his head with suddenness. He looked to his left and then to his right. He was like a man waking up from a deep sleep, from a puzzling dream.

He appeared confused, asking what had happened.

He was reassured by the group who down-played the experience.

SGT Roberts said, "I feel a little foggy. That hasn't happened to me in over a year."

He was able to converse normally. His physical appearance was now unchanged from the time he walked into the group session. He gradually became animated, walking and talking normally.

At the end of the 90-minute group therapy session, the group members took leave of each other, hugging and shaking hands in their customary manner.

SGT Roberts firmly shook hands with me.

He said "I'm fine now."

I judged him to be clinically stable when he left the group at 0930.

When I phoned to check on him that evening, he said "I'm fine, Dr. Brown. How are you?

Dr. Brown, I will say this. On the way home from the group session, I couldn't remember the number of my exit off of Interstate 295. I got confused. It took me a little while, but I finally figured it out."

Two weeks later SGT Roberts phoned me. "I need to talk to you about my civilian job." I detected anxiety in his voice. It was difficult for SGT Roberts to return to work following his deployment with his Army Reserve Unit.

"Dr. Brown, they moved me to a different job. I would be working by myself. That part is good. You know I don't like being around a lot of people.

But they said I might have to work some days more than 8 hours.

You wrote a letter to the Director of Human Resources. You told him I could not work more than 8 hours. I don't trust them.

Once I work an hour or two over 8 hours, I think they will expect me to work more than 8 hours all the time.

"What should I do, Dr. Brown?"

Calling him by his first name, I said, "Adam, I can't tell you how pleased I am that you were able to return to work."

I paused before I spoke again, weighing my words, not wanting to unnecessarily alarm him.

"My first concern is your safety."

SGT Roberts replied, "I agree."

"You have PTSD with Dissociation, the most challenging type of PTSD to treat."

Dissociation means "to split off some part or component of mental activity... ." The split off component of the mind then "acts as an independent unit of mental life."

Dissociation may be understood as a remarkable form of self-protection. In this sense, the mind has a mind of its own. Instantaneously, involuntarily, automatically the mind removes its attention from painful, unacceptable awareness.

It is thought, for example, that children being abused may "remove" themselves from the actual abuse, avoiding the awareness of the unacceptable experience, and even see themselves from above," as an out of the body experience. Here, again, dissociation is protective.

Imagine, however, how a dissociative episode might be incapacitating. Imagine how it might become a dreaded reality, one potentially fraught with danger, and seriously restricting one's life.

SGT Robert's dissociative episode in the group spared him from re-experiencing combat trauma memories of the "smell of human remains," the disturbing subject discussed by the Soldier seated next to him whose hands could not be cleansed of that unique odor a year after he encountered it.

I said, "Your first episode of dissociation, you remember, Adam, occurred when you were suddenly stressed at the VA Medical Center. Do you remember what happened?"

SGT Roberts quietly laughed.

"That's when I drove almost to Raleigh, North Carolina. I had no idea how I got there. I live in Northern Virginia. I was on my way home from the VA. I was going the opposite way.

I remember I called my battle buddy in Pennsylvania. He told me to get out of my truck and walk around it to make sure I had hit nothing. Then he told me to fill up my truck with gasoline, get back on Interstate 95, and drive back to Northern Virginia."

"Adam," I said, "I don't want you to have an accident at work. The Neurologist said your brain is fine, but you and I know that all your episodes of dissociation have been triggered by stress. I don't want you to be stressed at work."

"That's the reason I called you, Dr. Brown."

"When you come to the clinic next week for your individual psychotherapy session, ask your provider to invite me in so all three of us can discuss your work situation."

"Thank you, Dr. Brown. I will do that. Tell Mama Brown hello for me, will you?"

Combat Trauma Memories

Soldiers with PTSD are preoccupied with troubling memories of combat. Soldiers tell me, for example, "I remember everything from my combat deployments."

Often at unpredictable times, their memories become so real they are experienced as genuine, life-like reenactments of actual combat situations.

When the combat memories are intolerable, as in SGT Roberts' case, the components of consciousness separate, becoming disunited.

This involuntary complex of psychological and biological processes may be conceptualized as merciful, sparing the Soldier from consciously experiencing that which is unbearable.

The instantaneous speed with which re-experiencing a memory occurs may cause panic.

The vividly recalled memories are often associated with biological, psychological, and behavioral changes that terrify the Soldier and those nearby who witness the turmoil.

The recovery from an acute, unintended, powerful recollection of combat is unpredictable, lasting from minutes to hours to days. The improvement from one of these emotionally painful recollections invariably requires dealing with feelings of shame and feelings of depression.

The Soldier with PTSD struggles to avoid triggers that remind him or her of their combat trauma memories. These Soldiers are comfortable in fewer and fewer places. They become socially isolated "loners" whose range of feelings is stuck on "numb."

The widespread feeling of numbness may be difficult for the Soldier to recognize or acknowledge. It is what the Soldier feels, seldom directly observed by others except for those desiring intimacy. Its equal and opposite feeling, anger, however, is what is too often felt by the Soldier and observed by all others with whom the Soldier may associate.

From Panama to Ethanol

"I was only 19 years old.

I had only one day of relevant training.

It was my first major combat trauma.

We flew out of Fort Bragg to Panama.

Our mission, to overthrow their dictator, occurred in 1989.

When we got to Panama, we were flying low at 500 feet.

We were under constant attack from the ground. Our plane was flying evasively.

We jumped (parachuted) into a field of elephant grass. It was twice my own height and I'm 6 feet tall.

I could not see anything around me. The elephant grass blocked my view.

I could only move by pressing the grass down with my weapon.

We were attacked with mortar rounds and small arms fire.

I couldn't speak. It would give away my position.

I had no idea where any of my unit was located.

Eventually, I was able to form up with fellow Soldiers.

We found our way to the landing strip we had missed during our jump.

We were under siege for 3 days and nights without respite.

We had to mount a hill from a valley with only steep cliffs, making us easy targets for the enemy.

From day 4 to day 30, we were warmly greeted by crowds lining the streets.

The Panamanian Defense Force was intermingled with the crowds lining the streets.

They ambushed us repeatedly.

It was the first time I saw so much death...any death, actually.

We flew back to Bragg and jumped from our plane.

For the next 10 years, I drank very heavily. It was the only way I could rid my mind of death.

It was the only way I could sleep."

Traumatic Grief Group

Another said, "I let everybody down! I promised my unit I would bring everybody back home.

But I didn't keep my promise.

I sent a Soldier to his death...

It was nearly 10 years ago. I think of him every day. I feel unworthy.

I didn't bring my Soldier back.

I think of the decision I made, but I don't usually say anything.

I feel like I'm in a hole."

This is the Soldier's first Post-Deployment Traumatic Grief Group session. The rule of confidentiality was explained. He was welcomed by the five fellow group members, all of whom were unknown by him.

He was dressed in his ACUs (Army Combat Uniform), but he did not remove his outer jacket whose collar he kept turned up. He was almost hidden in his uniform, an impression worsened by his refusal to look at anyone or anything but the floor.

"The unit was called together. We were told by our command there had been an accident and we had lost someone.

Who was it?

When I heard the name, 'Frank Martin,' I went numb.

Everybody started crying. He was on our basketball team, one of our better players. The whole basketball team cried.

His girlfriend came over. She was also a Soldier. She was stationed nearby when she heard about his death.

It was my fault. I knew he had a drinking problem. He had to piss a lot from drinking the night before. He stood by the opened truck door while it was moving and pissed outside the truck.

He could not hold onto the truck.

He fell out the opened truck door. The trailer ran over him. It killed him instantly.

Later there were sneers from other Soldiers in the unit.

I think they were upset with me. I think I heard people saying things like 'maybe he should not have been on the road…rumors of alcohol.'

It should have been me. His parents don't have their son… maybe I don't deserve to live. Everybody loved Marty."

The Soldier held his face in both hands and wept.

The group members were silenced, knowing they could have easily been in his boots.

I walked across the room, took the seat next to him, and gently put my arm around his shoulders. I felt his body trembling in torment.

"Your tears are healing," I said. "Please share them with us. Your tears may help other Soldiers in this group find the courage to cry. Let out your sorrow and begin to heal."

These were the grieving Soldier's first tears in 10 years. He is taking the first step in a painful but necessary journey to remember his lost friend with less pain.

"I Lost My Faith"

Another said, "We were in the wrong place at the wrong time.

We were trying to get out of the kill zone...

Mortars were dropping on us.

The road block trapped us into a bottle neck.

Small arms and RPGs (Rocket Propelled Grenades) were fired from positions on both sides of the road.

We were trying to get out of there as fast as possible.

I was in a turret of an M-ATV (Mine Resistant-All Terrain Vehicle), trying to get out.

We were running convoy security.

Immediately after I shot, there was an explosion.

A mortar hit the top of a mud building 8 feet from us.

I felt the shock.

At times I see a weapon in the boy's hand. At other times I see no weapon...an AK-47.

At the time of the shooting I felt nothing. We had a mission. My adrenalin was up.

We wear protective armor all the time over there.

It was not until 2-3 months after I got home that I started having feelings about the shooting.

I started having issues at home...outbursts...angry outbursts.

I was telling stories...talking to the wife...that's when I couldn't remember if the boy held a weapon or not.

Before this deployment to Afghanistan, I felt I had a firm belief...in God.

I believed that what I was doing was the right thing.

But I lost my faith...somewhere I became very jaded and angry.

It was in JUN or MAY 2010 while I was deployed to Afghanistan... it was what I saw people did to each other in the name of God.

The way we treated them was very kind...the way they treated each other was....

I went with a desire to help them.

I felt pity for them.

Before every mission, I went to the PX (Post Exchange) and bought a bag of candy to give to the children...but I got tired of them throwing rocks back and trying to kill me.

I also bought ball point pens...if the Afghan children saw a pen in your pocket they wanted the pen. Ball point pens fascinated them.

Yes, I lost my faith when I deployed to Afghanistan."

Without his faith, SGT Bob Jennings' terrible feelings of guilt haunt him, inhibit grieving, and hamper his interpersonal relationships. His previously acceptable sense of worth as a person has been ruined, he told the group.

Two and half-years after his most troubling combat trauma, he could not bring himself to directly state that he shot a child.

His suffering is intense. It is observed in his stuttering, multiple tics, and nearly incessant, uncontrollable chewing movements of his mouth, including the chewing of the inside of his right cheek. Had he not been seated, his rapidly moving legs would have traversed 5 miles during our 60-minute session.

Thankfully, a brief psychiatric hospitalization significantly lessened his suffering, a good job awaits him upon completion of his medical discharge and he is heroically verbally expressing his hidden thoughts and feelings in weekly post-deployment group therapy.

Tuesday Morning Post-Deployment Psychotherapy Group

"You can't take away memories, Dr. Brown, so what good does it do for us to talk about them?"

The thoughtful question was asked by 1SG Barry Walker,

"Can memories be healed, Dr. Brown?"

The group of 8 combat Soldiers stared at me. They wanted a good answer to this good question. It is the question on the mind of every Soldier with PTSD.

I took a deep breath, exhaled slowly, and I looked into the eyes of each Soldier in the Tuesday Morning Post-Deployment Psychotherapy Group.

"Memories are biological," I said. "They are stored in our brains. Memories serve an important role in determining who we are, how we think and feel, and how we behave."

The Soldiers were listening intently, making no sounds. Everyone present was fully in the present moment, a state sometimes referred to "mindfulness."

"The biological storage of our memories in our brains has been known since the 1920's when Dr. William Penfield, a brain surgeon, made a fascinating discovery.

The patient was conscious for the brain surgery. When Dr. Penfield touched specific areas of the brain, the patient vividly recalled a concert she had attended years ago as well as a happy birthday party.

It was all there. Every registered memory could potentially be recalled when the brain was physiologically activated by his surgical instruments or his skillful hands.

Demented people, sadly, lose much of their memory. Alzheimer patients, for example, may appear much like they looked before their illness, but they are no longer the same persons.

In one important perspective, Soldiers with PTSD are perplexed by trauma memories they have difficulty 'forgetting.' In this sense, Soldiers with PTSD can't forget. Alzheimer patients, on the other hand, can't remember."

1SG Walker asked, "Will we get Alzheimer's, Dr. Brown?"

I replied, "I can say with confidence that there appears to be no causal relationship between combat PTSD and the development of Alzheimer's disease."

I sensed the Soldiers felt relieved, one less fear, among countless others, to worry about.

"Memories that are related to our survival are the complex set of 'instincts' that help keep us alive. I believe all combat trauma memories are survival memories."

"Dr. Brown, are you saying that our painful memories from combat kept us alive?

I don't understand what you are saying, Sir.

Am I just a dumb ass, Sir?"

"You may be a 'dumb ass,' my friend (group laughs, releasing some anxiety) but I am not an expert in making that call.

Except for the 'dumb ass' phrase, your question is a very good one. It deserves a better answer than I have provided so far.

Let me try to make it clear. Let's call it 'Combat PTSD Trauma Memories for Dummies and Dumb Asses.'"

The group applauds loudly…even whistles.

"You have all been Soldiers in the most dangerous places in the world.

No Soldier has been more persistently subjected to terrorism in all of history.

You have been deployed to operational areas where there are no rules. The only rules are the rules of engagement or constraints that determine how you, not the enemy, must function as a Soldier.

Each minute could have been your last minute to live.

You survived. Some of your closest friends did not make it.

Too often, your survival is not an occasion for celebration but a lingering mixture of images that are associated with guilt, remorse, self-loathing, and spiritual bewilderment.

You are told that you are different. 'You are not the person I married.' 'You are not the son you were before deployment.'

You misinterpret these unsolicited statements to mean you are no longer a good person.

Yes, memories are biological, but they are like all biological functions. They need to be balanced, nourished, corrected, and treated with kindness, dignity, and respect.

Your precious survival memories can become treasures when you work to see how they can be corrected.

When the distortions are minimized, the truth is discovered, new meanings can be found, and then memories can be understood and perhaps, most importantly, accepted."

1SG Walker said, "I was neglected in childhood. I learned to be a survivor...I struggled a lot, wondering who was against me.

I wake up in the mornings now back in garrison and I feel like I am struggling just like I did as a child."

Another Soldier said, "A hug will take me a long way...my little girl hugged me and said, 'Daddy, are you okay?'

How come I can't remember what I want to remember, but I can't forget what I don't want to remember?"

"Mood affects memory," I said. "We tend to remember sad or negative things when our mood is depressed. A sad thought may also lead to a sad mood.

Sometimes it is difficult to distinguish between being asleep and being awake.

SGT Frank Irby, for example, was a snare drummer in high school and college. He was asleep, dreaming of playing snares in a marching band when he was suddenly awakened by the sound of a text message.

'I answered part of the text message and then I started texting. I guess I was texting my dream.'

The confused recipient of his message replied, 'What band?'

This may be one of the first unpublished cases of 'sleep texting.' Soldiers with PTSD are likely to have sleep-related behavioral changes, known to include sleep talking, sleep walking, REM (Rapid Eye Movement) Behavioral Disorder, and now, possibly, 'Sleep Texting.'"

SGT Roberts, good at coining phrases, told the Wednesday Morning Post-Deployment Group, "PTSD is like Herpes...you have it and go on with your life, but once in a while it flares up."

MSG Johnson said, "The smell of gun powder after firing a weapon is highly stimulating…it will give you an erection.

The smell of diesel and a cup of coffee while you are in combat waiting for the vehicles to warm up is more than special…you are just sitting there waiting to go on a mission and that combination of smells is very special."

Every group member suddenly remembered the scene and in common agreed. "Puts me at ease, the smell of diesel and coffee, while the vehicle is warming up before a mission."

SFC Rob Lacey said, "But you can't erase faces." Silently agreeing, the group stopped talking.

Dream Interpretation Group

SFC Jake Kelly, hands visibly trembling, said "I'm having a bad day. I really feel off. Even my tongue feels heavy. My hands are swollen and I just feel swollen in general."

His individual therapist is prescribing Zyprexa, a medication that may cause carbohydrate craving. He admitted he has been snacking more on salty foods that are likely making his body retain fluid and cause swelling.

SFC Kelly has become more hypervigilant, but the vigilance is focused less on his environment, more on his body. He also doubts his mental processes. "I am paranoid and feel like I may be losing my mind."

I went to the whiteboard and drew the following different way to look at PTSD. P=Paranoia; T=Trust destroyed; S=Suffering; and D=Depression.

Pointing to the whiteboard, I addressed SFC Kelly. "You are not losing your mind. You are just having a wonderful case of PTSD. Try not to despair. Help is on the way."

COL Robert L. Stewart, former co-leader of the Dream Interpretation Group, a combat-experienced Clinical Psychologist, correctly pointed out that the symptoms of PTSD may appear suddenly, unexpectedly, often after a long delay, and recovery follows an up and down course, not a straight up one to recovery.

Within 15-20 minutes, SFC Kelly's mood was significantly improved, demonstrating the power of the truth presented in an educational format.

"I don't understand"

SFC Michael Ford was tense and discouraged while speaking to the Tuesday Afternoon Post-Deployment Psychotherapy Group.

"My MRI today was hell.

The neurologist wants me to have an MRI of my brain.

I freaked out in the MRI machine.

I don't understand. I had an MRI once before, and it was not a problem, but this time I failed 4 times.

The technician was very patient and kind.

It felt exactly like the roll-over I was in…a roll-over in an MRAP (Mine Resistant Ambush Protected vehicle)…flashing lights…claustrophobia…tied down.

I had a panic attack and I have not been able to get rid of the anxiety since I tried to have the MRI a week ago."

I asked if his first MRI, the uneventful one, occurred before or after his roll-over in Afghanistan.

"It was before the roll-over."

"Many people have problems with anxiety and claustrophobia in the closed MRI," I said. "That is why they have the newer, open MRI. Request the open one next time," I recommended.

"Do you see any connection between the roll-over and your experience in the MRI?"

"No, and I don't think a lot of people have problems with the closed MRI."

Addressing his fellow group members, I asked, "Do you see any connection between SFC Ford's roll-over and his 'freaking out' in the second MRI?"

The group members, almost in unison, said, "Yeah, the MRAP is a closed tube, too. You can't see out, you are strapped in around your waist and straps go up and down in the vehicle. You can't see out. You have to trust the driver and there are explosives inside.

It is frightening when an MRAP rolls-over."

The group agreed that SFC Mike Ford had a flash back triggered by the similarity between the MRI and the MRAP.

SFC Ford still felt demoralized and discouraged.

With cognitions clouded by marked anxiety and perhaps also by mTBI (mild Traumatic Brain Injury), SFC Ford will require ongoing encouragement and more reasoning before discovering the truth of his situation. Then he will be ready to deal with the truth.

SFC Ford said, "I am constantly watching."

"What are you looking for?" I inquired.

"I am just being pro-active.

I want no surprises.

Knowing that I am not in combat now ... that I am back in a safe military fort in the US ... and still having PTSD symptoms, makes me feel even worse."

SGT Tommy Edwards said, "We all have our ways of dealing with things. I avoided everything. Drinking alcohol was a way to forget. I was the life of the party when I was drinking and then my liver went bad."

"SFC Ford, I'm Mike. I have little confidence in myself. I don't want to go to work so I have to put on this face every day.

I returned from Afghanistan in January and my house was basically empty. My wife and kid were gone. I had no internet, no cable, no TV and that's the way it is now 5 months later.

I learned some coping skills in Anger Management, but I do lots of sweating and I really hate the way I feel.

I just want my confidence back...things really hit me in Iraq in 2006."

SGT Edwards said, "My self-confidence was taken away...that investigation...made me feel awful guilty...one of my men was destroyed by an RPG (Rocket Propelled Grenade)...

The trauma was bad enough but the 15-6 (Official Army Formal Investigation) tore away any confidence I had left...

The crazy thing was they found me to be at no fault....even gave me a Bronze Star...

It was too late then...the emotional damage had already been inflicted."

One-hundred per cent of those present in group therapy reported their loss of self-confidence.

I wonder if this is related to their loss of trust. How can lost self-confidence and lost trust be restored?

SGT Edwards said, "I feel like I am stuck in a time-zone I can't escape."

SFC Ford said, "I told my wife that I am sick. She wanted to know if it was physical, like cancer. She does not understand why I can be psychologically sick. That hurts. Our own wives don't understand why we got PTSD."

Wednesday Morning Post-Deployment Psychotherapy Group

When I walked into the group therapy room two slices of bacon on a white paper plate were on the side table next to my chair. It may have been a gift not unlike the Drummer Boy's gift in the Christmas carol, a present from a group member fond of bacon.

The task today was accomplished with such success that I told the group at the end of the session I was very pleased and proud of the way they nurtured a new member into the group.

"My Medical Record was thin ... until recently"

SGT Billy Dawson, a light-skinned, married, 38-year-old Soldier with a full head of black wavy hair, looking 10 years younger, joined the Wednesday Morning Post-Deployment Group. It was his first session.

Anxiously staring at the floor, right hand over his mouth but mostly failing its purpose to hide his face, he said, "I had three back-to-back combat deployments. When I came home my father, an alcoholic, died of brain cancer, my grandmother died of stomach cancer and my grandfather died.

I'm worried about my health. I keep getting medical tests and they are always normal.

It is like I am paranoid about my body.

I have been in the Army going on 16 years. My medical record was thin ... until recently. Now it is thick. I hate that.

I have been married 14 years. When I came home at mid-tour I found out that my wife was pregnant with our son.

I already had a daughter, but when I went back to theatre after the mid-tour break, I got real anxious...I don't know why but ...it was like I really needed to live for my son.

I love my daughter, but it was different to be thinking about having a son.

I have been faithful to my wife, and I trust her, but I have been asking to be tested for STDs. There is something wrong with me, and I don't know what it is, but I don't want to give it to somebody else."

Does he have PTSD?

SGT Billy Dawson continued. "I am a 91 B, Mechanic. On the recovery team, I saw lots of bad stuff. I have been told I have anxiety."

Speaking to the fellow group members, I asked, "What do you need to ask him to find out if he has PTSD?"

MSG Kenneth Compton said, "Did anything really bad happen to you while you were deployed?"

SGT Dawson said, "We had just gotten into country...on a coalition force post...lots of people were milling around. We were setting up...lot of Bradleys (tanks).

My friend and SGT Harold were conducting checks on top of a M88 recovery vehicle. I heard a loud boom. SGT Harold yelled my friend's name, shouting, "Don't look down...don't look down."

I ran over toward him. The back of his leg was missing and it was cauterized.

The back of his leg was being held on just by the knee cap section.

Somebody had gotten into a Bradley and accidentally fired the cannon. It struck a tall metal pole and the shrapnel flew off the pole and struck him in the back of the leg. The heat had sealed the wound. He did not feel a thing.

SGT Harold was holding him. He finally looked down and said 'Oh, not my leg...not my leg,' and went into shock.

I was told later the leg was going to be removed, but a doctor saved his leg."

SFC Lacey said, "I worked in Bradleys (Bradley Tank) for 5 years. Those weapons have an electric and a mechanical safety. Somebody released the safety. When that happens, the weapon loads and fires automatically...that must have been horrible.

Do you think about it a lot?"

SGT Dawson said, "I went to Behavioral Health in theatre, but it stays on my mind. I dream about it."

"Do you avoid things that remind you of it?" I asked.

"Yes, but most of the time I get anxious or have a panic attack for no reason."

"There is always a reason," said SFC Lacey. "You have to learn what your triggers are and then you will get more control over your anxiety."

SGT Allen Burch said, "You need to keep coming here. Come every week. It is not easy in the beginning, but you will get better. This group has done more for me than anything else I ever tried."

MSG Compton: "Do you feel different now than you did an hour ago when you first came in here?"

His hand still covering the right side of his face, still anxious, hesitating, he replied, "...I think so."

"He is still anxious," I said. "Tell him how to reduce his anxiety. He needs to start feeling better now."

Laughter: "Hell, Doc, we all need to know that ourselves!"

"What about breathing exercises," I asked. (CO_2, hyperventilation, brown bag discussed; Cognitive Model of Anxiety discussed).

SGT Burch: "I learned to relax in here. I look forward to this group…but I still get anxious when I leave here…you will have to learn to relax in here first."

SFC Lacey said, "I felt more relaxed in combat; I would rather be down range right now. In combat I had my weapon 24 hours a day. I had plenty of ammunition. I had my protective gear. I had my buddies. You know you are needed. We become a family down range.

Here, the Army really doesn't need us any more. Being killed in action is possible, but it causes less anxiety than being crucified here."

"I believe we come closer to all those conditions you stated, SFC Lacey, in our weekly Post-Deployment Group Therapy Sessions than anywhere else other than combat," I said.

MSG Compton: "Stupidity, that's what caused your buddy to nearly lose his leg; somebody jumped in a Bradley and fired a round. I get very upset when and wherever I see stupidity."

"Memories are more acceptable when distortions are minimized, when the truth is drawn out of the suffering Soldier (not leading but encouraging him/her) in a trusting relationship," I said.

At home, these Soldiers do not feel valued by our nation, by the new units to which they are too quickly assigned, and often by their families who do not understand the degree of inhumanity they have witnessed.

What can be done to help the nation value our Soldiers? This book's principal objective is to help this happen and to have it become sustained and lasting.

What can be done to help the Army value the relationships formed in combat, to help continue these special relationship after redeployment, and to keep these Soldiers together for at least 12-18 months after they return from combat? These relationships/attachments are crucial. They remain one of the most important requirements of recovery.

What can be done to help families value their Soldiers? This is a challenging dilemma; horror stories will not be understood, accepted or necessarily disclosed. Education about PTSD may help families appreciate, value and love their Soldier more and more, just as I have come to admire, appreciate and respect these Soldiers and their sacrifices.

Suffering is stressful, particularly if it is witnessing the suffering of others and even if the witnessed suffering occurs in the comfort and safety of a fine military medical center in the US.

"Generals cried at the bedside of seriously injured Soldiers"

SGT Virgil Adams said, "For 5 months as the NCOIC (Noncommissioned Officer in Charge) at WRAMC (Walter Reed Army Medical Center), I tracked every Soldier admitted from Europe and the Middle East.

It was more stressful than combat. I had to see every wounded warrior every day and I had to contact their family within 48 hours of their admission to the hospital.

I had to make all the arrangements to get their family to WRAMC.
Generals cried at the bedside of seriously injured Soldiers.
Some patients had families that could not speak English.
Some of the Soldiers were in a coma.
I can't stop it when these memories come into my mind.
The memories are as painful as the reality."

"What it means to be a Soldier"

CSM (Command SGT Major) James Hall shared his thoughts with the Tuesday Morning Post-Deployment Psychotherapy Group.

CSM Hall said, "What is the meaning of the experience of being a Soldier?"

When I sit in this chair (recently retired, awaiting evaluation for VA Disability Rating for PTSD) and look at the chair I used to sit in, it has no meaning now. Once a Soldier, always a Soldier, but the system tells you that you are not a Soldier now.

You must retire.

You are thrown to the side, a retiree, no longer essential...

No one wants to die abroad or alone. Everyone wants to die at home...

These Soldiers who die in combat are a real loss to me...

The suicide rate is up in the Army because this is difficult stuff to deal with...

Where do I belong now?

I don't belong anywhere."

His sentiments had a ring of truth to them. Over-powered, the group did not know how to reply.

SFC George Gibbs, a chronically depressed Soldier, was the first to respond.

"In Landstuhl Regional Medical Center, busses came in every day loaded with injured Soldiers.

Some are burned over 90% of their body...you know they will never recover...

Some have both legs blown off."

CSM Hall spoke again.

"I convinced myself I would willingly give my life for my Soldiers in combat, but when I got back home, I don't get the respect I expected.

I feel denigrated...so now I care less about people."

As I sat at the top of a semi-circle of Soldiers in group therapy, listening to their heart-wrenching stories, the following image came vividly into my mind:

Chirping baby birds, crowded closely together in their nest, pale yellow featherless skin absorbing sun rays, with their mouths open wide, starving for respect and recognition and a place to feel accepted (beloved) so they can get back their identity, their normal memory and their self-respect so they can learn to fly. How sad and unfair it is that so many Soldiers who gave so much in the 21st Century War to save American lives are now feeling useless, unvalued, and unrespected!

7

A Soldier Suit for Christmas

World War I

The first 10 years of my life were influenced by World War I, a war that ended 13 years before my birth.

There was no TV. My family first bought a TV long after I went away to college.

I don't recall WW I's persuasion in the infrequent times I was taken to the movies.

There were no WW I radio shows we listened to as a family.

As I write this chapter of my life, the first 10 years and the highlights of the second decade, I remain puzzled, therefore, just how WW I became such a major inspiration, significantly molding what I thought, felt, and did.

Oddly, without explanation, I have vivid recollections of visual images of American Soldiers in trenches in France in WW I. I see brave, exhausted Soldiers fighting severe winter weather, deep in mud.

I see Soldiers severely injured by shells, infections, and Mustard Gas.

Hand to hand combat with German Soldiers captures my mind's eye.

The skeptic may argue that I received ample exposure to scenes of American Soldiers bogged down on the Western Front in WW I as widely depicted in modern movies.

The chances were slim, but I could have seen WW I movies while accompanying my mother to LOEWS Theatre on Granby Street on her Mondays downtown. Her avowed interest, however, was more in movies of Frederick March or Spencer Tracy in love than in movies of combat.

Within the limits of my imagination, I re-enacted and re-experienced WW I, dressed in the most realistic facsimile of the handsome WW I American Army uniform.

I envisioned Soldiers fighting in ditches in France, the use of deadly mustard gas as a weapon and battle field amputations of gangrenous infected legs. WW I was meant to be the "war to end all wars."

The stories of atrocities and heroes were dramatized in my impressionable childhood mind. Other children may have played "cops and robbers" or "cowboys and Indians," but I reinvented WW I.

There were two empty city lots behind my house at 1231 West 47th Street. The lots became fields of battle.

In the fields formed by the empty lots, I dug trenches, striking sand no more than a few inches beneath the surface. Wearing an imaginary gas mask, I endured the dreaded Mustard Gas.

I was particularly influenced by the Army uniform worn by our brave Soldiers in WW I.

It was the WW I uniform that I begged Santa Claus to bring me each Christmas. The brown jacket looked sharp with a wide leather belt around the waist and a thin brown leather shoulder strap.

Christmas was the most important time of the year for my family.

It mattered little to me from what source our Christmas presents were received. It must have been difficult, however, for my proud mother, a Beale, to be given baskets of fruit from a church, clothes from the Welfare Department, or surplus government food such as hard cheese and hard-to-dissolve powdered milk.

I will never know how my family afforded to buy a Soldier suit for me for Christmas 1938.

How strange, in retrospect, that a seven-year-old boy's heart could not have been more pleased or more satisfied than the Christmas morning he discovered his Soldier Suit under the Christmas tree.

Being a Soldier was one of the earliest and continuous dreams of my life. Being a Soldier required being in uniform.

No Christmas present ever outshined my Soldier suit. It meant more to me than graduation from West Point or a Bronze Star.

When my brother, Randolph, outgrew his Western Flyer bicycle, his initials, RTB, were replaced with mine, RSB. My father repainted the bicycle, a fine royal blue trimmed in a glossy white, and it became my Christmas present, 1940.

The Western Flyer, free of fancy gears typical of more expensive models today, was hard to pedal, but it helped build strong legs and healthy lungs.

I rode my Western Flyer from the fifth grade through high school.

It was a useful and much appreciated Christmas present, but it paled in the glory and brilliance of my Soldier suit.

My mother made Christmas the most wonderful time of the year. Because of her, I still believe in Santa Claus. Poor but proud, my mother never burdened her children with finances. We were never told we were poor. We were never permitted to believe our plight was gloomy. Hope prevailed. If sacrifice was necessary, it was quietly assumed by my mother.

All Things Army

Norfolk, Virginia, my home town, is a Navy town.

The largest natural harbor in the world is defined by Norfolk's coast line. One could stand on its shores on March 8-9, 1862 and observe, up close, the celebrated Civil War naval battle between the Monitor and the Merrimack, the most important naval battle of the Civil War.

Norfolk and the US Navy had a love-hate relationship before WW II. I recall seeing a painted sign prominently displayed in front of a professional office building in the 1930's warning, in bold black letters on a white wooden post, that read, "Dogs and Sailors Stay off the Lawn."

If Active Duty Soldiers were stationed in Norfolk before WW II, they were seldom, if ever, seen.

Nonetheless, my military interests were in all things Army.

We had old Army blankets, uniquely Army brown; these were prickly woolen blankets. I have no idea where they came from, but I was the Soldier in the family permitted to fashion them into an Army pup tent in the side yard.

The Army blankets lasted longer than my childhood despite their rough treatment. Nail holes were required to fasten the Army blankets to the tent poles created from scrap wood.

Many nights were sleeplessly spent in my Army tent outside of which the Star Spangled Banner waved with the summer breeze.

I had a brass Army bugle. I could play most of the Army bugle calls before I was 10 years old.

Neighbors were defenseless. Loud, startling Army bugle calls were inevitable. A passerby approaching 47th Street would easily mistake the neighborhood for an Army installation.

The Army headquarters of the "Blues" was located not more than 3 city blocks from my house. I believe it was an Army National Guard Center.

My knowledge of the "Blues" is very limited. My contact with them was entirely indirect.

Uncle John A., my mother's younger brother who lost his left arm as a City of Norfolk employee in a motor vehicle accident, spoke about the "Blues" with reverence, pride, and untrammeled respect. In a melancholy manner, Uncle John A. missed the "Blues" in which he served briefly before the tragic loss of his arm.

When the "Blues" returned from summer camp, their surplus food supplies were shared with local families, including mine. I recall happy summer days when a sizeable section of our yard was covered with their generous gifts of edible feasts.

Uncle Richard Brown

I believe my father's brother, Richard Brown, rode a motorcycle as an American Soldier in France during WW I. I cannot say this is factual, but I remember that each time he visited us, he promised to make a side-car for my bicycle.

He worked for a sheet metal company located on Colley Avenue in Norfolk, as I recall.

My father was proud of his brother. He often encouraged Uncle Richard to tell me what it was like in the War. His stories were forgotten long ago, but they captivated my childhood imagination. I rarely saw Uncle Richard. His influence on my interest in World War I could not have been more than trivial.

For a long time, I kept hoping Uncle Richard would keep his promise to make a side-car for my bicycle. It is not likely he ever will.

If he made a shiny metal side-car for my bicycle, it was never sent over to me from Atlantic City, his neighborhood in Norfolk. Sadly, both Uncle Richard and Atlantic City passed away long ago.

My Father's Family

If we visited my father's family in Atlantic City, it was not often and the visit was made over the protests of my mother. For whatever reason, my siblings and I were not encouraged to get to know my father's family.

Atlantic City was a neighborhood close to downtown Norfolk. During my childhood, Atlantic City may have been held in less repute than Lamberts Point, a debatable point.

A copy of my paternal grandfather's marriage certificate hangs on the wall of my bedroom. It came into my possession several years ago. It came to me in the old-fashioned copy system of white print on black paper, a legal document produced for a special need of my father in his advancing years.

Photographed and framed, the marriage license is as appealing to observe as it is interesting to read. Benjamin Franklin Browne, age 30, married Missouri Brady, age 18, on 24 October 1883, in Norfolk County, Virginia. He was identified as an "Oysterman."

The spelling of my last name gradually changed from Browne to Brown. To my knowledge, it was not the result of court action, merely disuse. Of note, however, years ago, our second son, David, had his last name legally changed to David Milton Browne. It happened about the time one of my sons, an adolescent, threatened to run away. As I recall, it was a difficult period in my life: one son threatening to run away and another son changing his name. Thankfully, it all turned out happily.

I never measured it, but the distance from Atlantic City to Lambert's Point cannot be more than a few miles, probably less than 5 miles. The emotional distance, however, separating my mother from my father and his family must have been close to the distance between the planet Earth and its moon.

I met my father's father, but I never knew him. I encountered him not more than 2 or 3 times. I may remember one meeting.

I could not have been more than a 5 or 6-year-old. Dad drove us to his father's home in Atlantic City. My grandfather's house was large and plain, occupied by several generations of Browns.

John Dunn, a large, friendly, pleasant, out-going man in his mid-thirties, was an "adopted" son reared by my father's parents. His friendliness stood in marked contrast to my grandfather, who appeared disinterested and annoyed by our surprise visit.

Feeling awkward, unwelcomed and subservient, we drove away intending not to return. My dad did not speak to me on the way home.

Most of what I know about my father's father was told to me. It would fill a post-card, leaving enormous space.

Ben Browne, my paternal grandfather, always wore a black suit. He was tall and thin.

He had a stern demeanor and sterner personality.

He "always purchased the first car Ford produced and made available in Norfolk each year."

He lived to be well into his 90's, just as my father lived to be 93.

I never knew how he made his living.

I never met or heard about his wife, Nancy Missouri Browne, my paternal grandmother.

Two of Richard Brown's children, Wilbur and Tilton, the best jitter-bug dancer in Norfolk, occasionally came to our home to visit my brother Randolph and my sister Edith.

Tilton was affectionately known as "T." He and Edith won every dance contest they entered. The ones that I attended were conducted at Nolde's Bakery on Hampton Boulevard. These well attended social events took place during World War II. The bakery served refreshments.

Mainly, sadly, I never knew why I was not ever to know my father's family.

I Loved My Mother...and My Father

It now occurs to me for the very first time, that my mother's marriage at age 14 to my father at age 21 lasted until she died at age 71 probably because she would never break a promise.

I never saw my mother treat my father affectionately, but she was a loyal wife, and a dutiful mother of 6 children and 4 grandchildren.

Theirs was not a bickering relationship. There were no memorable boisterous arguments. Dad hung out behind the house at his work bench.

Most of his life, my dad smoked a pipe. Prince Albert tobacco, his favorite, came in a small bright red can. Long before our present regulations banning smoking in public places, my mother never permitted him to smoke inside the house.

If I have created the representation of an unhappy marriage, an unhappy childhood or an unhappy family, then I have failed to be honest. Ours was a busy household, and I don't believe we ever considered our lot as unfair or unhappy. It was a family inspired with hope.

It may be difficult to accept that my mother was unaffectionate to my father, but she was not indifferent towards him. She never devalued his talented handiwork. He fixed all that was broken around the house from frozen water pipes to plumbing or electrical problems.

None of us children ever treated my father with disrespect.

He taught me how to tie my shoes. I remember his patience, something I learned slowly.

There were no displays of affection from him towards us, but many times I saw him pushed aside when he tried to put his arm around my mother.

I remember when he was arrested for making bootlegged beer during prohibition. He stored the home-made brew in a crawl space under the kitchen floor. The kitchen linoleum covered a trap door leading to the forbidden, clandestine, golden liquid treasure.

Tall, angry, aggressive officers of the Norfolk Police Department came with a warrant, banging loudly on our front door on a dark, cold night. I remember their black shiny boots and gruff manner.

The Police officers went directly to the hiding place. They left with the evidence, cases of beer in dark brown bottles. My father's trembling hands were cuffed painfully tight behind his back.

My father was shoved into one of the several police cars strategically positioned in front of 1237 West 47th Street. We stood helplessly watching, barely understanding but painfully aware that something ruinous was happening to my father.

The police cars sped away rapidly, appearing to be in engaged in a fight to the death. Their flashing bright lights and loud, haunting sirens left none of our neighbors unaware of their mission.

The Wild Cherry Tree

A large wild cherry tree stood in our backyard on 47th Street. Its long branches were bent toward the ground with its rich fruit. The many friends and neighbors who came to visit were treated with the fermented form of the wild cherry.

One wild cherry homemade wine festival stands out distinctly in my memory for a very good reason.

Those who have sipped at the fountain of wild cherry delight will recall that it is both potent and sweet. It is so sweet that serious wine drinkers leave a sizable amount of the beverage in the bottom of the glass, unable to force down every drop.

The remaining deep purple reddish aromatic unconsumed wine is not likely to go unnoticed by an adventurous 4 or 5-year-old boy.

This little boy's family and their friends and neighbors, fortified with the fruit of the cherry tree, found their way into the front room to talk and to act sober. They left the remains of the treat on the dining room table whose white table cloth emphasized the attractive colors of the wine.

I remember standing next to the table on my tip-toes, barely able to inch each glass to the edge of the table, and ridding all the glasses of their remaining contents. The stealth with which the feat was achieved kept my secret.

I am ashamed of what happened over the next few minutes.

I removed all my clothes and went outside, standing naked on the back porch for the entire world to see.

The vertigo was nearly intolerable and more disrupting than the nausea and vomiting.

"Lord in Heaven, child," said my mother, "what has made you so ill?"

Edith, my older sister, shouted, "Bobby is drunk. Smell his breath!"

When all the evidence was collected, I was found guilty of stealing wild cherry wine, drinking under age, and drunk in public. At the most, I was only 5 years old.

Nearly 80 years have passed since the wild cherry wine festival. Thankfully, I have never again experienced such physical and emotional turmoil and misery. It was a trauma I will never forget.

"Not this day, Our Father!"

My mother was the primary care-giver to all her children and to all her grandchildren. She was a strong disciplinarian who lived by inflexible rules and expected those she loved to live by the same rules or face the consequences.

She never smoked a cigarette, never drove a car, and she never flew in an airplane. God bestowed upon her an enormous strength of will and an even stronger strength of character.

She went downtown on Mondays for a ham sandwich and a movie on Granby Street.

She washed clothes on Tuesdays and dried them in the fresh air and sunlight of our backyard.

She ironed on Wednesdays.

Dishes were washed in the kitchen sink and dried with a "cup-towel" after each meal.

I learned early in life never to attempt to negotiate or bargain with my mother. Once her mind was made up, it would not be changed.

"Not this day, Our Father!" was her last word on any matter under consideration with which she disagreed. My request for her permission to walk to nearby Tayloe's Garage, for example, may be declined by my mother with "Not this day, Our Father." For me, it had the strength and reverence of a biblical Commandment.

On Saturday nights, my mother made rolls containing yeast. She covered the rolls with a clean cloth, letting them rise over-night. She baked the risen rolls on Sunday mornings, filling the house with an unforgettably delightful aroma that remains one of my favorite smells.

Bright yellow butter oozed out of the warm rolls as they were eaten in a devotional-like ritual around the kitchen table. The silence my family creates today while consuming desserts reminds me how quiet all the Browns were while enjoying my mother's "hot rolls."

My mother was a Beale. The Beale's heritage, I am told, can be traced back to Germany and England. My mother cleaned house and baked like a German.

Her multi-layer chocolate marshmallow white batter cake was delightful and short-lived.

Her meals were tastefully prepared and served. Sadly, little was known in her day about the relationship between nutrition and heart disease. For example, my mother considered the fatty portion of meat to be a delicacy, often saving much of it till the end of the meal to savor as one savors expensive port or Cuban cigars.

My Mother as Healer

I remember people coming to see my mother about their health.

John was a middle aged man whose interest in another man's wife was painfully and dangerously costly. He came to my mother with his right arm in a home-made sling fashioned out of a pillow case.

With singleness of purpose and the confidence of a Mayo Clinic clinician, my mother approached her patient skillfully.

She was nonjudgmental. She asked no questions about the behavior causing the injury.

She carefully removed his shirt. His hairy back was peppered with buck-shot. His right forearm was black and blue with bruises and more buck-shot.

She cleaned the wounds with soap and warm water.

She sterilized her surgical instrument, also known as eye-brow tweezers, with rubbing alcohol and held the blue flame of a match to the working end of the tweezers.

She seated her patient in a kitchen chair which his legs straddled as he faced its back.

Amid his cries for mercy and shouting, "Lord Jesus, Louise, don't try to kill me," each removed buck-shot made an unforgettable high pitched, tiny sound as it landed in a cereal bowl.

He looked worse when he left than he did when he arrived.

He returned every day, however, for weeks for wound care.

Gradually, he regained the use of his right arm. Most importantly, he was free of any evidence of infection.

She removed foreign objects from the red eyes of adults and children.

I recall seeing my mother removing broken glass from an injured, barefoot child, undeterred by its screaming.

Her bedside manner was calm and confident. We all knew she cared for the people she took care of.

My mother never complained about her life.

I never heard her say she ever seriously considered health care as a career. Her formal education ended in the fourth grade, but she was a life-long learner. She was the person to whom people turned when they were in trouble or unwell.

All Things Musical

Beyond the importance of the American flag, my mother expressed little interest in my love for the Army. I recall no childhood encouragement from my mother to be a physician.

Her encouragement, indistinguishable from a mandate, was singular and unwavering.

My mother wanted me to sing country music and learn to play the guitar. I wanted to make my mother happy.

Singing came easily for me. Learning to play the guitar was more difficult than I ever dreamt.

"I like to hear you sing, Bobby," my mother often told me. "It lets me know you are happy." Her words rang in my heart. I often sang while playing in the yard whether I was happy or not because I wanted to please my mother.

Each time I learned a new song, my mother would call me inside the house to sing for visiting relatives. I had to stand up straight with shoulders pulled back and squared. The song was secondary to the posture of the singer.

I faced my audience, sensing we were all captives of a strong personality. My performance occasionally was pleasing, even entertaining if I danced along with the song. The dancing was identical to Elvis Presley, 25 years before he was discovered.

Still under 10 years of age, I met a kind and gentle middle-aged neighborhood man with whom I walked from his house to the bus stop each morning. I sang his favorite songs. He usually paid me several pennies for singing. My income was not reportable to the IRS.

Guitar lessons were started early in my life. Edith's former boyfriend, Buddy Brothers, played handsomely on his attractive guitar. "Buddy" was painted smartly on his guitar's name plate. Somehow I ended up owning Buddy's guitar. I believed Buddy pawned his guitar before leaving town.

When my guitar lessons were started at the Levy-Page Temple of Music, located on City Hall Avenue in Norfolk, my mother paid one dollar per lesson. The largesse from which this expenditure was obtained remains a well-kept secret. My weekly guitar lessons were paid faithfully, inflicting further indebtedness to my family during the Great Depression.

I cannot recall my age when my guitar lessons began. When the guitar case stood next to me, however, it exceeded my height by several inches.

The little boy and his big guitar case attracted the attention of Sailors who crowded the street cars that transported me to the Temple of Music.

"Play us a tune, young man," was the Sailors' usual request. After my brief recital, Bobby's guitar with "Buddy" adorning the name plate was passed around and Sailors strummed a wide variety of warm tunes.

Often, I hardly had time to return the guitar to its brown case before departing for my anticlimactic guitar lesson.

In the sixth grade at James Madison Grammar School I competed in a talent contest. I am very fond of Hershey Chocolate Candy Bars, the consolation prize. I ate my prize on the walk home. It was a tasty disappointment.

I broke my mother's heart when I refused to continue my guitar lessons. If I had learned anything from the years of lessons, it was not how to play the guitar.

At Blair Junior High School, I walked on the stage, faced the judges and the audience with visible insecurity and announced, "I am going to sing, 'Without a Song.'" To my surprise, the audience broke out in loud laughter that lasted several minutes. I had not intended to be funny. The anxiety melted and I got a "Superior" rating from the judges for my baritone solo.

I sang in Sena B. Wood's Fifth Bell Chorus at Maury High school for three years. The most talented singers in the large high school were selected by its demanding director. It was a fulfilling, satisfying musical assignment, rich with many pleasant memories.

Because of its lasting positive effect, I mention, again, Perry Como's "Chesterfield Supper Club," the fifteen minute radio show that instilled romance into my relationship with Dottie.

As a ritual, we listened to Perry Como's soothing love songs from our homes just a few blocks apart. I lay on my back in the front room of my house at 1321 West 39th Street. Dottie lived at her grandmother's at 1326 West 27th Street.

Every lyric went straight to my heart.

When the show ended at 7:15PM, as I said earlier, I immediately called Dottie and sang Perry Como's songs from the show to her.

If it were possible to plagiarize the voice of a renowned vocalist by making one's own voice sound indistinguishable from the gentle singer himself, then I would be guilty of attempted impersonation.

With my best friends, Baxter and George, I went to choir practice at Burrows Church every Thursday night and sang in the choir for the Sunday morning and evening church services.

Much later in my life I came to appreciate classical music, for which I am indebted to my loving wife, Dottie.

A compact 45 record player was the first gift I received from Dottie. Dvorak was the first composer that attracted my attention.

All the 45s she gave me were recordings of the great classical composers. I feel discontented when I am forced to go a day or two without hearing the good classical of Mozart, Beethoven, or especially Mendelssohn. The effect of good classical music restores my soul.

The old guitar was not totally abandoned. Occasionally, I strummed and sang "In the Pines where the Sun never Shines" for the entertainment of our children.

Framing my history in terms of guitar lessons presents an intriguing mystery.

I really wanted to learn to play the guitar. I really wanted to make my mother happy, but mine was a generation too soon.

Our youngest son, Clinton, picked up my old guitar when he was very young. He never put it down. Without lessons, my guitar, as last, yielded music in his masterful hands.

Nothing is more important to Clinton than music.

Mother, he would have pleased you beyond the telling of it.

All Things Athletic

I had athletic skills before I was aware of them. Basically, I could run fast, faster than any student at James Madison Grammar School.

I was more aware of my lack of self-confidence than my athletic skills.

I repeatedly declined Mr. W.P. Sullivan's requests to join the school basketball team. He was an attentive principal at James Madison and its basketball coach.

Mr. Sullivan judged me to be a potential asset to the school team. I knew little about basketball at 12 years of age. Extremely sensitive, I feared public embarrassment.

Paul Decker was the father of athletic opportunities for the underprivileged in Norfolk. He oversaw the James Madison Community Center.

When Paul Decker moved to an administratively higher position, he retained J.T. Shellnut to replace him as its director. J.T. Shellnut brought along Jimmy Clark.

Any child who had a heart for sports was given the opportunity by these good men.

At 14 years of age, I helped organize a football team, the Lamberts Point Rangers. We played in uniforms made available by the Norfolk Recreation Bureau.

We suited up at the James Madison Community Center and jogged 6 or 7 blocks, in cleats, to Dunn Field. Dunn Field was near the Lamberts Point Coal Pier. Now it's part of ODU.

I stopped by my house at 1321 West 39th Street to show off my football uniform to my mother. My sister Edith said, "Bobby, put a penny in your shoe (cleats) and it will bring you good luck."

I wrestled off my shoe and was furnished a copper penny to bury under the white sock of my right foot. I then ran down the concrete street to Dunn Field. The excitement of my first football game left no room in my awareness for the copper penny.

It took more than luck to succeed in Community League Football. We did not win a single game. Truthfully, we did not score a single point the entire season.

The following year was a different story. Coach Jim Collins conducted our daily practice sessions and coached every game. The Lamberts Point Rangers were undefeated, untied, and unscored upon.

Our performance attracted the attention of Tony Saunders, Maury High School Football Coach.

We played an exhibition night game at Foreman Field. Coach Saunders came to the game and invited us to play for Maury High School the next year.

Nothing was more important to me in high school than playing football. Coach Saunders, a retired Naval Officer who fought in WW II, was a good coach and a good man.

Bill Story was Assistant Principal at Maury High School. He had been head football coach at Granby High School, our rival.

Bill Story was a remarkable Southern gentleman. He was tall, handsome, and distinguished.

I still have a letter Bill Story sent in which he congratulated me for my performance on the football field, urging me to perform as well in the classroom.

A "football scholarship" arrangement made it possible for me to attend the University of Virginia, a chapter in my life described elsewhere in this text.

All Things World War II

WW II was a major influence on the second decade of my life.

There have been no shortages of war and, sadly, no decade of my life has known lasting peace.

I fought tirelessly, in my mind, in my thoughts and in my emotions, next to my brother, from the Japanese attack on Pearl Harbor in 1941. I was beside him in his fourteen major battles in the Pacific. I went over the side with him twice when his ship was torpedoed.

My brother Randolph, before his death at age 87, gave me his military ribbons, testimonials to his honorable service during WW II. His ribbons, a cherished gift, hang attractively in a frame in my office.

Alvin Smith's mother invited me to have an after-school treat with Alvin at their home on West 38th Street. We were classmates in the sixth grade at James Madison Grammar School.

As I walked up their steps I could see the Gold Star Flag symbol in their front window announcing the death of a service family member.

Alvin, a quiet child with dark, crew-cut hair, was quieter today than usual. Mrs. Smith, a frail slender woman, with graying hair, and gold colored thin metal rimmed eyeglasses, needed to be brave.

She quietly served us her home-made peach cobbler. It was very delicious, but it was like eating at a funeral. I still remember the sadness from 7 decades ago.

The silence of sadness surrounded and pierced all three of us. As an 11-year-old boy whose brother daily faced the reality of death in WW II, I had no words for my feelings.

As elementary school children, we knew we were at war. During Air Raid Drills at school, we recognized the signals of alarm. In an orderly manner, we went to the school basement, remained silent, and sat on the floor with arms raised to cover our heads.

We knew the meaning of "Black Outs." Air Raid Wardens searched for light leaking out of our windows covered by shades and masking tape.

We knew the meaning of rationing because we saw rationing books for food and gasoline.

We heard the incredibly loud explosion from the Norfolk Naval Base that shattered some of the windows in our school ten miles from the base.

Shortly after the end of WW II, my great disappointment was unspeakable when, at age fifteen, I read in the Norfolk Ledger Dispatch, in a small article of no more than one-hundred words, that the Communists in China were starting an armed rebellion against their government. I suspected another war was on its way.

Like Jack and the Bean Stalk, wars great and small, always costing life and limb, appeared to pop up almost overnight in most of the world.

It meant to me, even as a 15 year old, that the US must remain strong and battle-ready and the likelihood of war, if not war itself, was a permanent reality.

A child's interest in a "Soldier Suit" for Christmas may have held major implications, none of which entered my thoughts then.

Now that interest makes all the sense in the world to a retired Army doctor racing against dotage.

I love the military more every day. I respect and admire the one percent of our entire population that defends our nation. Their heart-felt stories inspire me every day of my work.

My mother taught me as a young child to honor the American flag.

"That's our flag," she would tell me. "Men have given their blood for it; never forget that, Bobby."

If the Soldier carrying the flag in battle got shot, then another Soldier grabbed it quickly. "Our Soldiers always need to see the American flag waving in the air," my mother would tell me. "The flag kept them fighting. They never gave up as long as our flag was held up in battle."

We had a flag pole in our yard on 47th Street in Norfolk, Virginia, where I lived the first decade of my life. It was a free-standing, official appearing flag pole constructed and erected by my dad. Weather permitting, the American flag was raised each day in our yard. Our neighbors were not members of the military at that time. It was unique to have a flag pole in our yard.

If there was anything in our house we respected more than the American flag, it was the Bible. They were handled in similar ways.

As a child, the only thing I wanted more than an American flag was a Soldier suit. My mother purchased a small American flag for me when she had the means.

I can't ever recall as a child going without an American flag for more than several weeks. The flag possessed magical qualities for me!

It stimulated exciting thoughts about military battles, all leading to victory. In this vast imaginary land of military struggles and conquests, I always carried the American flag, leading the troops from the front of the line.

I reenacted military campaigns with neighborhood peers, portraying American Soldiers in battle. We were mightily equipped with sticks as rifle substitutes on our shoulders. We proudly marched as an elite military force comparable to Special Operations Forces or Navy Seals today.

My soldier suit for Christmas was never ornamental! It was worn in battle until it was torn and tattered. Each hole or discoloration proudly signified a successful battle against an evil force that outnumbered our forces by an unimaginable number.

The present day British Army Officer uniform, but much more modest, closely resembles the WW I uniform I craved each Christmas.

We once had a photograph of yours truly, maybe at age nine, wearing his WW I Army uniform standing behind his Western Flyer bicycle.

The photograph depicts a boy with head piece tilted back, exposing his forehead. He is standing neither at attention nor at ease but leaning unmilitarily forward. Worst of all, the young Soldier is smiling. It is enough to make a real military man or woman cringe.

Christmas, I repeat because of its importance, was the most wonderful time of the year for my family, poverty be damned.

Mother's recipe for hot egg nog called for a dozen egg yolks, heavy cream, light cream, and milk. She slowly heated the special mixture in a large open pan on top of the old gas kitchen stove.

Several spices, but mainly nutmeg, and generous amounts of bourbon and rum were added.

Finally, the beaten dozen egg whites were blended into the concoction before it was poured hot into a coffee cup and served with pride and a warm "Merry Christmas."

Neighbors and some family members not seen for a year would brazenly visit on Christmas morning just as the aroma of mother's egg nog filled the house, if not the neighborhood.

Mother's hot Christmas morning egg nog was a strong family tradition, unbroken until her Christian values were significantly realigned by a major change in her life described elsewhere.

The Values of My Childhood

My mother was the hero of my life. It is to her that I attribute my most deeply held beliefs.

Hers was a philosophy of hope. "We will get by."

"We fight legally for what we need if it is not provided."

"We keep our word."

I made a promise after school to an older child taunting me to fight. "If you don't beat me up," I promised, "I will give you a boat my father made."

I described the boat, an attractively hand-fashioned wooden vessel, painted white. The bottom of the boat was painted a deep red color.

It was a row boat, about two feet long, with oar-locks and functioning oars. It was sea worthy.

My father had made the boat for me. He loved boats and always wanted to own a real boat himself, one of his unrealized dreams.

The bully's interest in the boat magnified as we walked together from James Madison Grammar School to my home at 1231 West 47th Street, 10 city blocks away.

My plan, poorly contrived, was to dash for the back door, leaving the bully empty handed in my back yard.

I ran up the steps, raced through the door, slammed and locked it behind me.

My mother looked at me suspiciously.

As the bully pounded on the back door, I ran upstairs.

My mother opened the back door, listened to the story, and called for me.

When I came downstairs to the kitchen, my mother said "Where is the boat?"

I returned with the boat.

My mother said, "Give him your boat." Protesting her decision would have been futile.

I don't remember ever seeing the bully or my boat again.

"We do not lie."

"We do not steal."

"A promise is sacred. Make few of them. Keep all the promises you make."

"Don't mess up a good girl."

"We treat others the way we want to be treated."

"Family comes first."

"We are proud. You are a Beale. We get on our knees first, and then we get on our feet and fight."

"Never forget who you are."

"Never forget where you came from."

"We are not yellow (cowardly)."

"Work for what you want."

"God will guide you if you seek His will in prayer."

"Stand up straight."

Should my mother be here to add a conclusion to this chapter she would remind me that faith conquers fear, that love is everything, that I must dream and my dreams will come true.

A good mother is God's special gift. I had a good mother.

8

WAR ON INTIMACY

Drama of Combat Trauma: Scene One

THE TRAUMA OF terrorism is a complex subject. In keeping with my plan of sharing with you what our Soldiers tell me, however, I do not wish to oversimplify this defining, essential, and organizing theme of our story.

Using a pedagogical approach called imaginal exercise or practice, I want you, dear reader, to create a picture in your mind of our Soldiers combating terrorism in the Middle East.

"Imaginal" or "Prolonged Exposure," a modification of imaginal exposure, is one of the treatments for combat-induced PTSD approved by the Department of Defense.

Imagine that you are attending a dramatic presentation on the stage of your local theatre. The performance you are now anticipating starts with the opening of the deep maroon colored, heavy velvet-like curtains.

The lights are lowered. The drama begins.

It is very early in the morning of a very dark night, a night as black as you have ever beheld.

You feel the cold of the desert night, surprised by its stark contrast with the unbearable heat of the day to follow in just a few hours.

The silence is broken by the noisy sounds of diesel engines starting, accompanied by the familiar smell of diesel exhaust fumes.

The hazy image of Army vehicles slowly becomes clear, changing from silhouettes to three dimensional trucks of great size. Now you see smaller vehicles as well, each with a 50 Caliber gun turret on top.

Hushed voices are receiving a safety brief at an SP (starting point). The Soldiers have been up since 2200 or 10:00PM, preparing for an early morning convoy that leaves at 0430.

Some of the Soldiers, gathered voluntarily in small groups, pray together for safety and for the successful completion of their mission. Their convoy of vehicles will carry food and medical supplies to an Iraqi village where starvation, injury and illness are constant realities.

You fight back tears, anticipating danger signaled by a queasy, noisy, embarrassing churning of your stomach.

These are our sons and daughters, brothers and sisters; some are mothers and fathers, spouses, neighbors and friends. They come from towns and communities we know, now only hours away from us by jet flight, but they are in places as foreign to us as distant planets.

You are startled, much to your surprise, when the piercingly loud deep voice command is shouted by the convoy commander, "MOVE OUT!"

The sun, more mighty than Zeus, mercilessly beats down, pounding the helmeted Soldiers whose 80 pounds of protective gear silently begins to absorb the heat.

The visibility is now perfectly clear. There is sand as far as you can see. You notice the heat.

For the first time, you imagine that you are drenched in sweat. Soon it will be 140 degrees Fahrenheit in the shade.

You are casually dressed for your night out at the theatre, but on the stage the Soldiers are garbed in uniforms and protective gear.

You feel empathy and want to help. What can you do?

"This is what I can do," you say to yourself. "I can watch. I can be a witness. I can learn. I can become more informed about the emotional cost of combating terrorism."

You are silently asking yourself, "How soon will I have to fight terrorism here in my home town? When will terrorists strike us again? How wide-spread will their attacks be in America?

"Thank you, Dear God, for our Soldiers! They are keeping the unthinkable from happening to us now."

You make a promise to yourself, a resolution stronger than stopping smoking, or losing weight.

"I will never again pass a Soldier on the street and feel the same way. I will not give up on those who have not given up on me. I will remember MSG (Master Sergeant) Keith L. Johnson's comment, "War is easy; coming home is Hell."

Thank you, MSG Johnson, but let me see if I can make your sentiment more accurate.

"War is never easy and coming home will be less of a Hell because we are going to express our appreciation for our Soldiers in the most meaningful ways conceivable."

Drama of Combat Trauma: Scene Two

The presentation is not over. The imaginal exercise continues.

Suddenly, the entire scene turns orange.

What is this? You ask.

The Soldiers shout "Sand Storm! Sand Storm! Cover your mouth and eyes. Seek cover!"

Tiny grains of sand, almost the consistency of powder, driven by a mighty powerful and destructive wind, penetrate every clothing fiber, every canvas truck top and wherever it can stab and infiltrate.

Time stops. This could go on for hours, you assume.

Now you imagine that you are not only hot or hyperthermic beyond your tolerance, but you can barely breathe. You experience an orange, uniquely orange, blindness.

The sand storm stops as suddenly as it started.

The large trucks and the smaller gun trucks slowly start the trip.

However, it turned out to be a dry, very dry run, a rehearsal for a night convoy to take place in sixteen hours, an unexpected change in orders.

The Soldiers take turns sleeping. In shifts, some Soldiers sleep while others stand guard.

You jump with a start, involuntarily, reflexively, to the sudden and very loud sound of mortar fire or "in-coming."

The enemy attack, lasting several hours, destroyed several important targets, ignited fires, and widely scattered debris.

Small arms fire has a characteristic high-pitched, whistling sound and metallic "ping" striking a vehicle. It is aimed at our Soldiers. Today, thank God, it missed its targets.

You stare blankly as a rocket-propelled grenade has transformed an unoccupied smaller vehicle into a flaming metallic skeleton.

In-coming mortars, small arms attacks, and rocket-propelled grenades were launched by invisible enemies, leaving no trace of their strategically changing locations.

You want to leave the theatre. How much more of this can you take? You have never felt this hot, this uncomfortable, this estranged from your comfort zone.

You don't leave your seat because you know our Soldiers do not leave their posts.

Drama of Combat Trauma: Scene Three

The scene on the stage changes, Thank God.

The new scene looks like a quiet, small, peaceful village. There are small buildings and shops.

Women with their young children are shopping, walking slowly down narrow dirt roads in front of shops fashioned out of tents and corrugated sheets of rusty metal.

Three American Soldiers drive up in a small gun truck. Two other gun trucks accompany them.

A Soldier slowly dismounts. He calmly and kindly offers a black and white soccer ball to an Iraqi child. The Iraqi child is eight years of age. He is standing close to his mother.

From under her dark burka, his mother snatches an AK-47 rifle.

Before she can fire the weapon, however, it is knocked out of her hands by the Soldier.

In an instant, six American Soldiers drew their weapons upon the woman.

The Iraqi woman grabbed her son's little hand and fled. She disappeared into the crowd that appeared instantaneously as if from nowhere. The crowd transformed itself into a human body guard.

The sun, its work completed, vanished into the scorching sand.

In the dark cold night, the convoy of nine vehicles, noiselessly as possible, slowly starts its trudging journey of mercy, its headlights turned off.

The second vehicle out of the gate of the FOB (Forward Operating Base) hits an IED (Improvised Explosive Device).

Blown high into the air, the vehicle miraculously landed back safely on the ground. Its five Soldier occupants sustained no apparently significant injuries.

Accountability is taken. "All Present and Accounted For" is the precious response the convoy commander prays to hear when each Soldier's name is called.

The convoy rolls on into the dark night.

A "day" in the life of American Soldiers in Iraq, sanitized for publication, ends for you.

The curtain drops.

Intermission

You are glued to your seat.

Sweating, cold, heart pounding, abounding with the strongest emotions you have ever felt, you are paralyzed with fear.

Overtaken by undeniable paranoia, you cautiously look around with suspicion at the others in the theatre.

No one is leaving.

Here is a gigantic chunk of the problem for our Soldiers combating terror in far off nations:

It is not on a stage.

It is not on a battlefield.

It is not against uniformed Soldiers.

It is not against an enemy that accepts the Geneva Convention for the humanitarian treatment of prisoners of war, or any other civilized, conventional rules of warfare.

The terrorist takes enormous pride and delight in the performance of dastardly deeds which the civilized world finds detestable.

There is also a daily painful irony in our 21st Century War in Iraq and Afghanistan. It is an irony that makes the death and injury of American Soldiers even more sorrowful.

This irony eclipses every step taken by combat boots on the firm feet of our Soldiers and by every combat boot on the mind of their loved ones.

Our Soldiers are primarily in Iraq and Afghanistan freeing these countries from their own terrorist leaders, building schools and hospitals, feeding the starving, producing fresh drinking water, performing innumerable acts of kindness in the ugly face of dangerous terrorism.

You may ask, what motivates America to shed its blood for the ungrateful? Ulterior, selfish, monetary rewards from our decade of burdens for Iraq and Afghanistan are not perceptible.

Yes, we would prefer to fight terrorism there instead of here. This undeniable truth, however, is dwarfed by the benevolent, charitable, and mercifully consistent self-imposed conventions that have guided our Soldiers during the longest war in our history.

In this war, we gain no new territory, no booty, and no riches.

In this war we lose. We lose our young men and women. We lose our economic stability.

Sadly, we lose our memory. Our nation has forgotten, if it ever actually knew, the cost of human suffering our Soldiers volunteered to incur.

You can be traumatized by merely observing the trauma as an observer of a staged dramatic production.

Imagine how our Soldiers are exposed to crimes against humanity and the ensuing trauma, a principal objective of terrorism.

We must defeat the effects of combat-induced terrorism on our Soldiers. Terrorism close up in the midst of battle is deadly. Terrorism cognitively re-experienced in the quietude of home years after combat, as in PTSD, can be no less terrible.

The response to this challenge is greater than military medicine can handle alone.

It must be conjoined by an informed public moved with the weapons of love and knowledge.

It is a marvel that only fifteen to seventeen percent of our Soldiers in the 21st Century War are found to have PTSD.

Drama of Combat Trauma: Scene Four

After the brief intermission, the curtain waits to rise again.

Glued to your seat, you are shaken emotionally and mentally distraught by the realistic reenactment on the stage of "A Day in the Life of 21st Century American Soldiers."

Paranoia holds you down, pressing you even deeper in your already uncomfortable theatre seat. A prison dungeon could not be worse or more confining.

Your heart is broken by the senseless sadness you witnessed. Your thoughts race from rage to marked fear.

The deep maroon colored heavy velvet curtains again slowly open, not to a stage this time but to a silver movie screen. You are going to observe one of the most powerfully loving and encouraging stories of a lifetime. It is the antidote for the poisoned play you just watched.

Two Soldiers, their weapons snuggled up close to their cheeks pressed against the darkly shiny metallic barrel of their rifles, are deeply asleep. On their unshaven, unwashed faces, undeniable contentment is preciously present.

A third Soldier sits at the base of a 50 caliber weapon, methodically scanning one hundred and eighty degrees. The back of the three Soldiers is protected by a thick concrete wall.

The hours, "marked by the changes in the face of mother nature," pass slowly.

Quietly, the guarding Soldier awakens one of the two sleeping Soldiers. They soundlessly exchange positions. The third Soldier, undisturbed by the changing of the guard, peacefully sleeps on.

These three Soldiers have trained together and served together in the same unit. They have come to respect and trust each other with their lives.

They know each other's families. Their wives are friends. Their children play together. They have different favorite NFL teams. They argue over the World Series, but the strength of their attachment to each other is nearly indestructible.

Without a moment's hesitation or regret, these Soldiers would lay down their lives for each other, but only after they gave their last breath to fully protect and defend each other. This is not the exception. This is the rule. It is the basic assumption by which they live. Psychologically, their relationship to each other is the best example of secure attachment. Their survival depends upon it.

It's daylight. Our three Soldiers are in their vehicle. The truck commander is seated in the right front passenger seat; the driver is concentrating on the road; and the gunner is standing in the rear, peering out of the hatch of the gun turret.

"When I get home," the driver speaking with excitement in his voice, "I'm getting on my Harley and open it up just to see what a twelve-month's rest did for that baby."

The gunner chimed in, "I'm going to a shack in the mountains where no one can irritate me…just to be totally alone."

"What about Gail?" the truck commander inquired.

"She will understand...Gail knows I shut down for a while before I leave for combat. She knows I shut down again when I return home from combat. We have an agreement. We've tried it the other way and nothing works."

Their feelings about coming home are punctuated by a long period of silence. Without warning, an RPG (Rocket-Propelled Grenade) sailed through their vehicle, striking no one.

More silence.

With each passing moment the attachment between these three Soldiers is deepening. You could tell it in their voices as they addressed each other. You could see it in their faces. You knew it in their words.

Three brave men knew they were where they needed to be. More than that, they were where they wanted to be. They were there for each other. They would prefer to be nowhere else in the world at this moment.

The familiar curtains close.

Inexplicably, you feel safer.

You smile. You admire these three fearless Soldiers.

You are so proud of them. You are proud to be an American. You are even more thankful for our Soldiers. You leave the theatre, but its impression will never leave you. You go home, safe.

"Are you ashamed of me?"

Charles and Katherine are married with 3 children under 6 years of age. Charles is a SGT in the Army. Three combat deployments since September 11, 2001, were difficult for Charles and his family.

Katherine is a full-time mother and house wife. They have been married 7 years.

Charles, a 30-year-old Soldier with sandy hair and hazel eyes, has PTSD. The details of his combat trauma have not been shared with Katherine.

At my request, Katherine has been coming to Charles' weekly psychotherapy sessions.

I often find it helpful to learn from the combat Soldier's wife how she understands the influence of combat on her husband. Their interaction in my office often illuminates my perception of the Soldier as a husband and father.

Charles, tall and lanky, is shy. His disposition was best described by a woman provider in our clinic as "sweet." Charles is sensitive.

Self-conscious of his tall frame, Charles slumps down in his chair. He speaks softly and wants to be accommodating and agreeable.

Charles has mastered the physical impression he wishes to make in public. He appears composed.

When I shake hands with him at the end of the session, however, his very sweaty palms suggest high levels of hidden anxiety.

Katherine is of medium height and weight. She wears blue jeans that emphasize her shapeliness. She tends to be assertive, readily stating what is on her mind. Like Charles, she has brown hair and eyes.

This couple has problems typical of Army families. They have been separated by Charles' deployments.

Charles missed his children's birthdays. "Those special occasions can never be restored," Charles said with regret.

Katherine has had to be mother and father to the children, even including important events.

A Soldier's psychological reentry into family and marriage after each deployment is precarious and risky. It may be as hazardous as the return to earth by an astronaut after circling the earth in space.

Their frequent separations are caused by multiple, lengthy combat deployments.

The nation hears little about separations taking Soldiers far from home to arduous pre-deployment training centers in the US. The war-like training before combat deployment has proven value, but it is yet another cause of separation from family. One Soldier said, "I am either deployed or I am in pre-deployment training."

This couple has been stressed by changes in Charles from combat and even more stressed by changes in Katherine that are apart from Charles.

Katherine plunged herself into a vigorous fitness program, improving her health and her appearance. She had frequent cell phone conversations with an old friend.

Charles grew uneasy and jealous. He was hurt and confused. His trust of Katherine weakened.

Worst of all for Charles, Katherine recently spent a weekend attending an out-of-state conference with a girlfriend. However, Charles discovered that she did not attend the conference.

Katherine denied interest in another person. She provided a plausible explanation of her whereabouts.

With months of counseling, Charles' disappointment and anger subsided. He is more at ease in the relationship now.

Their "Chief Complaint," the commonly used medical term with which each treatment session begins, was, "We are good… good…we are communicating much better," Katherine said. Charles, quiet as usual, nodded his head in agreement.

"What shall we put on our agenda for today's session," I asked.

Charles continued his silence.

Katherine said, "Charles is getting promoted next month…I am very proud of him."

Charles minimized his promotion, saying "I have been waiting 6 years for this and I only got it because they dropped the required number of points needed from 700 to 499."

"I don't think it is fair the way the Army does promotions," said Katherine. "Some people get promoted fast and they do half the work my husband does."

More silence from Charles whose pleasant facial expression could be said to have a formed a tiny smile.

"If Charles has nothing to talk about…do you, Charles?… then I want to bring up something I don't understand and it hurts my feelings."

More silence from Charles.

"We went to a Christmas party at our gym. We took our kids. It was crowded...a lot of people filled the small basketball court.

Every time I turned around, Charles was not there. I felt he was avoiding me. It has happened before. It happens every time we go out.

I just wonder...Charles, are you ashamed of me?

You never say I look pretty when we go out. Once in a while, a woman likes to hear that kind of thing from her husband. You never say anything like that to me."

Charles moved restlessly in his chair. He is gawky. It is difficult for him to hide restlessness with his long legs repeatedly crossing and uncrossing.

Finally, Charles said, "I was focused on the children, honey... they went off in different directions. It was crowded.

I am sorry. I did not mean to neglect you."

"I agree that it was crowded and I know you are more conscious of danger for our kids...maybe sometimes too conscious when I am not...but I still don't understand.

You do it whenever we go out, whether the kids are with us or not. At the gym you were always standing off to the side, not talking to people...just leaning against the wall."

"Let me see if I can help you understand, Katherine," I said.

"As you know, Charles has PTSD.

His symptoms are often worsened by social situations.

He is not ashamed of you.

He is ashamed of his symptoms.

In many emotionally painful ways, Charles resembles nearly every Soldier with PTSD.

Sadly, they see themselves as failures because they have returned from combat with symptoms they believe will ruin their relationships, their career, and their future if they fail to conceal them.

Crowds were dangerous in Iraq and Afghanistan. Soldiers are trained to keenly observe every situation for potential enemy action.

The enemy exploited crowds to hide suicide bombers, some of whom were involuntarily strapped with explosives and shoved into our convoys.

Our Soldiers change their ZIP codes when they return from war, but little else is changed.

Their deeply held beliefs about safety and survival are imprinted indelibly.

For you and your children, the Christmas celebration at the gym was a fun-filled event.

For your husband, it was another dreaded mission fraught with the danger that every crowd had for him in Iraq. He bravely completed the mission, never divulging his intense fear and dread."

Katherine reached for the box of Kleenex and carefully wiped away tears streaming down her cheeks.

Charles remained silent. He stared at the floor.

Katherine was now as quiet as her husband, Charles.

"Are you all right, Katherine?" I asked.

"I just feel so sad for Charles. I am so sorry."

"It's okay, honey," he reassured her. "It's okay. I'm all right. You don't have to worry about me. I'm fine."

Sometimes a party or celebration is not what it is meant to be.

Another Army Family

Tom and Mary, husband and wife for the past 7.5 years, are unhappy with each other.

Tom is a SSG (Staff Sergeant) in the US Army.

Mary is an administrative assistant, mother to three children, all under 6 years of age, and a house wife.

Tom is a stocky, assertive, at times aggressive, man in his mid-thirties.

He keeps his head shaved.

His unchanging facial expression depicts a stern, angry, infelicitous, sad, and disappointed Soldier.

Mary is a short, no longer physically fit woman whose dark eyes, short black hair, and infrequent but beautiful broad smile, suggest a lady who was likely more attractive several years earlier. Now she is tired, discouraged, and frustrated.

Physical attractiveness is less important to Mary than reducing the tension in her life as the wife of an active duty Soldier with PTSD.

Mary, too often disappointed in counseling, agreed to attend one, and only one, of Tom's psychotherapy sessions.

Tom's PTSD was not responding to therapy.

Addressing her in a kindly manner, I said, "Mary, what changes have you noticed in your husband? It may help me to make improvements with Tom. Can you describe the changes you observe in Tom as a result of his combat deployments?"

According to Mary, the changes in Tom get worse and worse after each combat deployment.

Tom, trying to appear resolute, was determined to listen to Mary, not to rebut her statements.

"He is more aggressive…even over little things…anything… chicken nuggets…he threw his nuggets at our 5-year-old daughter when she asked if she could have one of his when no others were left.

His sleep is very disturbed. He jumps all night in his sleep like the bed is a trampoline."

In his defense, Tom said, "I can sleep only if I am exhausted."

"Alcohol is a problem. His father was an alcoholic and his uncle died of it.

He is even more aggressive when he drinks alcohol.

He thinks he is superman.

He is always right and everyone else is wrong.

He got up to a 12 pack every night of the week and then hard liquor on weekends."

Tom, violating his resolution, said, "I need to take the edge off, doctor."

Recently, Tom has been talking to ASAP (the Army's Alcohol and Substance Abuse Program), "but I am not actually enrolled."

"His alcohol consumption went up with each deployment.

He lies even about meaningless things…lies… lies… lies."

Tom added to the list of changes himself. "Doctor, I am a colder person. I am short-tempered.

Before my combat deployments, I was a warm person."

Mary was not yet to the end of her list.

"Trust is hard to get and easy to lose.

He has lost my trust.

I found pictures of him and some girl in a bathing suit sitting on his lap."

Tom spoke up in his defense.

"Doctor, it was nothing. We had a green Soldier in our unit. He never had a girlfriend.

We promised him when we got back home we would get him a girlfriend.

We even ran an ad on Craig's List. We looked at the pictures of hundreds of girls before we found a good one for him."

Mary was bored with his unacceptable answer. She immediately changed the subject.

"He is really, really, really selfish!

In Iraq they traded him for a twin and sent home the bastard. I got the bastard." Mary was not attempting to be humorous.

Mary continued. "When he was in Iraq, he called home. Every phone call got shorter."

Tom, no longer defensive, confessed. "These are the ugly truths about me, Dr. Brown."

Mary, unimpressed with Tom's acquiescence, continued.

"He does nothing in the house.

He takes off his dirty shorts and leaves them on the floor.

He never takes out the trash.

I do everything.

And he expects me to be intimate in bed.

No!
I have gone without so long it makes no difference to me.
Maybe it's different for men.
For women, we have to get our mind wrapped around him.
In the past 4 months, maybe we have been intimate once.
Of the 7.5 years we have been married, he has been home for a total of three years."

Sadly, Tom returned once or twice for therapy, never with his wife. Then he stopped coming for treatment of PTSD. Phone calls were not answered.

"I Did a Lot of Crying over the Holidays"

Another Soldier, physically muscular, in his mid-forties, comported himself as a man's man. Physical strength exuded from his presence. Sadly, sitting in front of me, today he was not feeling like a man.

The details of his combat are too gory to forget. Many innocent lives were taken in an instant on 21 DEC 2004. The number of dead and grievously wounded ranks the trauma as one of the worst days for our Soldiers in Iraq.

"It just makes me feel so helpless to think about it.
I can't stop thinking about it this time of the year.
Why am I here?
I haven't bought a Christmas present for the past 8 years.
Janice says I don't smile any more.
My mother said, 'I can see rage in your eyes.'
I get in that zone. I don't know what I am thinking about.
I have used Testosterone cream for three years. Now that I am off of it, I feel weak.
I have completely lost interest in sex.
It's like sex doesn't matter any more.
I haven't had sex in months.
I could feel it coming on because sex started to feel like a chore.
I just do it for her. There is nothing in it for me."

"I Believe in Love"

Another Soldier in his mid-thirties appears much more youthful. He loves his wife, but the expression of his love for her has been altered by combat trauma.

One day, he witnessed the senseless deaths of many children, the intended target of insurgents. I am told that Afghan nationals, too friendly with American Soldiers, are "taught a lesson through brutality."

"We were celebrating the opening of a well. It was a cooperative project between our engineers and theirs. It fixed their water system. Everyone was in a good mood.

We were pleased.

American Soldiers gave out candy for the kids.

We had clothes for the kids.

All children are special. The Afghan kids are beautiful…their eyes are so blue…

We were excited and thrilled. Something good was happening.

It ended in an instant. I have never seen anything like the explosion.

Body parts came down from the sky on us…scraps of bones were stuck in a tree.

We cried."

The Soldier was reporting horrific, inconceivable agony, entirely without feeling.

"All my emotions are gone now.

I became hardened. I am numb. I feel nothing…nothing except sadness and anger.

I called my mom and I was without emotion…cold…without emotion.

It was so hot…the explosion. I smelled the blood.

It was 3 VBIEDs (Vehicle-Borne Improvised Explosive Devices)…car bombs. Smoke went up 20 feet in the air. All those children were killed.

I go from numb to the return of my feelings all of a sudden. Then I go numb again.

My body feels like it is moving 100 miles per hour. I guess it's nerves.

I was in the hospital for depression and PTSD.

Sex is the last thing on my mind.

My wife wants to have a baby.

It is not easy for me. I want to please her, but my heart is not in it.

It's a job for me, a job I don't like, but a job I feel I must do." He ended the session wanting silence from me.

"Emotionless Sex"

Gene is a good Soldier, a caring husband, and a proud father. At age 40, Gene will soon retire at the rank of SFC with 20 successful years in the US Army.

Gene, a quiet, modest, Puerto Rican Soldier, is recovering from severe combat trauma of the most unimaginable type.

"The things we went through in combat were absolutely brutal.

In combat, I slept with the sling of my rifle wrapped around my arm, with the rifle beside my leg. You never knew who might come in the night and try to take your weapon.

In the beginning of the war we ran out of food. We ran out of water. Everyone thought the war would be over soon.

We bought chickens on the side of the road and boiled the meat.

We killed goats. We were hungry."

Gene is a thoughtful person, a gifted teacher, and he generously shared his "deep thoughts" on the effects of combat on the Soldier's potential capacity for intimacy upon returning home.

"Sometimes you don't feel affectionate.

Sometimes you don't want to share affection.

After combat you can't be lovey-dovey.

I don't get the urge to be intimate.

I try to be intimate, but I can't.

It stems from combat. There's no sensitivity in combat.

Every day for many months, you are told in combat to 'Man Up.'

Where do you get love, sensitivity, and warmth from in combat? You don't!

When you come home from combat, your mind and your body are so used to being numb that you feel little if any emotion. You are numb to that emotion…the emotion of intimacy.

In combat you are vigilant. You can't let yourself feel emotion.

When you leave combat on a jet, you are home in a matter of hours. The stark contrast is overwhelming.

When I got home, I felt very confused. The first morning I woke up at home, I could not find my weapon. Oh my God, I thought, I'm in trouble because I can't find my gun. I thought I was still in theatre.

You can't turn a knob and bring back your emotions.

As a man, I wanted to have sex, but I just couldn't.

It is so hard to let people in…

Our spouse expects the same guy we were when we left for combat.

We are changed people. We are changed human beings. There were so many losses…so many things happened to us.

We are not the same body. We are not the same emotional state.

The woman is not the same, either. She has to feel loved.

It has gotten better for me.

Even on Levitra (medication for erectile dysfunction), it was a job for me to try to please her.

It was a job more than love.

Levitra was a way of doing it. It was done without emotion. It was done without intimacy.

Now it is emotional sex, passionate sex.

For the first 3 years, it was emotionless sex.

It started getting better when I started getting desensitized to combat.

When I knew I was being taken care of, it started building my confidence; the doctors are taking care of me.

When combat became secondary...not primary...in my mind, then my family became primary.

Laughter helped.

I started to accomplish things. It built my confidence. My emotions returned. I was able to love...

It took three years before I got that tingling sensation inside, the tingling of lovingness.

At first, she thought I was cheating.

You have to go through her battles...the blaming of cheating for my lack of interest.

You have to go through her psychological mind set.

We went to a couple of marriage counseling sessions at Fort Hood. The woman counselor blamed me, too. She was young, she had never been married, and she did not know anything about PTSD.

My wife and I took a course in "Love Languages" at our church. It was good.

Women are emotionally attached to us.

When a husband shows less interest in his wife, the public says another woman is involved. That was not true in my case.

It is very troubling for the Soldier's wife when he loses interest in her. When it happens to her friends, the husband has been unfaithful.

I have to fight her emotional stress.

Her love language is affirmation. She has to hear it from me. My wife has to be told that she looks good...that her cooking is good.

Therefore, you have to learn your wife's love language.

My love language is different. I like it when my wife cooks for me. She makes my dinner with love.

You have to make love to the mind. It brings in passion. Please the emotional state and the physical state will come in.

Please the mind first." The session ended on a positive note. The patient and doctor felt better.

The Healing Truth

LTC William Anderson was a college football star before he enlisted in the Army. A rugged linebacker and defensive end, he was known as the "Brick Wall." If he did not stop the opponent's runners in their tracks at the line of scrimmage, he nailed them to the turf before their legs left their stance.

Bigger than his brawn was his brain. He was intelligent and handsome at six feet 2 inches and 185 pounds. His body fat was immeasurable. The cleft in his chin disappeared and his light brown eyes twinkled when he smiled.

Despite his popularity, Bill Anderson was a quiet, reflective man. He had a kind face with an intriguing expression that I found difficult to describe. He appeared apologetic while his angular jaws, unsmiling lips, and staring eyes painfully communicated "it is not my fault."

Bill was the elder of the two sons of a Vietnam War veteran. His father was affable, fond of women, and found relief from his terrible but undiagnosed and untreated PTSD with alcohol abuse.

Unannounced, Bill's mother, a school teacher, took their two very young sons from their home in Alabama to reside with her in New England. Bill was six years old.

Bill had no contact with his father until he returned to live with him as an adolescent, too difficult for his mother to manage alone.

Until his father's recent death from alcoholism, Bill spent his life drawn by love between his parents, traveling from one to the other.

In the Army, Bill ranked among its best Soldiers. An airborne paratrooper, he served in Special Operations with numerous combat deployments, most of which remain unspeakable because they are still classified.

My own Top Secret Clearance has expired. Bill could not share with me most of his self-shattering combat traumas.

The healing truth, in his case, must remain undisclosed, a potential obstacle to regaining his mental health. The narrative that follows, however, is unclassified and brought relief to Bill after he recounted and revisited the trauma in a recurring dream.

"The Enemy gets a Vote"

"I have been having these intrusive thoughts.

It's hard to identify the thoughts because it is a mixture of thoughts that run together.

I have been having a dream in which I feel helpless.

It is a strange kind of dream because I know what is going to happen. I can't do anything about it.

In the end, people die.

I have had the dream almost every night for the past 2 weeks.

In the dream, I can think. I am conscious of being in a dream.

It is a crazy feeling to wake up from the dream: I'm aware; I'm very emotional; I can't describe it but I still feel connected to the dream.

I have a feeling of profound hopelessness…of having the dream, of not being able to stop it, of being aware of what will happen; of feeling I can't stop what will happen in the dream. The dream has to play itself out.

It is around midnight when I wake up from the dream.

I get up and see what's on TV.

I go back to bed around 0330."

Bill described his recurring dream. It is an exact reenactment of a traumatic combat experience.

"I am in a convoy.

The vehicle in front of me hit an IED. It was catastrophic. Everyone in it was lost.

I watch it.

I know what will happen. Here it is coming. I know it will happen. I want to say "Stop" but I don't.

I feel the impact.

I feel the guilt.
We are driving armored SUVs.
The truck is totally destroyed.
Everybody is burning.
Everybody is instantly killed.
The truck is burned to the ground.
One American Soldier and three Iraqis were in the vehicle.
The American in the truck was one of my Soldiers.
I didn't know him that well, but he was a good Soldier.
I didn't know him on a personal level, but he was a good guy.
We drove right around them.
I had an Iraqi Brigadier General in my truck. He was the target.
I was his advisor. I was a Captain at the time.
I was with a MITT Team. A MITT Team is a Military Transition Team, responsible for training and advising the Iraqi Army."

Bill appeared relieved. He had shared the dream. It was the means through which he could also share the combat trauma.

Half-smiling, half-puzzled, Bill said, "I'll tell you what's weird about this. At the time this happened, 2004, I did not feel traumatized by it. I felt I was in control.

I saved a Brigadier General's life.

I delivered him to his destination without delay.

The convoy was hit. There was an explosion, but I got the general where he needed to be. That was all that was required of me. That part of it went flawlessly.

I know what is going to happen, but I don't have the ability to save another life.

The enemy gets its vote. Rationally, I know I can't prevent the enemy from doing his action.

At the same time, I wish I had known how to prevent it from happening."

Bill dropped his head in sadness.

"Another kid will not have a life.

To grieve for all that I saw die would be overwhelming. A multitude of people I knew were killed or seriously injured. I don't even know how many. At first I kept up with the number. Then I didn't want to know the number of losses any more.

You feel sad for the ones you know…especially if they have kids…like my kids. It's got to be extremely sad for them.

I do my best to avoid personal recollections.

Recently, they required me to take a Casualty Assistance Course. It was too much. I walked out.

I found it hard to take the Iraqis seriously. We were propping them up. No matter what we taught them about democracy, it made no real difference. They always had one question, 'Who is in charge?'"

Bill is now 43. Soon he will complete 20 years of honorable service in the US Army and retire. He and his wife love their children and want what is in the best interests of their children when his wife divorces him.

"My wife definitely thinks we should divorce.

She doesn't trust me.

I have never committed adultery.

She thinks the contact I have with other women will never stop.

She feels betrayed by my contact with other women.

I needed Viagra. It is like a cast for a broken leg.

My wife is a black or white thinker.

My wife says she should have left me a long time ago. She believes she has given me too many chances.

Maybe divorce is for the best…but I don't like it.

I feel bad for my children.

I feel guilt.

They won't have a family together."

Hope for Bill and his Wife

I am hopeful that Bill's story will not end here, not end like his own childhood, strained by separation and divorce.

Bill's "contact with other women" started in Iraq.

He did not turn to alcohol like his father, unsuccessfully self-treating his combat nightmares.

Bill's "contact with other women" did not take the form of pornography, a potentially addictive distraction that other distraught Soldiers temporarily find diverting from combat stress.

Bill's "contact with other women" did not include finding other women in combat with whom to consort.

Bill's "contact with other women" arose from his own childhood struggles of which he is mostly unaware.

Never feeling secure, never feeling understood or accepted by his mother, he was sent back to his father at a time in his life when he longed for recognition and approval.

Bill must have wondered why his mother kept his brother safely by her side, but sent him back to live with his father.

"How could she send me back to the man for whom she had lost respect, even despised? How could she send me back to a man broken by the Vietnam War?"

As an unruly teenager, Bill loved his father, but he fought against the natural inclination to identify with him, an alcoholic "ladies man." Bill did not completely win his battle to be unlike his father.

"Everywhere I went, people knew my dad. He was known by all the bartenders.

Even in the small, nearby towns, people knew my dad as the Vietnam War veteran whose weakness was women and alcohol.

My dad was married 5 times."

Bill's "contact with other women" emerged creatively from the depths of his unconsciousness in a time of great stress, the bloodiest time of the War in Iraq.

Bill could not have survived the act of infidelity.

Bill needed something more enduring than meaningless sexual encounters.

Bill needed to know if he were loveable.

How could Bill answer the most important unanswered question from his childhood?

Cyber science provided what Bill thought was the safest way to answer his question.

No one will be hurt this way, he reasoned. However, he failed to appreciate its meaning to his wife were she to discover it.

Bill went on line in Iraq. He initiated a relationship with a woman unknown to him. Casual, insignificant conversations slowly grew over time into intimate discussions. Eventually, a meeting, never intended to be kept by Bill, was planned.

Bill never met a woman he contacted on line.

Once the cyber date was set, Bill quickly broke off the "contact" with the other woman by abruptly ignoring all contacts from her, only to start up a new on-line "relationship."

In its most simplistic form, it was a "She loves me, She loves me not" experiment.

At its deepest, saddest, and most painful level, it was a symptom of a disturbed, unfulfilled step in maturity.

It took on a "doing and undoing" quality described in psychiatry as a "repetition compulsion."

Totally unaware of the cause of his behavior, Bill repeatedly tried to gain mastery over the trauma of his disrupted childhood by ingeniously creating situations that were remarkably similar to his childhood.

Sadly, one never gains mastery over a conflict of which one is fundamentally unconscious.

The inevitable occurred. His cyber relationships were uncovered but not understood by his wife.

She felt betrayed.

He felt confused.

Resisting the temptation to blame and thereby rationalize one's responsibility for one's behavior, I respectfully offered an explanation that may restore hope to Bill and his wife.

Bill's wife's acceptance of his intolerant, unacceptable behavior has understandably reached its limits.

Up to the time of this entry, Bill has declined my frequent appeals to have his wife join us in his treatment sessions for PTSD. I wonder if his shame is over-riding his judgment.

The reader may ask, 'What role, if any, does Bill's combat trauma play in his repetition compulsion that may well cost him his marriage?"

Bill's problems did not begin in combat, but the repetition compulsion began in the pitch of the Iraqi war.

It began while he was separated from his wife.

It began while he was separated from his children, from all those who loved him.

The stress of overwhelming grief, the loss of more friends than he is willing to count, the abandonment of all emotion required of a military leader in combat, in combination or alone, created the openings in his emotional armor through which his problems sought daylight.

I continue to appeal to Bill to let understanding have its opportunity in his life.

I appeal to him as an athlete to keep trying.

I appeal to him as an officer in the best Army in the history of the world to never surrender.

I appeal to him as a loving father to continue to be loving.

I appeal to him as a husband to continue to be faithful to his wife.

I appeal to Bill's wife to read this chapter, a recommendation made by my own loving wife.

I remind Bill's wife, whom I wish to get to know, that marriages are like multiple choice exams. The first choice is usually the best choice. Don't change your answers.

9

Mondays and Tuesdays

"It must be Monday"

In the pre-adolescence and early adolescent years of my life, every Monday, until my mother was "saved," she went downtown. Except for a rare emergency, none of which come to mind, she never went downtown on any other day of the week. When it was possible, I accompanied my mother downtown on Mondays. I don't recall that we said much to each other on those missions.

We took the street car from its designated stop at 46th Street at its intersection with Hampton Boulevard. The twenty-five minute ride ended at our destination, City Hall Avenue, at the Penny Arcade.

She had a ham sandwich on white toast with lettuce, tomato and mayonnaise and a "fountain" Coca Cola at George's family run restaurant on Monticello Avenue. It was located near its intersection with City Hall Avenue in Norfolk, Virginia. Ham was not my favorite, but without complaining, I ate mine.

After lunch, with some "window shopping," she went to the NORVA or LOEWS Theater. Both are located on Granby Street, previously known as "downtown" Norfolk, but on opposite sides of the street.

She had her favorite actors, but I believe she more often went to the LOEWS no matter what movie was playing.

One of my most distinct memories of these expeditions was air conditioning.

Signs in front of theaters graphically advertised just how frigid one might feel inside, no matter how blasted one felt from Norfolk's incomparable humid, torturing summer heat. I was a college graduate before I experienced air conditioning, except in a movie theater, in any house in which I lived.

"I was prone to car sickness"

I was prone to motion sickness, often worsened by the unpleasant exhaust fumes from a bus, the alternative mode of transportation should the street cars not run.

I was less likely to throw-up on a street car than a bus. It was called "car sickness" when I was a child. My car sickness angered my parents, who failed to understand that the brain's complexity, not the child's willfulness, produced the undesirable symptoms.

In some, at most small, way, the child admits that he was rightfully found at fault. This was a proud child.

I recall that my mother was hospitalized at the Norfolk General Hospital. At 5 or 6 years of age, I had no understanding of the reason she was ill and needed hospitalization.

One evening, my dad took me on a bus from our home on 47th Street to visit my mother in the Norfolk General Hospital. The short trip took not more than 20 minutes of exposure to the unpleasant exhaust fumes.

I was wearing a navy blue Pea Coat, thick and heavy, buttoned up to my neck, to keep out the cold.

We were seated on the right side of the bus, near the front. Exhaust bus fumes stimulate nausea and vomiting for me faster than a merry-go-round, a near second best sickness-trigger.

Overcome by waves of nausea, looking proudly ahead, saying nothing to my dad seated next to me on the bus, I emitted the recognizable gagging sounds of one thus afflicted, then threw up all down the front of my navy blue coat.

"Why didn't you bend down your head and throw up on the floor?" my disgusted dad asked.

"Why did you mess up your clothes?" He did not say it but I felt the rest of his sentence to conclude with "You stupid child!"

It was one of the very few occasions that my father was annoyed with me.

I always associate the strong odor of ether with the Norfolk General Hospital. It was the most popular anesthesia in the 1930s.

My dad took me to a nurse when we reached the Norfolk General Hospital. It may have been called the Protestant Hospital in the mid-1930s. He did not want to alarm my mother with the evidence of my car sickness.

A kind nurse did her best to scrub the vomitus from my coat. Its odor, however, was stronger than ether. Soon my mother was more concerned about me than about her own illness, whatever it was.

"The Yearling"

I remember seeing "They Died with their Boots On," at LOEWS Theater, with my mother on one of her inerrant Monday's downtown.

Several years later I would wear the blue and gold usher uniform at the LOEWS Theater.

In my fine-looking usher's uniform, I saw my favorite movie, "The Yearling," so many times I memorized most of its lines. Unaccountably, some of those lines are remembered even today 66 years later.

The tenderness between Gregory Peck, the father, and his young son, touched me.

When his son returned home after running away, grieved over the loss of his fawn to whom he was devoted, his father, lying in bed physically injured, welcomed him home with the love we all seek.

"It must be Tuesday"

Tuesdays were wash days.

Sweat poured down my mother's brow as she mastered the dangerous wringer washing machine.

"Don't put your hands near the wringer, Bobby," was my mother's command to me.

Our kitchen on 39th street was where we lived and ate our meals. On Tuesdays our kitchen was transformed into a (I search for the words) "laundry." Water leaked from the washing machine.

The old, round, wheel-mounted Maytag washing machine's black drain hose was attached loosely to the kitchen sink. Two or three large galvanized metal tubs were staggered around the Maytag.

The sequence from one tub of water to the next was important, but I do not exactly recall the sequence now.

I remember "bluing" was performed in one of the tubs.

Another tub was for soaking.

The last tub held the laundry from the wringer before it was carried to the back yard clothes line. There they were dried by God's fresh air and bright sunshine.

We were in a terrible dilemma, should it rain on Tuesdays. The washing ritual was conducted as usual, rain or shine, but the drying became an indoor proposition.

Clothes-lines were strung sturdily throughout the house and unhung items were placed over wooden chairs to dry.

We stood in several inches of water that hatefully leaked from the washing machine and tubs. The water completely covered the red flower-designed linoleum. It was an awful experience. I dreaded Tuesdays. It is even unpleasant to recall, worse when I contrast it with today's washer and dryer.

Later that day and every Tuesday, we mopped up the water. We got down on our hands and knees and scrubbed the floor.

Also on my hands and knees, I waxed the floor with Johnson's Floor Wax until I could see the reflection of my face in the linoleum. If I failed the reflection test, it was done all over again.

Tuesdays were as distasteful as Mondays were pleasurable.

In a curious way, I recall Mondays with my mother at the movies much more often than I recall Tuesdays with my mother and her Maytag and our water-soaked kitchen floor.

Truthfully, I had completely forgotten Tuesdays until I recently watched an old episode of "Matt Dillon" in which Chester scrubbed the federal marshal's office wood-plank floor.

"The Silent Treatment"

I can't say Mondays at the movies with my mother were carefree or happy occasions. If my mother spoke to me on these Monday missions downtown, it was only as necessary.

Mysteriously, my mother was prone to be solemn, if not taciturn.

Until much later in my childhood, there were few exceptions to my mother's characteristic way of communicating with me.

I look back now trying to understand my dear mother's preference for action over words.

There were many things on my mother's mind to worry her in those days that I record.

Like our neighbors, we felt the gnawing effects of the Great Depression.

My brother left home for the US Navy under less than desirable circumstances.

My mother's widowed father, whom she loved very much, was confined to the City of Norfolk TB Sanatorium on Water Works Road, Norfolk. He lived in a white frame "cottage" shared by 4 men also afflicted with TB. I remember his building and several of identical size, color, and shape as clean facilities occupied by old, never smiling men. We often visited my grandfather on Sunday afternoons. I waited with my dad in the car while my mother went inside to visit her father.

Her youngest brother's wife was admitted to a state mental hospital.

Her youngest sister was abused by an alcoholic husband.

Two of her daughters were physically and emotionally abused by their husbands. Both these daughters lived within her view.

Words of a country song come to mind: "It takes a worried man to sing a worried song. I'm worried now but I won't be worried long."

My mother was not worried long. She was never worried into inaction. I never recall her worrying aloud.

No upper lip in all of the British Isles was stiffer than my mother's.

It was to my mother that her extended family and her needy neighbors came for help.

She turned no one away empty handed or emptied of hope.

My mother was never glib.

She always meant what she said.

She always expected that what she said would be taken seriously.

Creeping melancholy is finding its way into my awareness now, a thought and its feeling I have not known consciously for decades. It is sad and emotionally raw.

It was known in the British Public Schools as being "Sent to Coventry."

It is a harsh form of discipline in which a student is shunned. No one is permitted to speak to the student being punished.

This is a unique form of verbal solitary confinement.

I can tell you from personal experience, with my mother, it is more disturbing than being locked in a dark closet, even one said to be visited by ghosts. It is worse than being beaten with a belt.

"When you are training a dog," said my good friend John Sanderson, "you turn your back to him when he needs discipline. It is what the herd did naturally to rid itself of unacceptable behavior."

Thank God I was not often sent to Coventry or shunned by my mother's back, but I recall its devastating effect.

My pleading for her to speak to me perceptibly angered my mother, further prolonging the chastisement with which I was being shrouded.

Strangely, I cannot recall a single guilty incident with which I provoked my mother to inflict her punishing silence upon me.

The "silent treatment," as she called it, however, caused perplexing self-doubt, even psychological disorientation. The return of its memory today is a recollection of sorrow and anguish.

"Please Deliver Me from My Tormentors"

These recollections lead me now to a slowly emerging insight.

There was something in me as a child that drew taunting and jeering from other children and perhaps even from my own mother.

I scared easily. When I was frightened, I expressed my emotions intensely. Helplessly and involuntarily, my degree of emotional despair and anguish were unmistakable.

I begged like a Charles Dickens' urchin in an English foundling home, not begging for "some more, Sir," but for mercy and deliverance from my tormentors.

I went through a stone throwing stage.

Senselessly, not out of anger, I threw stones at everything.

When all one has is a stone, everything looks like a good target.

Usually missing my target, I threw stones at passing cars, at stray cats, and even at houses.

An elderly Dutch couple lived in a darkly stained cedar shake shingled house adjacent to the field in which I participated in WW I maneuvers behind my house. Their window shades were always closed.

One of my stones was thrown perfectly, as if it were a hand grenade, crashing through the window of the elderly Dutch couple's house.

It was both the best grenade I had ever thrown on an enemy building and the worst unlawful act of destruction of private property with the intention of inflicting bodily harm with a stone missile.

Dressed in my WW I Soldier suit I was capable of performing infrequent but important heroic acts for my country while still only 7 years of age.

Regrettably, I was an immature warrior, a poor logistician, incapable of imagining the enemy's response to my attack.

My basic and advanced individual military training had not adequately prepared me for emotional hardening.

I did the unforgiveable.

I cried in front of my troops.

In fact, I cried all the way home.

When I reached Headquarters, I was greeted coldly by my commanding officer who was also my mother.

"Bobby," she sternly reminded me, "I told you to stop throwing stones. Now the police are on the way for you."

Picture a fully uniformed American Soldier, crying copious tears, all but on his knees, piteously imploring his mother to keep him out of jail.

The words of an old country music song come to mind. "I'm not in your town to stay, said a mother old and gray. I'm just here to get my baby out of jail." Yes, warden, but in this case it seemed that the mother was sending her son to jail, not requesting his release from jail.

His superior officer gave one command: "Stand in the corner until the police arrive for you."

The youthful Soldier, shaking with fear, obeyed the command, but continued to cry.

A subtle signal was communicated to my father. He left the house.

There was loud banging at the front door.

"The Police are here, Bobby," said my mother.

"I hope you have learned your lesson.

The police will know what to do with you.

Go to the front door.

Goodbye."

She could not have been more grim.

Samson's grip could not have been stronger than the 7-year-old WW I Soldier clinging to his mother.

"No, Mother," the Soldier cried. "Please don't let the police take me away…please…please. I will never throw another stone."

It was almost dark outside.

It was late winter.

It was unknown to me, but my father was a part of the team to teach me at last to cease and desist from stone-throwing.

My father banged loudly once again on the front door.

He then came through the house laughing.

He had colluded with my commanding officer.

The police had not been called.

I never heard from the elderly Dutch couple.

I never threw another stone.

"Yellow Jaundice"

The fear of impending incarceration, for the wanton destruction of property, even in the line of military duty, as described above, gripped me another time in the early years of my childhood.

My fear in this second instance tested the sanity of a 5-year-old. I marvel now at the lifespan of intense fear. Is it ever really forgotten?

Unlike my usually active, very active self, I lost my energy. I remember falling sleep on the front porch in the morning, preferring sleep to all other possibilities, including playing with my favorite toys.

"Bobby, how well did you sleep last night," my mother inquired. "You seem tired all the time, Bobby. Are you sick?"

I did not feel "sick." I felt tired.

"Go pee in a bottle and let me look at it," my mother ordered in the same way a physician orders a urinalysis.

Our bathroom at 47th Street was an addition to the original 2-story frame house.

To enter our bathroom, one stepped down one steep step into a cold, poorly lit bathroom, devoid of windows. It was also devoid of, and uncluttered by, the customary facilities one expects to find in a residential bathroom.

On the dirt floor, covered by a thin linoleum rug, stood a commode with an oak flush box connected by water pipes running down from a white porcelain reservoir near the ceiling.

A wide, white porcelain sink to the left of the commode completed the furnishings except for several glass milk bottles and a small stash of little bottles of patented medications.

Knowing where to find the appropriate receptacle, I returned to my mother with the specimen in hand.

"Just as I thought, young man; you have Yellow Jaundice. I'm calling Dr. West."

"Yellow jaundice" sounded ominous. I knew only that it must be a condition to be feared.

Dr. West was called only when a diagnosis required treatment surpassing my mother's armamentarium.

The "calling" of Dr. West was no small feat itself. The nearest telephone was at Tayloe's Garage on Hampton Boulevard. Neither my mother nor my father had ever spoken on a phone.

"Frances," my mother ordered, "go to Mr. Tayloe and tell him we need Dr. West for an emergency. He will look up the number and make the call for you.

"You tell Dr. West that Bobby has Yellow Jaundice. I want him here today.

"Randolph, put Bobby to bed. Then wash your hands and come back downstairs to me."

My mother called the family together. Everyone but me attended the family meeting.

I have no first-hand knowledge of what transpired at the family meeting. Six members of my family lived together in the small dwelling at that time at 1231 West 47th Street.

The house had two fates. First, it survives as a sturdy structure in my memory. Secondly, it was bull-dozed years ago, a victim of the enlarging embellishments of Old Dominion University.

Dr. West of the City of Norfolk Public Health Department walked up the steps of our small front porch.

Dr. West knocked at the door within an hour of my mother's urgent message. He was accompanied by Ms. Anderson, a Public Health Nurse.

Dr. West, dressed in a navy blue suit with a navy blue vest, was a tall, quiet man with a fair complexion. His receding hair line, rimless spectacles, soft grey eyes, and pointed nose permitted the impression of an older middle-aged man given to seriousness. His hair was soft and white.

He shook his head after pulling down and peering into my lower eye lids and pushing firmly on my abdomen.

My mother stood with sturdy anticipation at the foot of my bed. "What is it, Dr. West," she asked.

"It's not good, Mrs. Brown. You did the right thing to call me.

"Bobby has infectious hepatitis. He will have to be hospitalized today."

Hospitals scared me. Doctors scared me. "Infectious hepatitis" was unknown to me, but it really frightened me. Quietly, unobserved, I started to cry.

I did not feel well before Dr. West arrived. Now I felt decidedly worse and worried.

"What hospital are we talking about, Dr. West," my mother asked with deep concern in her voice.

"It will have to be the City Hospital on Water Works Road," said Dr. West without equivocation.

My mother came to the side of my bed. She took my hand and said, "Bobby, I thought you had Yellow Jaundice, but Dr. West thinks it is something else. He thinks it is something people can catch from you."

Dr. West said, "Mrs. Brown, you call it Yellow Jaundice. A lot of people say that because the patient looks yellowish. 'Jaundice' also means yellow.

Doctors call it Hepatitis. It's the same disease. Bobby has the type of Hepatitis that is infectious.

Anybody with close contact with Bobby can catch it. I don't like to say it in front of the boy, but it can be (whispering) serious."

Dr. West and my mother went down stairs to talk. Ms. Anderson, the Public Health Nurse remained with me.

"You will like it at the hospital, Bobby. We will take good care of you there until you are well again."

Ms. Anderson could have been an angel, gently reassuring me.

What happened next is vividly recalled, but my written portrayal may fail to impart my marked degree of emotional tumult.

It was my first entry into an abyss from which I feared I could not be retrieved.

My bed stood in a small alcove connected to the room in which my brother Randolph slept. He would have been 15 at the time "Yellow Jaundice" raised its ugly head in my life.

My uncontrollable crying started in the alcove immediately upon hearing my mother through the thin walls of the house, addressing my father, "George, get the car started. Bobby is going to the hospital."

I can't imagine what frightened me most about the Norfolk City Hospital. The thought of being separated from my mother, however, was intolerable.

I cried until I could barely breathe. My body shook with sorrow. I see myself on the floor, now downstairs, clutching my mother's legs. I earnestly begged my mother not to send me away. I prayed for mercy.

Dr. West was impatient, uninfluenced by my "performance," as he called it.

"It is a matter of law, Mrs. Brown. My hands are tied.

You placed an urgent call to me to see a sick child. He is a very sick child. He can pass his sickness onto others."

If I could not be consoled before Dr. West spoke, then I was now beyond the point of inconsolability.

"Get up off the floor, Bobby. You are going nowhere," my mother declared.

Dr. West was no push-over.

He said sharply, "I can get a court order, if it takes it!

You cannot defy the law, Mrs. Brown."

Ms. Anderson, the blond-headed, blue-eyed angel posing as a nurse, not more than 22 years of age, spoke calmly, encouragingly, and softly to Dr. West.

My mother, my father, my sister Frances, my brother Randolph, and my sister Edith stared at Ms. Anderson in disbelief as she spoke.

"If you will agree to my treatment plan, Dr. West, I think we can make it work for Bobby and his family."

"And what 'treatment plan' might that be, Ms. Anderson?" Dr. West nearly shouted.

"We can quarantine the Brown family. I will bring the signs to nail to the front and back doors. I will visit Bobby every day for the 21 days of quarantine.

I will give you a daily report of Bobby's condition, Dr. West.

If you are willing, you can visit Bobby weekly until he is well.

Of course, Bobby's parents and his family will have to agree to be confined to this house, as small as it is for 6 people, for 21 days."

My mother spoke first. "Thank you," were her only words. Tears fell silently down her freckled face.

Dad said nothing, but nodded his head.

My siblings were not leaping for joy. They also nodded their heads.

Dr. West spoke. "I see I am outnumbered, Ms. Anderson."

Soon the large yellow signs were nailed up on the old house.

The yellow signs cautioned everyone in our neighborhood to refrain from entering 1231 West 47th Street for the next 21 days.

My pleas bypassed my mother's clinical judgment. They went directly to her heart of love.

The quarantine ended 3 weeks later.

No one else in my family became ill.

My family never discussed my "Yellow Jaundice" again.

My inspired energy gradually returned; it never subsided.

I will always remember the angel dressed in the navy blue Public Health Uniform.

Dr. West's fine disposition returned with each house call, gaining my lasting respect.

The decision maker, my mother, gave never ending power to the meaning of love.

"I learned to be humble"

The distance between being scared and being humble is a short one for me.

When I am not obnoxiously conceited, one of my most distasteful states, perhaps another trait attracting dethroners, I am attractively humble, if not needy or emotionally disadvantaged.

I don't want to be like Charles Dickens' Uriah Heep who took great pride in his humility, often reminding others of his great moral virtue.

I learned to be humble by growing up in an internal community of fear.

Humility rooted in fear is genuine. We are told in the Bible to "fear God." I understand this means to have reverence for God.

"The first and greatest commandment is to Love God with all your heart, all your soul, and all your mind; and to love your neighbor as yourself."

Fear, love, humility, and reverence are complexly related, a most fascinating topic that we best leave to our learned theologians and philosophers.

"Sublimation," on the other hand, a term meaningful to psychologists, suggests that we do a good thing when we knowingly, willingly, and consistently try to convert our negative personality features into socially acceptable behaviors.

How much of this process is fully conscious?

How does one become less irrationally fearful?

What role in this important, ongoing process is played by the circumstances in which one finds him or herself?

How important are the people we respect in overcoming a lifestyle unduly influenced by fear?

How does a fearful person find courage to leave his or her comfort zone?

Several memories help me understand, retrospectively, how I found, modified, and continue to find acceptable answers to the important questions raised above.

First, honestly writing about one's life, starting early and continuing late in one's life, consciously avoiding flattery and excessive demeaning, can be unusually beneficial in discovering the people and events that sharpened one's concepts and one's sense of self, sense of others, and sense of the world.

"I was told I could run fast"

In the spring of 1942, the early phase of our nation's WW II, I was in Ms. Bailey's fifth grade at James Madison Grammar School.

Looking at old photographs taken of me at age 10, I had a full head of brown curly hair, brown eyes, and a thin profile.

In a long sleeve white dress shirt and tan shorts, I lined up with the other boys in my class to run the 50 yard dash.

Ms. Bailey kept a record of the event on a large sheet of white paper, thicker than writing paper. We were given the impression that it was an important event.

Without much effort, I easily won the race.

I was told that I could run fast. It came as a surprise to me, not knowing its advantages.

I believe the extent of my running had been limited to "Keep Away," a game boys played on the school playground at recess.

The object of "Keep Away" was to run with a soccer ball, broken-field style as in football, darting in and out of a mob of ball-thirsty opponents resorting to hook or crook to steal the ball from the runner.

"Keep Away" was unsurpassed for ruining clothes, scraping knees and elbows, bloodying noses, and was at its best alienating class mates from one another.

Teachers and parents alike hated "Keep Away." We loved it.

After learning I could run fast, I ran faster and more care-free while playing "Keep Away."

I became the 10 year old boy who could run fast. I also remained the threat-sensitive, shy 10-year-old boy.

In the 7th grade I could run faster than anyone at James Madison School, but I declined the school principal's invitation to join the school's basketball team.

Winkie Marable

In legal terms, I was an "attractive nuisance." A more perfect target to "pick on" or "bully" by other boys could not be found.

Winkie Marable, one year my senior, often invited me to fist-fight him. To his credit, he was not one to give up a project easily or leave it uncompleted.

"Knock this rock off my shoulder" or "Give me a push with your hand" were among Winkie's favorite invocations to initiate the encounter.

Winkie always found me after school on 38th Street between Bowden's Ferry Road and Blue Stone Avenue. He also always found me meekly declining his summonses to fight.

If I spoke to Winkie at all, it was a barely audible plea to be left alone. I did not want to fight.

Had Winkie been my pupil, I would have failed him in "deportment."

He generally looked unkempt, "a mean and hungry look," perhaps intending to emphasize his meanness. His light brown hair was full in the front, often falling down, covering his brown eyes.

His chiseled jaws matched his determined style of approaching life. This facial feature contributed immensely to my fear of him. I sensed he lacked empathy.

Thus I was tormented every afternoon on my way home from school for the entire 6th grade. It was a well-kept secret, guarded by shame.

Imagine my relief when Winkie was promoted to the 8th grade. He went to Blair Junior High School, several miles away, and I remained in safety at James Madison School.

Imagine my shock and grave disappointment when Winkie continued to keep his uninvited appointments with me each afternoon, even after he attended Blair Junior High School, as I walked home from the 7th grade.

Incredulously, I never knew why Winkie favored me as his most worthy fist-fighting opponent. I never knew Winkie in any other context or anything about his past or future plans. Frankly, I never knew how surprised I would be by what finally transpired.

Spring had arrived in Norfolk in 1944. With spring came a change in a 12 year old boy who had been told he could run fast.

Winkie walked up behind me on 38th Street. Putting his hand on my right shoulder, he pulled me around to face him.

Up to this moment in our lengthy affiliation, Winkie had never touched me. He had demeaned and belittled me, but Winkie had never touched me.

I dropped my school books to the ground.

In a flash, I pounded Winkie's surprised face with a force previously unknown to me.

Over and over, I struck Winkie unmercifully.

Blood trickled from his nose.

If he swung back at me, Winkie never landed a blow.

Covering his face with both hands, Winkie fell to the ground, crying loudly.

Something came out of me that sunny spring afternoon on 38th Street that I have come to identify as a turning point in my life.

I still don't like to fight.

Now I know there is within me the capacity to fight, but I still call upon it as a last resort.

The capacity to fight, refined by time and good coaching, made football my favorite sport.

I beat up Winkie. I whipped my fear into a smaller place in my life.

I never saw Winkie Marable again.

I hope Winkie knows I bear him no ill will.

I would be enormously pleased if Winkie's life turned out meaningfully for him.

Thank you, Winkie, for being one of the teachers of influence on my life.

Winkie, you helped me learn to be humble.

The Provocative Paper Boy

In 1945, our Norfolk evening newspaper, the Ledger-Dispatch, was delivered to our front steps at 1321 West 39th Street by a teenage "paper boy" on a bicycle.

A large, dirty white canvas bag carried the large daily supply of specially folded newspapers on the front of the paper boy's bicycle, its straps sturdily wrapped around its handle bars.

With experience, a good paperboy could continue riding his bicycle while tossing his newspapers accurately on the porches or front steps of his customers, barely slowing his pace on his trusty bike.

With "mens rea" or evil intent, a spry teenager with a good arm, and strong legs for pedaling his bike, could strike targets other than steps or front porches. An otherwise boring task might be enlivened by occasional acts of treachery.

In the 1940s milk tasted like the delicious and healthy beverage it was intended by nature. Milk came in returnable glass bottles. It was not homogenized. Rich cream filled the neck of the glass bottle.

The Browns faithfully washed and returned its empty glass milk bottles for the early morning milk man to replace and replenish with the new order.

It was for the milk man that the glass milk bottles were placed on the brick front steps each evening, not for the paperboy to improve his paper pitching skills.

In several respects, it was a nearly perfect crime because there were no witnesses.

For several weeks, the paper boy's annoying act of breaking our glass milk bottles went unseen, even unsuspected.

The delinquency was committed while my mother prepared the evening meal. The kitchen was located in the back of the house, a considerable distance from the front porch.

My dad, in his 1932 Model B Ford Coupe, was usually en route home from Colonna Ship Yard where he joined a large painting crew maintaining WW II ships when the misdeeds occurred.

Several crime scene discussions regarding the broken glass milk bottles dominated the evening meals. My father suggested, "It could be the cat."

"Nonsense, George," my mother retorted, "Boozie has never broken a bottle in his life."

"What's for dessert," I inquired, showing no interest in the offense.

"We are discussing our broken glass milk bottles, Bobby," my mother firmly replied. "I want you to start cleaning up the broken glass out front. Maybe then you will take an interest in this problem."

As an after-thought, my mother gave an order commanding me to find its cause and eradicate the problem. As usual, dad submissively added, "Do what your mother says."

It was an uninteresting assignment. My heart was not in it. No matter how I felt, I was on orders.

My parents, using the income from dad's steady work at Colonna Ship Yard, in combination with sweat and persistence after an 8 hour work day, completed the renovation of 1321 West 39th Street.

Glossy navy gray paint covered the newly decorated front porch floor.

My mother could "see" the hovel they purchased for $1300 blossom into one of the most attractive homes in Lamberts Point. It was her vision of the finished product that guided every act of carpentry before my father drove the first nail.

I recall now that my mother's ability to visualize or see into the future was a special gift from which I was a beneficiary. "I can see you running out in front of the team carrying the football, Bobby. You are wearing a bright white football suit."

My mother's vision of her 16 year old son running with a football was shared with me on the first day I tried out with the Maury High School football team. Our all-white practice football uniform was a fact neither she nor I knew in advance.

The front porch was the Pent House portion of our home. Colorful green canvas awnings, purchased from Hogshire's in Norfolk, added the perfect finishing touch. A green and white glider moved listlessly with the summer breezes. A wooden rocking chair was reserved, of course, for my mother.

Henderson Beale, nick-named "Brother," was my mother's brick-laying younger brother. He built the fireplace that brought much pleasure and pride to our family. Brother also constructed brick steps for our front porch.

The front porch was the social center during the late spring and summer months in Norfolk. It is where family members gathered to relax at the end of the day and where the otherwise unemployed hung out.

The front porch was also easily engaged as an observation post, a place where all that happened on 39th Street could be observed and, if necessary, corrected or provided great resource material for gossiping.

One late June afternoon, I went to the front porch to relax. I liked to lie flat on the front porch deck. It was an ideal place to daydream.

The sound of breaking glass startled me. I sat up with a start.

The paper boy was smiling at his handiwork. Broken glass milk bottles strewn over the brick steps awaited their bare-foot victims.

The paper boy was seated on his bicycle in front of our house. His legs, straddling the bike, were planted on the ground. His undelivered load of Norfolk Ledger Dispatch newspapers bulged in his dirty white carrying bag.

He was in no hurry to complete his appointed rounds. A smirk on his face invited my attention.

"Did you break our milk bottles," I inquired.

"Does the Pope read the Bible," he replied.

It was an interesting answer because, among the very few things I knew about the paper boy, 2 years my senior and several significant inches taller, was his Catholicism.

"I believe you broke the bottles on purpose. Do not do that again," I spoke with authority.

The paper boy, in the mood for breaking noses as well as glass milk bottles, carefully placed his bicycle on its side, not wanting to spill his undelivered newspapers. He quickly approached me with tightened fists and glaring mean anger.

I sensed that verbal communication was his unchosen means of conveying his feelings at that moment in time.

The speed with which my fists found their bottom line created mixed feelings in me that I can recall precisely even after nearly seven decades.

I was surprised at how unaccomplished he was in manliness. In a word, I found, to my disappointment, that he was physically frail. He collapsed in defeat like a balloon suddenly depleted of its air.

Worst of all, I felt very sorry for this milk-bottle-breaking young person.

I helped him up. He rode away in silence.

The intentional destruction of our glass milk bottles stopped immediately.

Feeling ashamed, I never shared with my parents how my milk bottle assignment ended.

Bill Story

When General Douglas Mac Arthur wrote the following words he was superintendent of the U.S. Military Academy at West Point, 1919-1922.

"Upon the fields of friendly strife
Are sown the seeds
That upon other fields, on other days
Will bear the fruits of victory."
General Douglas MacArthur (1880-1964)

General MacArthur had his words engraved over the gymnasium's entrance where, then, as today, they remind each cadet that the lessons learned in athletic competition, never forgotten, will ultimately contribute to a sense of success and triumph.

I learned the lines from Bill Story when he was Assistant Principal of Maury High School, Norfolk, Virginia.

I also learned the truth of General MacArthur's enduring thoughts.

Bill Story used poetry and quotations to inspire generations of young athletes. Bill Story coached Barney Gill, a University of Virginia football star and West Point Assistant Football coach, who later delivered the Army game films to MacArthur.

Bill Story extended his administrative position from the principal's office to Blair Field where Maury High School practiced football.

Coach Tony Saunders was a recently retired Naval Officer who had served in WW II. He was our excellent, cigarette-smoking, Head Football Coach at Maury. He expressed no objection when Bill Story assumed unofficial football coaching duties at Maury.

Bill Story added flavor and distinction to our sport unlike anywhere else in the South.

I memorized General MacArthur's lines. They found lasting meaning in my life. I found their truth to be applicable to most endeavors of my existence.

One of my unfulfilled childhood dreams was to attend the U.S Military Academy at West Point. Doc Blanchard and Glenn Davis, football stars at West Point in the mid-1940s, were my heroes.

The next best thing to attending West Point is to share the combat trauma narratives of the remarkable people who wear the West Point graduation ring. Although they always understate the importance of their military achievements in combat, my bubbling enthusiasm for them cannot be hidden.

Bill Story's poetry and quotations found a mind already prepared for something that inspires, for good ideas, and divine influence.

First, I liked to commit things to memory and to be "tested" on it. When I developed the emotional strength to attempt to assert my will, from 8 or 9 years of age, I refused to take a written list of needed items when sent to a nearby grocery store.

My oldest sister, Christine, for example, a second mother to me, might need 5 or 6 articles. "Bobby," she would say, "Take this list to Liebowitz's. Here is the money you will need."

"Just tell me what's on the list," I begged. "I can remember it; I promise," I would reply.

Liebowitz's was safely within the area in which my mother permitted me to perambulate.

I liked memory games before I knew how to safely bring home the remembered items from the assigned mission.

Evening was falling upon me, as I raced home from one of the memorable errands for Christine. I was returning home with food and supplies needed for the supper she was preparing for Frank, her husband, whom I feared. His gruff harshness, of note, was never directed at me.

Things went well until I started crossing the field behind our home at 1231 West 47th Street. Next door stood the two-story frame house occupied by Christine and Frank.

I removed the fresh loaf of bread from the brown paper grocery bag. Walking speedily, left hand carrying the groceries, I placed the loaf of fresh smelling bread on top of my head with my right hand.

I coordinated the rapid pace with which I walked with an equally rapid backward and forward motion of the loaf of bread on the top of my head. Soon the bread, ejected from its package, formed itself beautifully into a neat configuration on the ground, repeating the pattern in which it had be packed.

Had the loaf of bread been perched on a serving plate, instead of on the ground, it would have been a culinary delight.

Racing against the increasing darkness of the night, I scooped up the bread, returned it with care to its original container, and arrived in time.

I usually had little to say all those nights I ate dinner with Christine and Frank. I sat quietly to Frank's right, always feeling scrutinized. For a very good reason, I feared Frank's scrutiny on the night recorded here.

If Frank said a word during that meal, I don't recall it. On some nights, like this one, Christine anticipated his needs, provided them, and the palpable tension was tolerable.

"I'm going to talk to the Liebowitz's," Christine announced at the end of the meal. "I believe they sold us a loaf of bread with tiny pieces of grit or gravel in it."

Little Bobby Brown, the kid who enjoyed memory contests, knew that the 5th Amendment protects citizens from being forced to incriminate themselves, or should in cases like his. That night he ate no bread. He also ate no crow.

Poetry

I started memorizing poems early in my life.

An inspiring poem, part of an old calendar, hung on the kitchen wall on the 39th Street house. It hung next to back door for years because my mother believed in the wisdom expressed in its simple rhyme.

"Sitting and wishing won't change your fate.

The Lord provides the fishing but you have to dig the bait."

I memorized poems that meant a lot to me such as George Herbert's "The Pulley," A. E. Housman's "The Cherry Tree," and a German poem about Strasburg's long history of saddening the hearts of mothers and fathers whose sons died for their country in combat.

For as long as I can remember, I write poems for family members on their birthdays.

As a student in Maury High School, I wrote a poem entitled "Eternity," a copy of which is placed at the end of this chapter. It came to me as a rhythm that beat in my head for hours, forcing me to write down the words one night before I could sleep.

My English teacher read "Eternity." She and another teacher called me out into the hallway. They wanted to know how I was feeling. Bobby was feeling fine.

"No, Bobby, we want to know how you were feeling when you wrote the poem."

It took a while to convince the concerned teachers that my zest for life was bounding. If my poem conveyed a disinterest in life, then the poet had failed.

Eternity

Today, my friend, I come to you to tell a tale that is very true,

About a Man that lives in the trees and flies around like the birds and bees.

He eats from the flowers and drinks from the sky and sleeps in branches that grow very high.

He needs no clothes to warm his bosom; the sun does the job and does a very good one.

I saw Him myself one warm spring day. He was chasing a butterfly that never got away.

He threw a glance into my face and I prepared for a nice long chase.

But instead of a chase, He tipped his hat and on a log we sat and began to chat.

We talked about the situation the world is in today and He began to cry as He listened to me say.

Oh Man of the Wilderness, You are fortunate to me. You have not a worry. You are Eternity.

But I am life and live I must do, but why in a world that is greatly untrue?

There is stealing and killing in this place where I dwell. There is no spirit of giving. They always sell.

There is cheating and lying and rumors of war. Yes, since the beginning we have gone very far.

The Man stood up and to my heart He said,
    To live with me you must be dead.
    And this cannot help the situation the world is in today.
    It needs your help, my son, and so I let you stay.

Robert S. Brown, 1946

Part Two
Middle

CHAPTERS TEN THROUGH sixteen encompass the Middle Section of <u>Sacred Ground</u>. It examines the spiritual impact of 21st Century war on our Soldiers.

The loss of the Soldier's sense of self, the "pre-traumatic self," is first noticed by loved ones soon after the Soldier returns home. It is followed by grief, poorly identified but nearly constantly present and inadequately understood. Soldiers refer to this loss in terms like, "I left an important part of me over there," and "I need to go back,"

After reading <u>Sacred Ground</u>, one Soldier asked, "So how do I deal with this new me ... the one that doesn't seem to fit in any more ... the one that feels awkward and feels rage within?"

"Rage" expresses strongly the influence of combat on temperament. If I understand the Soldier's use of this word in this context, it is not a cause for alarm. Contrary to widespread misjudgment, Soldiers with combat-induced PTSD are peace-loving, unlikely to behave violently and are not to be feared.

I have heard many combat Soldiers identify their feelings of rage, but it is a feeling more frequently described in response to frustrations after redeployment.

Soldiers with combat-induced PTSD often tell me, "I have no tolerance for incompetence." This feeling is best understood as a result of survival training for combat in which incompetent decisions can have a life altering or death-causing consequence.

An incompetent or inconsiderate store clerk may invoke feelings of rage, fortunately rarely commented upon, for example, in a Soldier with combat-induced PTSD impatiently waiting in a long check-out line in a store.

The loss of basic trust is the major hurdle to recovery that Soldiers address on a daily basis.

Trust may also be appreciated in spiritual terms. Twenty-first Century war gnaws away at basic trust.

"I trust no one and nothing," is what I have come to expect every Soldier with PTSD to acknowledge. If there is an exception to this declaration, it is the Soldier's trusted combat battle buddy.

When a redeployed Soldier is betrayed by a combat battle buddy, an extremely rare occurrence, the damage is severe and lasting.

The story-teller's life, powerfully transformed by his attachment to a high school teacher and her remarkable attention to his life-needs, begins a spiritual journey totally unanticipated, but results in remarkable dividends. Through the efforts of this teacher, the athlete becomes a hopeful scholar and the University welcomes him, albeit with some understandable reluctance.

10

WAR ON SPIRIT

"Is it a sin to kill in combat?"

"What I did was wrong. There is no forgiveness."
 "Is it wrong to kill in combat?"
 "Is it a sin?"
 "I asked my preacher. He said, 'I can't give you the answer.'"

Tuesday Afternoon Group

Sergeant First Class (SFC) Roscoe Bennett's face expressed deep concern. He sat motionless in group therapy like a condemned man awaiting the jury's sentence. Would it be life in prison without parole or would it be the death penalty?

SFC Bennett's expression that day still haunts my memory. His emotionally painful internal debate was too real to conceal, too tangible to ignore.

Regrettably, SFC Bennett, like many American Soldiers, is unaware that he is the designated convict, harsh judge, and hung jury. Without help, SFC Bennett will sentence himself to a lengthy, unjust, unfair and unmerciful life of mental imprisonment.

His fellow group members, all Soldiers who have been deployed to Iraq and Afghanistan, were touched by SFC Bennett's concerns. How often had they struggled over exactly the same questions!

"They tell us not to talk about religion to the Nationals (local Arabs). That's all the Nationals want to talk about," said SGT Peter Carr.

'Who do you pray to? Are you an infidel?'

I just tried to be nice, but I never answered them.

The worse feeling for me is not knowing …not knowing if you killed somebody."

Killing Children in Combat

"We were ordered to fire on a house. Inside the house we found body parts of children. That's the worst feeling of all.

I will never get over shooting a child in combat, even if he was trying to kill me with an AK-47."

"I ran over a kid in Iraq. He got up and ran away. What a relief."

SSG (Staff Sergeant) Bobby Davis, a thoughtful Soldier, 30 years old, seldom speaks spontaneously in group therapy. Today, however, moved by the discussion of killing children in combat, SSG Davis shared the following observation.

"They know how we protect children in America. They turn kids over there into soldiers.

Kids come out from nowhere over there. Just all of a sudden, you are surrounded by kids.

Big kids beat up little ones over candy…that's why we had to stop throwing candy from our vehicles to the children."

SGT Frank Kirby, dark-skinned, introvert, separated Soldier, has 8 months of sobriety. Last year, he got a DUI (driving under the influence of alcohol) on Post. A few months later, he got a DWI (drinking while intoxicated) in town.

SGT Kirby is attentive in group therapy, listening to fellow servicemen freely discuss their combat issues.

SGT Kirby spoke softly. He made no eye contact with his fellow group members, all combat-sharpened men.

Speaking as if in a soliloquy, SGT Kirby made the following statement:

"I was in a convoy in Iraq. We stopped. I was pulling security. A teenager ran out of a house with an AK-47. He ran right towards my vehicle. I unloaded on him. A bullet hit a lady who was standing nearby. The death of the lady bothered me most."

SGT William Elliott hides his feelings.

"I got hard after a while. Let a kid roll down here with a weapon...I'll show him. It doesn't bother me because they are born to kill. Over time, you get used to killing."

Remembering Bad Stuff

SSG Elliott spoke again.

"My wife hates it that I can't forget the bad stuff from combat.

After a while, all you think about is going home.

It's surreal. You go from killing in combat to flying home in a matter of hours.

When you get home, everybody asks, 'How was it over there?' That drives me crazy.

I know what they want to ask. They want to know if I killed anybody.

It's the first thing kids will say. They are not shy about it. 'Did you shoot anybody?'

I don't want to be bothered. I don't want to go outside my house.

My own kids asked me if I shot anybody. I don't answer. I change the subject or just do something with my kids."

"My temper came back," said SGT Kirby. "I yelled at my 5-year-old."

SGT Elliott said, "My kids keep me straight. My kids chill sometimes. They tell me I try too hard."

A sudden sadness came over SGT Elliott's face. "I missed my kids' first haircut. I missed their first steps."

SFC North had been very attentive but equally quiet, if not withdrawn from the group.

SFC North then said, "I've been thinking about the meaning my kids have for me. I believe it is their closeness, the connection we have, the interests fathers have for their children, their innocence." Almost as an afterthought, he said "and they don't judge us.

It is the thought of knowing what we did in combat that upsets us, Dr. Brown. Our children may not love us as much if they knew what we did in combat." Everyone looked painfully pensive; no one spoke.

"How many Soldiers in this group had a good relationship as children with their own father?" I asked.

Every Soldier dropped his head. No one said he had a good father-son relationship while growing up.

SFC North continued reflectively. "My daughter struggles with this question. I think she is angry with the military. She said, 'It is like you left me.' Yes, she blames the military."

SSG Davis, speaking as if he were thinking out loud, said, "I left my kid for deployment when he was just a baby. Will he remember me? Will he recognize me? That's what I kept wondering in combat.

My wife got used to me being gone from home more than my kids did."

SFC North added, "I agree with you, Bro. When we come back from deployment we disturb our wife's routine."

"Is it wrong to kill in combat?"

At the end of the 90-minute Post-Deployment Group Psychotherapy session, SFC Bennett felt no relief from the discussion until he asked his first question again.

"Is it wrong to kill in combat?"

The idea of a Greek Chorus came into my mind.

Would SFC Bennett feel liberated, delivered from his internal torture if a thousand voices lamented war?

Would SFC Bennett experience freedom from the captivity of his terrible recollections of the responsibility for the taking a life ... of taking more lives than he can count?

Is there a Greek Chorus in all of history that could soothe the Soldier's burning fever of guilt?

Would a Greek Chorus accompanied by a patriotic marching band remind him that a good Soldier follows orders?

Would a grateful nation, a supportive media, and the love from his community and love from his family release him from the guilt-driven nightmares that rob him of sleep?

SFC Albert North answered the question for the group.

"We all have the same question, my friends. In our soul we know that it was right to kill the enemy if it was the last resort.

Our rules of engagement protected our enemy more than it protected us.

We hate killing.

We hate war.

We went to war because we were ordered to exchange blows with our enemy.

Our enemy wore no uniform.

Our enemy used women and children to kill us.

Our enemy seriously injured more than 50,000 of our brothers.

Our enemy used deception and deceit to kill thousands of us with hidden explosive devices.

You asked is it wrong to kill in combat.

Let me speak for myself, and I hope this group agrees with me. Is it wrong not to kill in combat? I never shot at anybody who didn't shoot at me first." The session ended quietly.

"When is that going to stop, Dr. Brown?"

"This week, I was at a birthday party at work for one of our employees," said MSG Keith L. Johnson; "you know, one of those parties in the break room.

They had balloons and all that stuff you find at a party.

One of the balloons popped.

It caught me off guard.

I startled like a bitch. I tried to hide my reaction, but I jerked my back so hard I could hardly get out of bed the next morning.

When is that going to stop, Dr. Brown?"

"Keith, it will stop just as soon as you start feeling safe again," I replied solemnly.

SSG Wes Franklin carries the expression of seriousness on his face. I have never seen him smile.

SSG Franklin, married 12 years, was badly wounded in Iraq. He doesn't like to talk about his injury unless it is relevant.

With sadness and regret in his deep voice, SSG Franklin said, "I killed somebody over there.

It's on my mind. Sometimes, I think about it a lot.

It will flash before me like a movie when I get startled. Keith reminded me of it when he talked about being startled."

MSG Johnson, staring at the floor, hiding his face, said, "I'm ashamed of what I did in combat."

MSG Ken Compton spoke with confidence. "What I did down range . . . I never shot at anybody who didn't shoot at me first.

I agree with what was said, the enemy was somebody who was shooting at me." I was the next to speak.

"Do you experience a spiritual conflict with combat?"

I addressed the Wednesday Morning Post-Deployment Psychotherapy directly.

"Do you experience a spiritual conflict with combat?"

MSG Johnson was the first Soldier to answer my question.

"I was raised as a Baptist. I went to Sunday school and church. I even went to the Baptist Training Union.

We always talked about the Bible in my family.

My favorite Bible story was Noah's ark.

Over there in Iraq, I learned that Noah built the ark in Iraq.

I was told Noah's ark is on a mountain top in Turkey, not far from its border with Iraq.

It had a strange effect on me…knowing I was in a country with a strong religious history.

Abraham was from Ur in Iraq.

Daniel was in the lion's den in Iraq.

The wise men were from Iraq.

Did the rest of you guys have a bizarre feeling while fighting a war in a country that had been so important to our religious past?"

SGT Billy Dawson spoke. "I had the same thoughts, but I never said anything about it.

So many things in the Bible happened over there.

It was like knowing your own back yard.

Different religions started over there.

The Muslims say that Jesus was the Son of God or a prophet.

Saddam Hussein was rebuilding Babylon…restoring it with gold.

They told us not to talk to them about the ark on the mountain.

The U.S. made it a no-fly zone."

MSG Ken Compton said, "I was raised a Catholic. Christians and Muslims may not worship the same God.

I am confused by it."

SGT Billy Dawson said, "We get angry because we are all bothered by bad feelings about killing. It is our way of coping."

SSG Wes Franklin spoke convincingly. "I was on a convoy in Iraq. We drove most of the night. In the very early morning, we drove by some of the prettiest scenery I ever saw.

There was a long bridge we drove over. I was tired as shit. Sessions was my driver. He turned to me and said, 'look over there.' It was all burned.

"Over there is the Garden of Eden. Nobody can go there and live," Sessions said. "It is a forbidden area."

"It freaked me out as the moon shone on it…the Garden of Eden in Iraq.

It was near Kirkuk.

I definitely felt the effect of being in a place that was once a holy land.

Why are we destroying these people?

Why are we here?

I never expected this.

A lot of people's eyes were opened over there.

It stirred up their belief…killing in a place that had been holy."

MSG Johnson spoke seriously.

"It was a spiritual awakening for me.

Before I went to Iraq, I always thought Jesus was white. Over there, everybody is just as brown as me.

Killing over there had an impact on every Soldier.

The killing was worse because of the place we had to do it.

At first, I felt nothing about killing in a place that once had been holy. I just wanted to go home.

Later, I became more conscious of the history of Iraq.

Later, I became more conscious of the good Iraqi people.

We had an Iraqi truck driver who would give you everything he had.

He would roll out his blanket or rug, put all his food on it and signal you with his thumb and two fingers to come join him…just signaling 'come here…come here.'

On convoys we would see all their magnificent architecture.

God made those mountains.

The desert is the most beautiful place in the world when it rained. The way the flowers popped up was magical."

SSG Wes Franklin, his speech barely articulate from combat injuries to his face and throat, shook his head. "People have been killing each other over there for centuries.

We can't stop them.

Yes, the mountains are beautiful, but we can't stop the killing.

God's presence was very real, very real, but it was good and bad.

The life they lead is bad.

Iraq could be a great place. The people are hospitable.

They must be smart. They can put 50 movies on one DVD and sell it to American Soldiers. They even sold us new movies before they were released here.

Iraq could be a beautiful, rich nation.

I came home with mixed feelings."

Sadness remained in his voice just as it pervaded his face.

"Combating Terrorism is Spiritually Taxing"

Some of our most distinguished military leaders identify the spiritual values of our Soldiers to be unsurpassed in importance.

"Wars may be fought with weapons, but they are won by men. It is the spirit of the men who follow and of the man who leads that gains the victory." —General George Patton

"To this end, it is the duty of commanding officers in every echelon to develop to the highest degree the conditions and influences calculated to promote health, morals, and spiritual values of the personnel under their command." –General George C. Marshall

"Leadership is a potent combination of strategy and character. But if you have to be without one, be without strategy." –General Norman Schwarzkopf

The Army has long acknowledged the importance of the spiritual welfare of its Soldiers.

Perhaps because of a decade of combat in two countries, the Army has renewed its interest in matters of the spirit. In the recent past, for example, the Comprehensive Soldier Fitness Program gives preeminence to the Spiritual Domain.

It is also identified as a critical element of the Army Resiliency Program.

In "Scent of a Woman," an actor vividly depicting an Army officer with untreated PTSD from deployment to Vietnam, said with insight, "There is no prosthesis for an amputated spirit."

Combating terrorism is spiritually taxing.

For some of our Soldiers, it leads to painful despair that well may be partly spiritual, despair requiring support to regain spiritual health.

Ancient Greek Philosophy, from which our concept of democracy is derived, held a tripartite view of human beings, that each person has a mind, a body, and a spirit.

Our spiritual nature is difficult to define.

Our spiritual nature is too often neglected.

Sadly, our spiritual nature may bring us our worst misery, for example, when it is high jacked by the radically religious, by those who kill in the name of religious conviction.

On the other hand, "healthy minded religion," as defined by William James a century ago, in <u>Varieties of Religious Experience</u>, may be one of our greatest sources of joy.

"It is what it is" is one of the common sayings of our time. However, it is important to realize that the meaning we give to our experiences determines its effects on us, as stated earlier.

Despite what in jargon seems to make sense, it is never "it is what it is." It is always what it means to us.

Some of the most vital meanings we give to our encounters come from our spiritual values.

Post-Deployment Spiritual Domain Group Psychotherapy, co-led by a psychiatrist and a chaplain, may provide a unique opportunity for Soldiers to thoughtfully reflect upon:

(1) The impact of combat on their deeply held beliefs;

(2) The value of meaningful spiritual health; and

(3) The identification and application of resources to help reduce the inconsistency between what a Soldiers believes is ethically correct and morally right versus how the Soldier lives day to day.

In a word, Soldiers in Post-Deployment Spiritual Domain Group Psychotherapy may learn to soothe an injured or damaged spirit as they reestablish strong attachments to each other.

"It doesn't make much sense to me"

SGT Mike Goodson is new to the Tuesday Morning Group. That explains why he has said little in his first 3 weekly sessions and why he appears ill-at-ease.

SGT Goodson is a tall, muscular, shaven-headed, 27-year-old married man, father of 3 young children. His soft blue eyes surprisingly suggest an unexpected tenderness in this huge, strong, sturdy Soldier.

He is a quiet man by nature.

Militarily, SGT Goodson is an "11 Bravo." He is in the US Army Infantry.

"11 Bravos" form the foundation of combat arms, Soldiers most often directly engaged with the enemy.

SGT Goodson mustered up the courage to speak, overcoming the hesitancy common to PTSD Soldiers to interact socially. He came prepared to ask for help.

"I had a dream. It doesn't make much sense to me."

The group listened thoughtfully to SGT Goodson hesitatingly, straining for the right words.

"I was in the lead truck as the TC (Truck Commander). My job was to look for IEDs.

It was a convoy of MRAPs (Mine-Resistant Ambush Protected vehicle).

I had a small window to my right.

Traveling slowly, I looked down and saw a cardboard box. It was about the size of a diaper box.

One of my main tasks as the truck commander is to spot an IED. Inside the box there was a 2-liter Coke bottle.

I blew it off. It did not look like an IED to me.

The second truck called it in. They stopped and checked it out.

Under the box they found, buried in the sand, two 155 mm rounds (very large cannon rounds).

What if those rounds had gone off? Each one is almost as big as a Volkswagen.

Why does this bother me now?"

"Was your dream an exact re-enactment?" I asked.

"Yes, the dream is about exactly what happened in Afghanistan 2 years ago.

I feel horrible about it.

It comes into my mind too often. I keep asking myself why I did not check it more carefully.

I cannot explain why I just said to myself it is only a box."

SGT Goodson's face appeared grim. His corrugator muscle was stressed, making deep furrows in his forehead, just above and between his eye brows.

The dream provided an opportunity for SGT Goodson to make a confession to the group. "Will I still have the group's respect if they know what I did wrong?" he wondered silently.

SGT Goodson was doing what is most difficult for an 11 Bravo. He was divulging a weakness, a mistake, to fellow Soldiers.

He was haunted by his mistake. He was demoralized. He felt anguish at its most painful level, at the level of his spirit.

SSG Goodson rejected the group's first attempt to reassure him.

A fellow group member said, "There is redundancy. The system did its job. It was not a failure."

"I was pulled off the lead truck for 2 weeks," sadly said SGT Goodson, rejecting encouragement.

"The mission was not a failure, but I failed."

One of SGT Goodson's fellow group members is a Forward Sniper, a Combat Arms Soldier, similar to the Infantry but additionally trained in marksmanship. His combat experience is similar to SGT Goodson's.

"Let me get this straight," said SFC Tommy Kennedy, a bright, self-confident, no-nonsense Infantryman. "When one truck stops, the whole convoy stops. Right?"

SGT Goodson nodded his head affirmatively.

"The lead truck is a privileged position. Was your entire crew removed?"

"Yes, my crew and my MRAP were sent to the rear for 2 weeks," replied SGT Goodson.

The Forward Sniper, SFC Kennedy, continued. "You told us earlier that you were not sleeping well.

You are now dreaming. This tells me you are sleeping better.

You scanned your sector on this mission you are describing.

You lost your privilege of being the lead vehicle for 2 weeks, but it may not have been punishment.

If you did something to break the faith you would have been removed from the lead position forever, not for 2 weeks

You were sent to the rear with the gear for a rest, not for committing a crime."

SGT Goodson's eyes widened. Here is something, despite hundreds of rehearsals in his mind for the past 2 years, he had not ever contemplated. An entirely new idea was beginning to form in SGT Goodson's troubled thoughts. The truth was like a bright light.

"The front of the convoy is a lot more stressful."

SGT Goodson said, "I have been feeling horrible about it."

The Forward Sniper said, "It's just a feeling.

Feelings can be unreliable. It's a horrible feeling.

Every Soldier in this group knows what that "horrible" feeling is like. It is not based on the truth.

The horrible feeling has blinded you to the truth.

The truth is clear."

This was a special moment for SGT Goodson. It was like waking up from a very unpleasant anesthesia. He was prepared, long overdue, for the truth of his situation.

"The best Soldier was in the lead position," said Forward Sniper SFC Kennedy. He was making the successful closing argument with the confidence of a masterful defense attorney.

"The best Soldier needed a break. Sometimes, when a Soldier needs a break, he is the last one to know it."

The prosecuting attorney, unrelenting, was not giving up. SGT Goodson was still perplexed, still prosecuting. No expression on his face suggested relief. "I got my team pulled off the lead position," said SGT Goodson.

"I missed the IED (Improvised Explosive Device).

I was sent to the back for two weeks.

No one ever came to me to talk about it.

Why am I still dreaming about it nearly two years after it happened?"

The group silently, respectfully watched the dialogue between the Forward Sniper and the 11 Bravo.

The Forward Sniper, completely calm throughout the discussion, replied.

"I believe Doc Brown would tell you, like I did, it is good you are dreaming.

He would also tell you, as he frequently tells the group, that recurrent dreams tell us there is some unfinished business.

Your dream is the mind's way of trying to get it right, trying to correct some misunderstanding, trying to keep you focused on a conflict that must get resolved."

The Forward Sniper, seated as always by the door, the nearest exit, still working on his own painful conflicts, looked over to me for confirmation.

I confirmed what he said. "You are not expected to be perfect. The crew in the lead vehicle is not expected to be perfect. No one can tolerate stress indefinitely.

Even the best Soldier is not perfect.

Your command did what was best for the mission. There was no reprimand, no 15-6 Investigation, no blame.

In 2 weeks, you were back in the prestigious lead position of the convoy. You and your crew were rested.

The mission was accomplished. There were no losses.

Give yourself a break, Soldier."

SGT Goodson smiled broadly.

Hardly above a whisper, SGT Goodson, looking at the Forward Sniper, said, "Thank you."

I was the only person in the group who detected tears in SGT Goodson's voice.

The spirit of a brave Soldier was restored. The session ended. Will the melancholy end?

"How can I stop aching?"

It is difficult for Soldiers to keep intrusive thoughts of combat out of awareness.

"The idle mind is the devil's workshop." Reframed in the language of Soldiers returning from combat, "I can't stand to have down time. My worst thoughts take control of my mind unless I stay busy."

One Soldier put it this way: "I have to fill my mind like I have to fill my stomach."

What redeployed Soldiers most fear is the return of intolerable feelings that steal their precarious, unstable sanity.

Soldiers traumatized combating terrorism fear losing self-control. My words are woefully inadequate as I attempt to depict the awfulness they voluntarily endured.

The inhumanity and suffering our Soldiers witnessed and experienced in combat cannot be imagined or fully comprehended even by its eye-witnesses.

How feeble then are the Soldiers' efforts to lock the doors and windows of their mind to the intruding and inevitable memories and realistic physiological re-experiencing of every dreadful detail of combat!

Reliving the suffering is costly.

Reliving combat trauma impairs memory.

Reliving combat trauma causes irritability, distrust, and too often damages the Soldier's most important relationships.

Staying busy to avoid painful thoughts and unacceptable feelings is exhausting. Add this to unrefreshing sleep, typical of

Soldiers, and zombie-like creatures emerge, devoid of patience and empathy.

Can one's spiritual health flourish without the capacity to reflect and feel the full range of human emotions?

No one wants to be forgotten.

The losses sustained by our Soldiers can be grieved, a largely spiritual experience, only when they regain their capacity to normally grieve the pain of their losses.

The effect of 21st Century War has been most costly to the spiritual health of our Soldiers.

As a nation indebted to our Soldiers, we want to love these men and women back into spiritual health.

"I lost my faith"

"When I first started getting PTSD, I didn't know what was going on," said 1SG Barry Walker.

"I didn't understand."

1SG Walker looked around the group therapy room, speaking seriously. His fellow group therapy members respected this tall, physically imposing man with blonde hair and blue eyes. They also respected his rank.

"Once you go over there you are changed.

I came back from Iraq a different person.

Over there…it is not easy to explain. Sometimes it was like an out of the body experience…like I can't believe I'm actually here.

When I first came back I was detached. I had lost my empathy. I could not connect to people.

My brother died and I did not go to the funeral. I sent flowers because Dr. Brown suggested it.

No matter how hard you try to find the person you were before you deployed to combat, you will not find it again. The death of my brother meant nothing to me. I permitted myself to have no feelings about it.

I came back from combat angry, damaging my family relationships.

I was one of those Soldiers who have the hardest time with coming back. I didn't want psychological help. I kept telling myself I'll never get better. I lost time so that my mind was not going forward.

When I came in the Army, I believed in the Army values. I had confidence in Army leadership.

When my beliefs were challenged, I lost my faith."

1SG Walker paused, fighting back tears.

"What challenged your beliefs?" I asked.

"The circumstances of combat challenged my beliefs.

Seeing inhumanity in Iraq scarred my soul. The inhumanity of Iraqi people killing each other was more than I could take.

A VBID (Vehicle Borne Improvised Explosive Device) exploded in a traffic circle in Iraq. I was near the traffic circle when it exploded. It killed 130 Iraqi people…women and children. It was Iraqi people killing Iraqi people. I just happened to be there.

People were begging me to do something. I could do nothing. I felt hopeless a lot of the times over there.

I even questioned why I was over there.

I loved the people over there…the Iraqi people.

When I came back the first time, I checked in drunk.

The second time I came back, I just didn't care.

The whole reality of being in the Army changed drastically. I was not the same person.

Twenty years of military doctrine … I didn't believe any more.

I lost my trust in people.

I didn't know who I was…an identity crisis.

I couldn't get along with people."

The group remained quiet but attentive. They understood because they were readily recognizing themselves in what 1SG Walker said.

"One day in group, a pivotal point was reached. Dr. Brown said something and a light bulb went off in my mind.

Dr. Brown said you are not the same person after combat. It is a spiritual thing…like being born again. The old person is gone or dying.

I was looking for the old person and finding nothing. A lot of the time, I felt hostile.

I started looking carefully at what was on my mind. I had a lot of questions.

Did God turn His back on Iraq?

Why did they do such unthinkably destructive things to each other?

What was our role in Iraq?

I lost my Army values. I was changed. There was corruption in my MITT (Military Transition Team).

As a First SGT, I knew right from wrong, but in my MITT Team I was always in the middle. I lost my sense of right and wrong in Iraq. I lived in the gray area.

No creed, even the Army Creed, meant much to me any more.

I lost my faith.

My sense of truth was not the truth.

I felt like Adam and Eve after eating the apple. I saw the ugliness.

I liked the Iraqi people and they liked me."

The group agreed that the Iraqi people are often generous, hospitable, and likeable.

1SG Walker continued.

"Another pivotal point was reached recently. A man from my childhood died. I returned to my home in Louisville for the funeral. An amazing thing happened.

I grew up in the projects with a friend who did all the bad things I did as an adolescent in need of supervision. In a contest of the Most Likely to Succeed in Future Delinquency, my friend and I would be tied neck and neck.

We lost contact with each other for decades. I nearly fell over when my childhood friend walked in the church as the pastor to conduct the funeral.

He stared at me in surprise and included comments about our friendship in his sermon.

I spent hours with him after the funeral. He said a lot of things to me that made sense. I can trace the early steps of my journey to a new faith to my childhood friend, now my inspiration."

"I found a new faith"

The Post-Deployment Spiritual Domain Psychotherapy Group meets on Wednesday afternoons from 1400 to 1530. Some Soldiers dub it the "Bible Group." It is co-led with Dr. James E. Walker, former Post Chaplain. Dr. Walker was traumatized in the Pentagon when it was struck by terrorists on 9/11. He also served in Iraq.

1SG Barry Walker (unrelated to Dr. Walker) emerged as a leader in this group. It was encouraging to observe his metamorphosis into an empathetic being. He invited Soldiers to the group and to his church. He delighted in their response.

"I am so pleased that Jim Hicks," one of 1SG Walker's former Soldiers, also with four combat deployments, "is showing interest in spiritual things. He goes to church with me now. We sit on the front row. I looked at him last Sunday during the sermon. He was leaning forward, taking in every word the preacher said."

In an individual session, I spoke to 1SG Walker about his progress in conquering PTSD and his spiritual health.

"My mother was Pentecostal when I was a child. I was sent to a Christian School, but I was so rebellious.

I got into trouble for not knowing the Bible verses.

I didn't want to attend Sunday school.

I didn't want to go to church.

My mother would have to search for me in the neighborhood on Sunday mornings because I was not in church.

I started going to church when I was 8. When I was 15, I finally stopped going to church."

"1SG Walker," I asked, "How did you regain your faith?"

"I did not return to the faith I lost. The faith I had in the beginning was distorted. In that faith, I put my trust in man, in the military, and in society. Faith in man is going to be disappointing.

Now my faith is in God.

It is a new form of faith for me.

I still get stuck.

This did not happen overnight.

I gradually changed.

There was a period I spent in a psychiatric hospital. I was there for 7 weeks in a special treatment program for PTSD.

I started attending a nondenominational church. I was invited to church by a friend. Eventually, it clicked.

I started learning God's purpose for my life was more important than my purpose.

I went to Bible study.

I started reading the Bible and applying the Bible to my life.

First, I changed my beliefs. Then I changed my thought processes. Finally, my behavior changed."

1SG Walker could have been testifying under oath in front of the Supreme Court. In a certain, important sense, he was.

His eyes sparkled with the enthusiasm of passion. The harsh, irritable, revengeful 1SG with whom I had worked for the previous two years was psychologically AWOL (Absent without Leave).

"God can take the broken pieces of our life and put them back together, making them stronger than they were before they were broken.

The pastor talked about the importance of forgiveness after betrayal.

He said we are released from anger and frustration when we forgive.

The betrayal, even when forgiven, will leave a scar.

After a while, the scar, always visible, will no longer hurt."

"I feel like I'm on sacred ground"

The image of a scar after forgiven betrayal! What a valuable way to consider the concealed scars of combat-induced PTSD, scars that will stop hurting after a while.

How strangely contrasting are the effects of the hidden scars of combat versus the obvious ones.

Most of my work with combat Soldiers is limited to the indiscernibly scarred. To the untrained eye, the Soldier with PTSD may appear ordinary most of the time in most situations.

If there is anything that specifically characterizes the Soldier stricken with PTSD from combat, it is spiritless feelings of shame, disgrace, embarrassment, and even dishonor.

I treated a young Soldier several years ago whose combat scar was painfully apparent. The traumatic amputation of his right leg in combat in Iraq brought him honor, respect, and even pride.

He hid nothing about his loss. He minimized the courage it took to save others though he was severely injured and his blood loss was profound.

My work with the Soldier attempting to hide his or her "amputated soul," or mortified internalized, hidden scar, has a lot in common with the magician.

I am a magician with a different cape. Instead of making things disappear, I try to help the Soldier with PTSD to make the wounds of war appear. With the cooperation of the injured Soldier, I try to make the scars visible to the cognitive part of the mind in order that it can be understood and healed.

Also unlike the real magician, my work is not speedy. Here the hand is not quicker than the eye. It is like a slow motion film, shown over and over until the truth is discovered.

These victims of war on the soul come home, in the words of 1SG Walker, "disconnected."

They have learned to expect the unexpected and to always be on guard.

Attachment begins with trust.

Trust is often killed in action (KIA) in combat.

I tell each Soldier when we first meet in my office that I feel like I am on sacred ground when I hear his or her trauma narrative.

I speak from my soul to his or her soul.

The silence that follows indicates to me the Soldier believes he or she will be understood.

To be understood is to be immediately comforted.

Our work together is to restore his or her soul, the soul that the terrorists tried to destroy.

11

KITTY GARNETT

"A positive influence on me for the rest of my life"

I HAD LITTLE academic ambition until my last semesters of high school.

Having a substitute teacher was a welcomed day for me.

I did not expect to be called on by the substitute teacher.

My incomplete homework assignment would likely go unnoticed.

I could generally relax and forget just about everything except football.

Of course, I had no way of knowing, but today's substitute teacher would have a lasting positive influence on me for the rest of my life.

My memory is straining for the exact date that Mrs. Kitty Garnett entered my class room at Maury High School, Norfolk, Virginia, but it must have been a bright shiny day in the spring of 1947.

This woman, short of stature with short, prematurely graying hair and medium build, in a warm and kind way, said, "Take out your notebooks.

Write two or three paragraphs about your plans for the summer."

I took out my notebook. As my seat was the second from the front, in the row nearest the window, Mrs. Garnett could readily see my state of inactivity.

The substitute teacher walked slowly over to my desk.

"What is your name?" she inquired in a friendly way.

"Bobby Brown," I replied in an equally friendly manner.

"Why are you not writing?"

"I have no pencil."

"Why don't you have a pencil?"

"I can't afford one."

"Why can't you afford one?"

"I have no money."

"Why do you have no money?"

"I have no job."

"Would you like to have a job?"

"Yes."

"Would you like to be a counselor at a boys' camp?"

"Yes...but I never thought about being a counselor at a boys' camp."

"If I offer you a job as a counselor at Camp Greenbrier this summer, would you take it?"

"No, but thank you very much just the same.

No one has ever offered me a job," I announced in a thoughtful voice that conveyed gratitude.

"Why can't you take the job this summer?"

"I'm going to summer school this summer to take Algebra so I can play football next fall."

"Do you play football for Maury?"

"Yes. I'll be a star next year."

The class of about thirty students, some academically elite, were pleased with the distraction from writing. They laughed heartily at my immodesty, regrettably typical of my polished cover for deep feelings of inadequacy.

"I had my appendix removed last year; it held me back, but nothing will stop me this year.

Do you want to make a bet?"

"I will take the bet. If you are a football star for the Maury Commodores this year, then next summer you will be a counselor at Camp Greenbrier!"

I left my seat without permission, stuck out my chest, and sauntered up to the blackboard and shook Mrs. Theodore Stanford Garnett's hand, sealing the bet.

My classmates applauded.

Mrs. Garnett loaned me a pencil, a No. 2, yellow pencil with a brand new eraser.

In two or three paragraphs, I described how taking Algebra in summer school would be like taking Cod Liver Oil, a widely used medication that was effective as a medicinal as well as a disgusting medication form of punishment.

Nearly 7 decades later, as I write down these nostalgic thoughts, I suddenly become aware that I take its equivalent three times daily, the only supplement my cardiologist recommends, "Fish Oil."

The Maury High School Football Team

I worked hard to succeed in football.

I loved the game since I played for the Lambert's Point Rangers in a leather helmet, beginning in 1946.

On the offensive team for the Maury Commodores, I played wingback on the single-wing formation. We were coached by Tony Saunders, a good man mentioned earlier. I ran the "reverse."

I ran from my line-up position behind and to the right of our right end, Ed Stowers.

I ran undetected with my head and body down to take the hand-off from either the full-back, Stanley Tugwell, or the tail-back, Junie Floyd.

The reverse play was run either off the left tackle position or off the end position.

Once, I ran the reverse play from the left side of the line and threw a touchdown pass to Ed Stowers against Wilson High School at Ace Parker Field, Portsmouth, Virginia.

The plays were called by blocking back Billy Berry, later to become the CEO of Dominion Resources.

All summer, I worked out with my closest friends, Baxter Van Pelt and George Munden, traversing the streets in Lambert's Point as fast as we could run, for as far as we could run, mostly at night.

I even made a wooden device, the inverted rounded top of a chair, to hold the ball so that I could run from my measured position, replicating a hand-off as I grabbed the football out of the surrogate "player's hands."

As the result of the combination of physical fitness training and unwavering determination to play my best, I won the bet.

I mention one memorable game from that winning season. With 2 minutes left to play, we were trailing the Lynchburg Hill Toppers under the lights at Foreman Field. With excellent blocking, I ran the reverse for a touchdown, but we were still behind. I intercepted a Lynchburg pass and ran it back near the goal line. A fellow Maury Commodore ran it over for the winning touchdown. I believe Keats was referring to a winning touchdown when he said, "A thing of beauty is a joy forever."

I have never forgotten the sense of wellbeing with which I was infused at that time in my life. It is the goal that I repeatedly aim for as I try to remain physically active.

Regular physical exercise is the most robust antidepressant in all of psychiatry, a subject discussed exhaustively elsewhere in this text.

"Dear Old Camp Greenbrier"

Kitty Garnett's husband, Theodore S. Garnett, taught at the Norfolk Academy, one of the oldest private academies in America.

"The" (pronounced Thee) Garnett, Bus Male, Department of Athletics, University of Virginia; and Cooper Dawson, a retired naval officer and owner of the Penn-Daw Hotel, Alexandria, Virginia; jointly owned Camp Greenbrier.

Camp Greenbrier is one of the oldest independent boys' camps in America, a lovely natural beauty of several hundred acres on the Greenbrier River in Alderson, West Virginia.

I was privileged to work at Camp Greenbrier for five summers from 1949-1953, thanks to Kitty Garnett.

But the story continues.

Ms. Williams, a middle-aged woman, dark hair and dark eyes, mildly acerbic, academically mordant and uncompromising, taught Chemistry at Maury High School.

Her standards were high, her tolerance for poor students who preferred sports to scholarship was low, and I sensed her impatience with me personally.

It is not easy for me to record here that I received a final grade in Chemistry One of 46!

It would be unthinkable to be accepted by a college with a great pre-med program, like UVA, with a transcript blackened by a final grade of 46!

Even more unthinkable was being permitted to repeat Chemistry One while also taking Chemistry Two at the same time.

My class graduated from Maury High School in June 1949, but I remained another semester for two good reasons: to play another year of football and to take Chemistry One and Two.

Ms. Williams, "contrary to my better judgment," with great reluctance, shaking her head in disbelief in her own decision-making capacity and my audacity, taught me Chemistry One and Chemistry Two during the fall semester of 1949.

It was no cake walk. I took a full academic schedule of classes, continued to sing in Mrs. Sena B. Wood's Fifth Bell Chorus, acted in the senior play and played football. I was a disappointment to my football coach and to the player who wore Commodore Football jersey #40 who in earlier seasons was known as "fleet-footed wing-back."

How I learned Inorganic Chemistry

Let me tell you how Kitty Garnett's determination to encouragingly influence my life continued, even surpassing my own determination.

"Mrs. Brown, I'm The Garnett." The name of this remarkable man, the good husband of Kitty Garnett, was Theodore Stanford Garnett, hence the name "The."

It was a morning to remember. The cloudless sky of gentle blue was illuminated by the early June sun. A soft breeze off the Elizabeth River cooled the 1949 late spring morning.

"I've come to take Bobby to Camp Greenbrier.

I understand he has impressed my wife, and she makes few mistakes when it comes to sizing up people.

"Bobby, how are you?"

I had never met Kitty Garnett's husband, but he made us feel comfortable. He was a balding man, about 48 years old, five-feet 7 inches tall, medium build, piercing blue eyes, and notably energetic.

In retrospect, I doubt if Mr. Garnett had ever come to call on a family in "blue collar" Lamberts Point.

Mother politely greeted him. He grabbed my suit case; I took a box of remaining clothes, and soon we were driving to the ferry to cross the Elizabeth River, a first stop on a long trip to West Virginia. In those days, there were no tunnels under the river connecting Norfolk to Hampton or Newport News, Virginia. The pleasant ferry ride took about 45 minutes.

Barclay Sheaks, my favorite Virginia artist, in his 'Watchers on the Stern," depicts romantically the ferry ride enjoyed by a family feeding the large white sea gulls escorting the ferry on a bright summer day. It is the favorite of the ten Barclay Sheaks paintings that hang joyfully in my office and home.

Mr. Garnett and I arrived at Camp Greenbrier 10 days before camp opened to get the facility in working order.

We built a wooden dock and a mid-river dock, floated on 10 fifty-gallon drums and anchored securely in the Greenbrier River, about 50 feet off shore and attached to the base dock by strong ropes. The dock must have been 30 feet square, a substantial surface from which to dive.

The river was pristine; the clearest water I had ever seen, but it was cold. Soon trucks brought in green painted canoes and placed them on wooden racks near the dock. I could feel an increasing sense of excitement and adventure.

Other counselors arrived and then the boys came, almost always by train to the small depot in Alderson, West Virginia.

It was also fascinating to watch the trains at night, as their tracks were parallel to the Greenbrier River.

Each counselor was assigned a tent. I was responsible for 3 or 4 boys who slept in my tent, each on a single metal cot.

The canvas tents were erected on strong wooden foundations elevated 3 feet above ground.

Each day began with a military style formation, flag raising, followed by breakfast.

I was assigned Table 11. Ten campers sat with me at the round wooden table.

The food was the best, prepared by the best chef, Archie, who was also the chef for Beta House, a popular fraternity at the University of Virginia, located next to the Beta Bridge, Rugby Road.

After grace, it was traditional to have unwinnable contests of yells or coordinated raised voice singing chant-like, using some form of teasing.

Table 11 was easily the champion at each meal. We were the loudest and prickliest in our table yells.

Camp Greenbrier had some of the best clay tennis courts in the country. Tennis was one of the main daily activities, along with horseback riding, swimming, canoeing, baseball, basketball, track, rifle range, and crafts.

After lunch, everyone was required to take a much needed nap.

The Camp had a full-time nurse.

Doctors usually came and stayed for two weeks of rotating shifts.

We also had an Episcopal Priest who led Evening Prayers.

Campers and staff attended Evening Prayer each day at dusk.

Enter Ed Smoot

Ed Smoot, a man of great wit and wisdom, was in charge of the water front at Camp Greenbrier. He was an excellent swimmer and adored by campers and counselors alike.

Ed Smoot was in his early 50s. His physical similarities, though younger, with Benjamin Franklin, also an accomplished swimmer, were stunning.

Ed Smoot taught Biology and Chemistry at Petersburg High School.

Kitty Garnett had me bring the Maury High School required Chemistry textbook to Camp Greenbrier.

Robbing Ed Smoot of his daily nap, Kitty Garnett had him tutor me diligently every day in Chemistry, one chapter at a time.

It was not difficult to see that Ed favored rest over training and tutoring, but he did it faithfully.

When I returned for my fall and last semester at Maury High School, thanks to Kitty Garnett, The Garnett, and Ed Smoot, I made an A+ or 100 in Chemistry One and an A or 94 in Chemistry Two.

Enter the University of Virginia

I left home with a letter in my hand from A.B. Bristow, Principal of Maury High School, to George Ferguson, Dean of Admissions, College of Arts and Sciences, University of Virginia.

On a clear, cold January afternoon, 1950, I traveled to Charlottesville in a car driven by Kitty Garnett's nephew, Nicholas G. Wilson, III.

Several other young men from Norfolk, all friends of Nick Wilson, all UVA men, waited in the car. I took the last remaining seat, the rear passenger side. Given a choice, those with motion sickness would have rejected this seat.

Before Nick Wilson arrived, on my knees in our small living room, I joined my mother at her request, in earnest prayer for traveling mercy and for God's guidance and protection at the University.

In my suit case were shirts, and pants and coats donated by Kitty Garnett with the blessing of their former proud owner, her good husband, The Garnett.

It was the first time I ever left home alone, to the first destination previously unknown to me, and the first time the University entered my sense of myself. It still remains near the center of my spirit.

It is plain to see that Kitty Garnett, without fanfare or credit-seeking, fashioned me into a student acceptable to the University of Virginia.

I am unwilling to accept the notion that chance or happenstance account for a high school substitute teacher selflessly motivating a previously unknown student to dream of a future that she made possible.

Looking more like a middle-aged tomboy than an angel, Kitty Garnett, the substitute high school teacher, deserves angelic wings. Surely it was one of the great days in Heaven when her award ceremony took place.

I went to Camp Greenbrier in 1949 with a marginal academic record, but when I went back to Camp Greenbrier in 1950 I was a student in good standing at the University of Virginia.

However, there are, I admit, degrees of academic good standing.

First, and thankfully, I was not on academic probation.

I was one of only a handful of students admitted to the University in mid-semester.

I wanted desperately to continue to study Chemistry, but at mid-term or spring semester, January 1950, no one was admitted to Chemistry Two without having passed Chemistry One at the University.

The same was true of Biology.

I ended up with a dissonant set of courses during my first semester at the University.

The reader is asked to be the judge of my academic standing as I review the courses the young lad from Lamberts Point was permitted to take during the January to June academic session, 1950.

I list the courses below for the objective assessment.

My two most difficult courses were The Philosophy of Alfred North Whitehead, a level of discourse that is still well beyond my understanding, and Parasitology, an advanced Biology course.

Both courses were well taught by distinguished professors.

University Professor William Weedon taught the Philosophy course. Professor Bruce Reynolds taught the Parasitology course.

American History was no less difficult for me. The course was taught by renowned Professor Abernathy. It assumed a general knowledge of history that was taught the semester prior to my arrival in Charlottesville.

Instructor John Coleman taught English. It required a weekly written paper.

I walked into the English class room in the basement of Old Cabell Hall to find a sentence taken from my first written assignment in bold, large letters on the blackboard.

I did not know how to react to this surprise recognition. Did it foretell a bright journalistic future, I wondered.

"Gentlemen, take your seats," announced John Coleman, our gifted teacher. It was said that he had inherited the San Francisco Utility Company, one explanation for his self-confident, if not arrogant, chirpy manner.

John Coleman was an immediately likeable man, but one felt on guard in his presence owing to his intellect and brilliant command of the English language.

Dressed in a dark gray flannel suit, vest buttoned, carrying a long stick of white chalk, John Coleman left his stool in front of a table at the podium and lumbered to the blackboard.

He was known to throw chalk at unacceptably performing students in his class.

In this case, however, he loudly, repeatedly, unmercifully kept tapping the blackboard with his weapon, the long piece of white chalk.

I sat on the front row, not knowing what to expect.

Thankfully, it was a small class. All eyes were on the blackboard.

John Coleman could not have spoken louder or more angrily with a megaphone.

"This, gentlemen, is a 'comma splice.'"

I didn't know the term.

John Coleman's disgust was unmistakable.

It sounded as if he had been personally offended.

"I will not have a 'comma splice' in my writing class!"

"Is that clear, Mr. Brown?"

"Gentlemen, is that clear?"

No one responded.

John Coleman returned to the offensive tapping again, followed by circling my comma with deep, thick white chalk marks.

His face was getting red.

"Mr. Brown, a 'comma splice' is the separation of two sentences by a comma! Let it be your last comma splice or face the consequences."

It could have been yesterday, not six decades ago.

John Coleman was a down to earth academician with whom I developed a friendly and lasting relationship.

Before he retired, John Coleman taught my oldest son, Bob, Jr., at the University of Virginia.

My second son, David, now a permanent resident of New Zealand, majored in English at the University. Sadly, John Coleman by then had retired.

Happily, my wife, Dottie, my daughter Nancy, and my youngest son, Clinton, were all privileged to know John Coleman. We included him in many family and social events at our home in Charlottesville over the years following my graduation.

John Coleman's English class was the only course suitable for a student with my limited exposure to the realm of sophisticated education.

Kitty Garnett Continues

Unhappily, my supportive contacts with Kitty Garnett were limited to holidays and summer camp. I struggled.

The Korean War started in 1950.

The Selective Service Act was in full force and a number of Camp Greenbrier counselors were called up to serve, leaving behind those of us who had student deferments.

Four years later, I enlisted in the U S Army Reserve, launching a military career spanning many years about which I will have more to say later in this book.

Kitty Garnett opened a world to me I would never have known.

It is difficult to imagine why she took the time, repeatedly made the effort, and brought so many fine and good people into my life.

Her father, Dr. Nicholas G. Wilson, was a saintly physician. He had a full head of snow white hair. In a navy blue suit, he stood erect on the front row at the annual Preaching Missions, held at the Norfolk Center Theatre.

Dr. Wilson was a humble, devout, competent, much loved and respected person.

Dr. Wilson was a strong spiritual inspiration for me.

Kitty Garnett's brother, Nicholas G. Wilson, Jr., owned the Norfolk Door Engineering Company.

He used his income generously to help build the University of Virginia Alumni Hall, among his other notable contributions.

As a child, I had been to the Hague in Norfolk several times with my sister Frances. There we would meet the US Navy launch, docked at the Hague.

The US Navy launch carried people from Norfolk across the Elizabeth River to the Portsmouth Naval Hospital.

Ghent was the fine neighborhood of Norfolk in which the Hague was located.

Ghent was noted for its beautiful, spacious homes.

I had never been inside a large Ghent home, surrounding the Hague, until I was invited to meet Nick, Kitty Garnett's brother.

Like Kitty Garnett, Nicholas G. Wilson, Jr., was a kind but firm person, practical and inquisitive. He wanted to know why I wanted to attend the University and why he should endorse my application. The questions were unanticipated and my answers were not good.

In 1949, well before Alfred W. Whitehurst became the Honorable Judge of the Norfolk Circuit Court, he was a student in the College of Arts and Sciences at the University.

This learned man also had a remarkable influence on my life. He was an excellent athlete, several years ahead of me.

He became my Sunday School Teacher at Burrows Memorial Baptist Church.

On a cold fall day, on the James Madison playground, during a basketball pick-up game in 1949, Al Whitehurst offered me his ticket to a football game at the University.

I declined his offer because it seemed like Charlottesville was far away. I could not imagine how I would get there. I believe this was the first time I had thought about attending the University.

Later, Bus Male, a University coach, played a crucial role in getting me into the University on a specially arranged football "scholarship." I told Nicholas G. Wilson, Jr., that I wanted to study medicine. I told him I had heard only the best things about the University. I also told him I hoped to play football there.

Later, Kitty Garnett told me that her brother was impressed with me for one reason.

I had told him he should attend church on a more regular basis! Strangely, I had completely forgotten that part of my brief visit with him in his lovely home on a cold and dark evening in the fall of 1949.

The Personhood of Kitty Garnett

I regret if I have failed to capture for the reader the essence and personhood of Kitty Garnett. She was not "warm and fuzzy." She dressed plainly and could have been athletic in her younger years.

"Practical" describes a major part of Kitty's thinking and behavior. I frequently visited the Garnetts when I was in Norfolk on breaks from the University.

It was a first for me when I saw a slate or small backboard in their family room by their front door. A piece of chalk hung down on a string from the blackboard. Various things were written on the blackboard, reminders for those who would go shopping.

They lived on Claremont Avenue directly across the street from Taylor Elementary School.

"Young The," their son, destined to become an aeronautical engineer, and Maria, their daughter, were probably not more than 10 and 7 years old respectively when I first met them.

I never sensed jealousy or any feeling other than acceptance from the wonderful Garnett children.

It was a busy, happy home every time I went calling and it was always an unannounced surprise visit. "Young man," as Kitty always greeted me, "sit down and tell us what you have been up to."

"Integrity" best describes her character. Impeccably honest, she soft-pedaled nothing, and consistently treated others as having value and promise. Kitty Garnett, more than anyone I knew, was the best teaching role model I ever had.

"Letting down Kitty Garnett"

The next stage of my relationship with Kitty Garnett is told with more reluctance. It requires reviewing a phase of my life in which failure, regret, and shame are the painfully dominant emotions, even after many decades.

It seems strange to me now as I search for the words to tell it honestly that it really started much earlier than even I had imagined.

It really started on the playground of James Madison School, known then as James Madison Grammar School. Located on the corner of 38th Street and Hampton Boulevard, it was the educational center of Lambert's Point. My church was located one block West on 38th Street.

I walked to school with older children along Hampton Boulevard from 47th Street.

There were not many photographs of me as a child, although I remember one taken by Ms. Gray, my kind and gentle second grade teacher.

The photographs of each child in our second grade class taken by Ms. Gray were part of our Mother's Day Gift project.

Each photograph was glued to colorful construction paper shaped into a greeting card with an appropriate note for Mother's Day.

Forensic experts, interpreting my photograph at seven years of age, would likely have correctly described me as thin, passive, lacking strength, compliant, and threat-sensitive.

Is he a "momma's boy," they would ponder, with unkempt longish hair inauthentically styled to appear "curly," (my mother's wish), in a word, not likely to be athletic.

Should a legal question arise today regarding my past athletic ability, it would be the judgment of the court that "his accomplishments in athletics exceeded expectations but were at best modest."

Should a psychiatrist, however, testify at the same imaginary trial, he would state that "his courage in overcoming his fears sufficed on the "fields of friendly strife," and at other times it failed him."

In short, I was the object of, at times, unmerciful teasing.

When sides were chosen to compete in games, I was last or next to last chosen.

As mentioned earlier, "Keep Away," was a sport I played every day in the 6th and 7th grades at Madison. It surprises me today, looking back, how significant it must have been earlier in my life.

"Keep Away" combined English Rugby and American Football.

There were no goal posts. We all ran randomly.

The player with the ball literally ran away with the ball.

The objectives of "Keep Away" were not to get smashed, tackled, or simply lose the ball to other thieving players.

I ran the fastest, likely out of fear, and kept the ball the longest.

When lined up for gym classes to sprint 50 yards, surprising to others and to myself, I ran the fastest.

In the seventh grade, Mr. Sullivan, Principal and basketball coach, asked me to try out for the James Madison Basketball Team. I declined even though I was tall for my age and fast, but, sadly, I knew nothing about basketball. I needed to hide my ignorance, too easily embarrassed.

The City of Norfolk's Recreation Bureau operated a Community Center in the basement of James Madison Elementary School, an ingenious conception of Paul Decker, and later, J.T. Shellnut.

In this Oasis in the Desert of Lamberts Point, photographs of football, baseball, and basketball players lined the basement walls.

Bowling lanes were busily occupied.

Boxing matches were held Friday nights.

Equipment was readily available for all sports, and the salient features of each game were highlighted in the Norfolk Ledger Dispatch and the Virginian Pilot newspapers.

I played three sports in the league sponsored by the Recreation Department ("Bureau" was dropped along the way).

The most memorable of these teams was the Lamberts Point Rangers. We lost every game during our first season. I ran, passed, and kicked to no avail, but in 1946, coached by Chuck Collins, we were undefeated, untied, and unscored upon.

The Lambert's Point Rangers played an exhibition game during a special event at Foreman Field, under the lights. The Maury High School football coach came up to me after the game. "Why did you not try out for our team?" he demanded.

"I did try out for the Maury High School football team, Sir," I respectfully replied. "You said I was too small."

The coach, slightly smiling and slightly chagrined said, "You are not too small now, Bobby Brown. Show up for practice on August 25th... and don't be late."

The coach smiled as he walked off the field.

My years as a running back for the Maury Commodores were exciting and successful for the most part.

Football became an organizing influence in my life. It was almost as powerful as the influence of Burrows Memorial Baptist Church where I received a good Christian education from dedicated teachers.

Mrs. Clyburn was Chairman of the Sunday School Junior Department. I was a young adolescent under her tutelage at Burrows Church. Kenneth E. Burke, a quiet, scholarly person, was my pastor.

Every summer I worked closely with Bus Male at Camp Greenbrier. He talked to Art Guepe, Head Football coach at the University, and worked out the details for me to come to Virginia to try out for football.

The Virginia football team lived in the "football house," 504 Rugby Road, Charlottesville. The team also ate at the University Cafeteria on Main Street, an easy walking-distance from the "football house."

My "scholarship" gave me a bed in a room in the "football house," tuition paid for by a DuPont Scholarship, and a part-time job at Charlottesville Motors waxing new cars.

I would be looked at by Art Guepe and his twin brother, an assistant coach, at spring practice, March 1950.

Virginia had good football teams in the late 1940s and early 1950s. Returning WWII Veterans, taking advantage of the G.I. Bill, provided highly talented, strong and large players.

Johnny Papit, our All American Fullback, I can tell you, ran powerfully. Tom Scott, our All American as an end in football, was also an All American in Lacrosse.

Bob Pate and Bob Tata, both young players, proved to be superb running backs.

Rock Weir was well named and was immovable as a lineman. Tank Johnson stopped every play that was attempted over his position as tackle. What a privilege to be associated with these fine, talented men!

Graduating from Maury High School on a January Friday night and registering for classes at Virginia on the following Monday morning was challenging.

Another, even greater challenge, however, was leaving my home. On the same day, I went from my modest home in Lamberts Point to 504 Rugby Road. Using a line from my friend, Dennis Womack, I went from the outhouse to the penthouse, from a poor neighborhood to a good address.

It also reminds me of the then popular University drinking song, "From Rugby Road to Vinegar Hill I'm going to get drunk tonight."

"Vinegar Hill" was Charlottesville's Lambert's Point.

For the record, I did not drink.

I also remind the reader, as I mentioned earlier, that my departure from Lamberts Point was an event calling for prayer by my mother on bended knees in our small living room.

When Nick Wilson, III, and his friends delivered me to the "football house," night had already fallen and the January temperature had dropped.

As planned, I phoned Bus Male. He arrived shortly after I called, met me at the football house, and made sure I had a cot with bedding. Mine was the fourth cot in the room, near the window on the far left side of the room.

I was the new kid on the block in the "football house." I was among men whose proven athletic skills had already earned them a solid sociocultural position of strength.

Bus Male introduced me around the house and, being a man of few words, he left suddenly.

I won't recount all of the reasons that I was frequently heard to say, "That ain't right."

It became reflexive and, I think, largely unconscious. At any rate, it earned me the name in the house and on the field, of "Deacon Brown."

For short, I was soon known by the team as "Deac."

Football Spring Practice at Virginia in 1950 started on a cold, cloudy day in March.

Our locker rooms and equipment room were located in Memorial Gym. The football managers, not ever having known me or known about me, reluctantly, it seemed to me, gave me pads and a practice uniform.

"Do you have a locker, Deacon Brown?" a scruffy, older man inquired from behind a counter.

He already knew the answer to his question, assigned me a locker and gave me a key.

It felt good, once again, to be in uniform.

"I'm Charlie Harding," a tall young man with dark hair, a quarterback, said to me. "Would you like to snag a few passes?"

We walked out of Memorial Gym, around the reflection pool, across the street through a tunnel that took us under the railroad tracks to the football practice field.

"Just run out 15 or 20 yards and look to your left," Charlie instructed.

Like a feather, the perfectly thrown football met my fingertips as I kept running and it stuck like glue.

What a great feeling!

Over and over, Charlie Harding threw perfect passes.

Unfortunately, only a few players had made it to the practice field. No coaches had arrived.

Our stellar performance remained unwitnessed by those who judge talent.

Of course, I knew nothing about the Virginia offensive play book, but I wanted to show the coaches that I could run the ball.

"That's the best of broken field running I have seen," said Maury assistant football coach, Jim Hoffman, describing the way I returned a punt at Blair Field just a few months earlier.

Coach Hoffman, a former football standout at Virginia Tech, paid compliments sparsely, if not begrudgingly.

But it was not going to happen.

I was not going to show the coaches how well I could run the ball, my strength, my favorite part of the game.

I had less skill in defense and even less interest, unless it was pass defense from the position of "safety."

Art Guepe was putting his first string offense team through their courses. With some disinterest I watched, standing with a group of players near the side lines.

Suddenly, Coach Guepe yelled, "Brown, go in at safety."

At first, it caught me off guard.

I was pleased Coach Guepe remembered my name, but I wanted to run the ball.

"I said, Brown, go in at safety," the coach unhappily repeated himself.

It sounded reasonable to me. It was a position I played at Maury when the same players who played offense remained on the field to also play defense.

I felt that playing safety with 10 strong defensive players in front of me was going to be something I could readily manage.

But I was wrong.

Johnny Papit broke through the line and through the secondary like a bolt of lightning.

The goal post was to my back.

No one stood between me and the All American Fullback.

He was running low and fast towards me, much faster and much stronger than I had estimated.

We met in a clashing moment.

With my eyes closed, my arms reached around his thighs.

Instantly I was on my back, a kind of human mat on which Johnny Papit continued his journey to the goal line.

Johnny Papit trotted back toward me.

With encouragement in his deep voice, he said, "Good job, Deac. You made me fumble the ball."

To my surprised face, he said, "I mean it, Deac, you made me drop the ball after you hit me."

I really appreciated Johnny Papit's endeavor to be kind to me, but for the record, the All American hit me, not the reverse.

For the rest of spring practice, I stood in line to receive passes and to run laps.

Coach Guepe had given me the chance and I had failed it.

I tried to look like a football player at the University of Virginia, but something had been knocked out of my confidence.

The following summer I worked out with several good college football players at Camp Greenbrier.

Rufus Barkley, son of the Vice President of the United States, was a strong quarterback for Virginia. He threw me passes at camp. Bill Wade, a gifted quarterback for Vanderbilt, reassured me, as we worked out all summer at Camp Greenbrier.

Bill Wade nicknamed me "Thumper" because I tended to pound the ground vigorously when I ran fast. Later, Bill Wade would become the star quarterback of the Chicago Bears.

In the fall, I returned for the pre-season football practice. I found it to be very time consuming and it interfered with afternoon Chemistry Lab.

I met with Bus Male and told him I was quitting football.

Bus Male asked me to make no rash decision, to mull it over, and "talk to your academic advisor."

Bus had gone out on a limb for me, but I let him down.

I quietly moved out of the football house, feeling like a failure.

It is a decision I regretted for years.

The regret was worse on Saturday afternoons in Scott Stadium where I watched the game from the stands. I never actually played in a game for Virginia.

This was the first time I let Kitty Garnett down.

She never brought up the subject, though I worked closely with her at Camp Greenbrier for the next four years.

To be honest, Kitty Garnett had never said she wanted me to play football at Virginia.

Inexplicably, I always believed it was a part of the assumptions upon which Kitty Garnett built her increasing confidence in me.

"Disappointing Kitty Garnett a second time"

The second time I disappointed Kitty Garnett, even more painfully than the first disappointment, involves my life-long dream to be a physician.

I was able to graduate from Virginia in three and a half years with a BA Degree in Biology.

I made many wonderful friends at the University. With some of those friends I remain in close contact today.

In my senior year, I made the Dean's List of Distinguished Students, an academic honor.

I was blessed with a number of good part-time jobs in college. Working as a Dorm Counselor in Echols House for two years provided free housing.

I was a lab assistant in Biology for two years, working closely with Dee Runk, a remarkable man destined to become Dean of Students at the University.

A Florence Smith Scholarship from the Norfolk Foundation, now called Hampton Roads Foundation, guaranteed my major expenses in medical school.

During my second semester in medical school, I would leave notes for my bride: "Playing tennis. See you later. Love, Bobby," was typical of the notes I would leave for Dottie.

Dottie would find my notes when she returned to our house from her job as a bank teller in downtown Charlottesville.

The activity referred to in the notes I left for Dottie in our rented house alternated between tennis, golf, touch football, and handball.

I found a host of nonacademic pursuits to fill the afternoons for which no medical school classes were scheduled. Regrettably, those afternoons would have been better spent studying in the Medical School Library during my first year of medical school.

The reigning attitude I had during that period of my life was based upon my misguided, fallacious belief that I could pay close attention in class, skim the texts, and pass the tests by last minute cramming.

Of course, my scholastic method did not and should not have succeeded.

It is actually painful to believe now that I could have been so cavalier about the precious privilege to study medicine.

During the summer of 1954, Dottie and I lived with her parents at 450 Brickby Road, Norfolk, Virginia.

I was hired by the Norfolk Department of Recreation as a 1954 summer employee. I was a "Playground Instructor" at Willard School. Neighborhood children gathered daily at the school for supervised recreation, competitive sports, and craft activities. In a word, I was paid to enjoy the things I loved.

The phone call from Dr. Oscar Thorup, Assistant Dean for Academic Affairs, School of Medicine at the University, was made to my home on 39th Street, my address during the second decade of my life.

Dean Thorup, in my absence, spoke on the phone to my mother.

I shudder now. How horrible it must have been for my mother to bear the "bad news" alone. Even a "prayer warrior" has feelings.

The image of Daniel in the fiery furnace comes to mind. My mother would have unhesitatingly stepped in the blazing incinerator, taking my place.

A very sad irony at that moment was taking place. Her son was playing tennis at City Park in Norfolk, unavailable to the messenger of "bad news" from the University.

Fitful hours passed before I received the message from my mother.

"Bobby," mother said, "have you done something bad? The dean at the University wants you to call him right away. He said it was bad news.

"I told him you were a good boy and had never done anything really bad.

"He said he will only discuss it with you.

"Do you know what he may be referring to, son?"

I tried to console my mother.

I had done nothing bad.

"The School of Medicine's Committee on Academic Standing has denied your promotion to the second year, Mr. Brown." Dean Thorup sounded decisive, devoid of feeling as we spoke on the phone.

"You have the right to petition the committee, but I need to advise you that the committee is not likely to change its decision," Dean Thorup continued.

Dean Thorup granted my request to meet with him in Charlottesville the following day.

My anxiety worsened as I drove alone on State Route 250 West at 55 MPH. Nearing Charlottesville, my acute gastric distress was urgently relieved at a combined country store and filling station.

"That's where I stopped on my way to see Dean Thorup in June 1954. Will I ever forget that stop, I voicelessly ask myself. What a powerfully sustained infliction of my most sentimental journey."

"Mr. Brown, you are asking for a second chance. So many people are begging for their first chance to study medicine. Why do you think you deserve a second chance?" the dean drilled me.

Every explanation I humbly offered for a second chance was rejected by Dean Thorup.

"Believe me, Mr. Brown, I hear stories worse than yours, even from some of your own class mates, but they satisfactorily met all the academic requirements.

Based on my experience in this office, I have reached an important conclusion.

The difference between people is not their problems.

The difference between people is the way they handle their problems."

I felt ashamed.

I cried.

I shook hands with the dean and left his office.

My written petition to the Committee on Academic Standing was rejected.

Many, many years later, my son, Bob, Jr., was flourishing in the University's School of Medicine when he was approached by Dr. Thomas Hunter.

Dr. Hunter was the distinguished Dean of the School of Medicine during my brief tenure.

"Bob," said Dr. Hunter, "your father must have been very angry with me and Dr. Thorup when he failed out of medical school."

"I can honestly say, Dr. Hunter," replied my son, "that in all my life, I never heard my father express any angry feelings toward you or Dr. Thorup."

My mother lived another 17 years, long enough to know that I graduated from the School of Medicine, not in Class of 1957 but in the Class of 1967.

If Kitty Garnett regretted the investment of herself into the life of one of her students from Maury High School, she never conveyed it to me.

If the fortunate high school student whose life was magnificently formed by Kitty Garnett ever forgets her, he is to be pitied.

12

WAR ON SELF

Tuesday Morning Post-Deployment Psychotherapy Group

These Soldiers all speak the same language. They all know the wretchedness of terrorism.

Unfortunately, they don't all come home.

Few return unchanged.

Many Soldiers come home as "strangers" in their own home. They come home to a home that is changed.

Even home feels unsafe.

Group therapy provides a safe place for Soldiers.

The Tuesday Morning Group is one of six groups I lead at our MTF (Military Treatment Facility). The groups I lead are limited to Soldiers returning from combat deployment.

Each Soldier must first undergo a diagnostic evaluation by a Behavioral Health provider. Our providers include psychiatrists, clinical psychologists, physician assistants, psychiatric nurse practitioners, and licensed clinical social workers.

Soldiers who are considered likely to benefit from group therapy are offered an opportunity to join one or more groups.

Eligible Soldiers may choose between one of four Combat Stress Control Groups, of which the Tuesday Morning Group is an example. The principal objective of this type of group is to rediscover the sense of security and the strength of trust that develops from becoming re-attached to fellow combat Soldiers.

Specifically focused groups are also available at our MTF. The specifically focused groups include the Traumatic Grief Group, the Spiritual Domain Group, the Dream Interpretation Group and the Cognitive Behavioral Therapy (CBT) for Depression Group.

Anger Management Groups and Healthy Thinking Groups are led by other providers in our clinic.

Each psychotherapy group lasts 90 minutes.

The rule of confidentiality is inviolate: what is revealed in group must not be repeated outside the group.

Each group member also has an individual therapist.

The groups are technically called "open" and "process" groups.

In non-technical terms, new members may be added to the group as openings become available. Group process generally refers to what happens in the relationships between and among group participants.

Soldiers already socialized to educational groups used in military training and operations still find it initially difficult to disclose their emotional symptoms in therapy groups. Once Soldiers are comfortable in group therapy, however, they often sing its praises.

Soldiers who remain in our area who are medically discharged or retired may continue to participate in group therapy.

One member of the Tuesday Morning Group said, "Tuesday is the only day of the week that I go out of my house."

"I don't know, man. This is upsetting the Hell out of me"

SFC Gene Irving, a 42-year-old, married, fair-skinned African-American Soldier, works at the VA in a nearby city. He cannot regularly attend the Tuesday group because of work requirements. When he attends, the group expresses its admiration and respect for him.

SFC Irving is an intelligent, articulate, masculine, extraverted man of medium frame and an engaging smile. He is a most friendly, "take-charge" person.

SFC Irving, referred to as Gene, said, "I stayed busy to not face what we all have in our stomach.

I was a Combat Medic with an Infantry unit in Iraq. I saw the effects of combat every day.

I never said before that I was afraid.

Everybody is always running away from where we are running towards as medics. I'd get the truck ready and I'd do it again.

I retired 5 years ago...then my father died. My thought...let's get finished with this one and do the next one...it is not fair.

Then my wife's aunt died...same thing...no feelings, just get her buried and move on.

I haven't opened up here because I am afraid of opening old wounds...coming here off and on...acting like a therapist...never taking the patient's role."

SGM Hall (Sergeant Major), stocky, mid-forties, guilt-ridden over the deaths of Soldiers he hand-picked as his PSF (Personal Security Force), responded to Gene, saying, "You can't cover over excrement but so long."

MAJ Jake Kelly, depressed, 32-year-old-married father of two young children, said, "My father died, too...after I redeployed. I can identify with what you are saying. I did not grieve, either."

Gene: "I was a senior leader. We can't let troops see our feelings. I had 31 guys under me...all depending on me. How can you show them your emotions?

What we did affected us emotionally.

SWAs (Soldiers Wounded in Action) came to me in all conditions...legs blown off and placed beside them in the litter up here where the arms are...headless bodies."

The group never wants to hear the vivid, disturbing details of combat injuries and death. The silence was like sitting in a wake.

"I don't want anybody to see my emotions"

"Nobody expected what we saw," continued Gene.

"It is not normal to see what we saw."

"Gene, what is haunting you?" I asked quietly.

SGM (Sergeant Major) Sheldon McInnis, the NCO (Noncommissioned Officer) with a Ranger patch and alcohol issues, said, "A lot of times, I feel like the man who stuck his face in the cardboard cutout. You know, like the ones you have your photograph taken in. It could be a cowboy or whatever.

I don't want anybody to see my emotions. I don't want them to see the real me."

SFC Tommy Kennedy, a Forward Sniper, obsessed with devastating trauma, said, "I love Gene like a brother, but Gene, you are dancing around Doc Brown's question with generalities.

You are not answering the question.

What's haunting you?"

MSG (Master Sergeant) Michael Yoder, a perceptive and equally sensitive Soldier, said, "Gene has to chew that slowly, Tommy."

Gene is one of Michael's few friends, but Michael was unfamiliar with Gene's trauma. Michael's legs started moving up and down quickly. In an instant he was hyperventilating. He was visibly ill-at-ease.

Michael said, "I don't know, man. This is upsetting the Hell out of me."

Michael turned his head away from the group. Suddenly, he stood up.

Michael said, "I have to get out of here and walk in the hallway. I don't know. Let me come back."

Michael has a special relationship with Gene. Michael was becoming extremely uncomfortable by Gene's disclosures, saying things previously unknown to Michael.

They are close friends. I remember when Gene brought Michael to the group. "This is a good man, Dr. Brown. He needs your help, but he's afraid of coming in for treatment." It was several years ago. Then Gene left after introducing Michael to the group. Michael stayed and Gene just recently returned.

Their roles were reversed now. Michael was witnessing his friend's suffering.

Gene had brought Michael to the door of the group, but he had not entered the door himself. Gene had not taken off his own mask.

Michael did not know what he might see if Gene took off his disguise.

Michael did not know whether he could deal with Gene's painful revelation.

I credit Michael for his courage. He did not leave. He did not walk the hall way outside the group.

Michael sat back down.

The group tension lessened.

"Failure, that's what I have a problem with"

Gene spoke. "The only time I felt safe in Iraq was at 0200 in my concrete room."

Gene was finally going to answer my question, "What's haunting you, Gene?"

"Todd died right in my hands while I was performing CPR.

Another medic was giving the rescue breathing and I pressed on his chest to get his heart beating. It was two-man CPR.

Todd had been shot in the head.

The last time I pushed on his chest, brain matter burst out of the bullet hole.

Todd died in my hands.

I kind of feel responsible for his death. Did he die by my hands? We witness human fatality. We take responsibility for that life being gone.

Failure, that's what I have problems with."

The other members of the group sat in silence.

They could barely crack the door of their own emotional closet.

The vault, constructed of psychological concrete, in which they have secured their sense of suffering and the sensitivity to the suffering of others can only be opened when they recall their own combination.

The group members were all in one accord.

The group members joined together in one cacophony of screaming silence.

Feeling helpless in the presence of Gene's suffering, the group suffered with him. No facial expression or slumped posture could express greater anguish. It was the pictures of passengers waiting their flight having been told their plane had tragically crashed.

They were witnesses, not judges. Their witness could not have been more honest if swearing on a Bible.

"I put my hands on him"

"Gene, what happened right after Todd died?" I asked.

"The Colonel and the Sergeant Major left."

"What did you do, Gene?"

"I stayed with Todd."

"What did you do, alone there with Todd?" I asked.

Barely above a whisper, I thought I heard Gene say, "I put my hands on him."

"You put your hands on Todd?" I asked

Gene said, "Yes, I put my hands on him.

I thought about his wife and his kids and how we took photographs in Killeen, Texas, before we left just in case we didn't come back."

Gene suddenly burst into tears, covering his face with both hands like a person helplessly ashamed.

"I prayed for him. He was one of the nicest men I ever knew, a wonderful senior leader."

The group silence that followed was healing.

I wanted it to last.

SGM Hall broke the silence. "How do senior leaders heal?

They don't heal!" SGM Hall was answering his own question.

"When senior leaders stop being responsible, then the Army fails.

When I selected my team before my last deployment, I got SGM Mack Austin because he was the best combat medic. He was the best at what he did.

You get to a point where you are no longer afraid to die.

At one point, I believed the only way to show respect for the men who died is to die myself."

SGM McInnis said, "The fear of dying kept me going…but I didn't show it…until I was alone.

I would get so tired, but I didn't show it. I internalized it."

MAJ Patrick Kelly said, "I went numb."

SGT Tom Quincy, blown 25 feet into the air when his HUMVEE struck an IED in Iraq, said, "I owe my leg to a medic.

He stopped the bleeding when an IED blew me up and out of my vehicle.

The medic reacted really quickly.

I would have bled to death without the medic."

Gene said, "Yes, but we were trained to save lives. The medic who saved your leg did his job. I didn't do my job. I didn't save Todd's life."

"I watched MAJ Brown dying on the ground"

SFC Charles Lawson, quiet, introverted, serious-minded, married Soldier, spoke solemnly. "I watched MAJ Brown dying on the ground.

Dirt was all over him.

He did not look like the person I knew.

You lose something over there.

He died like a highly offensive, rejected dog." I could almost hear unintended growling among the group.

"I lost something. Maybe I am looking for what I lost over there."

The group's sadness was quickly changed to anger and resentment.

The suddenness of the transition from deep, helpless sadness to patent anger puzzled me. Then unexpectedly I realized this pattern characterizes their interpersonal relationships.

Sadness means helplessness. Soldiers cannot feel helpless. Anger means strength. Soldiers do not feel helpless when angry. When all else fails, Soldiers take charge with anger.

SSG Jim Morgan, soon to leave the group for deployment to Korea, a quiet, reflective man, said, "I don't think you ever get back the something you lost over there."

"You will get it back…that is what this group is all about," I said. "What you invested for your country you will get back with richly deserved dividends."

Unimpressed, SFC Lawson said, "It is like an annoying little brother, always picking at you.

That's what haunts me. At home I have these unwanted, annoying thoughts.

Why do I feel this way at home?

What is the purpose of life…to what end?"

Michael was calm now. Sitting quietly in his seat, he said, "We all have a purpose. Your purpose might be to be here for me."

Gene, no longer crying but looking sad, said, "I never feel like I did enough."

SFC Morgan said, "Like a lot of things took my innocence from me. They snatched a piece of my belief over there."

MSG Norris: "When does all this come to an end?"

Like the immediate action of a reflex, I said what I deeply believe. With the confidence of a commander, I said, "All this ends when you determine to make a new beginning."

The hands of the large satellite clock above the door, easily visible to the group members, rested on 1130.

I stood up. This emotionally powerful Post-Deployment Tuesday Morning Group ended.

I wanted it to end on a feeling of hope.

"Have a good week, men," I said smiling.

Gene walked over to me and extended his hand. A broad smile, the teeth-showing kind of smile, prominently adorned his face. A beautifully decorated Christmas tree with bright lights and a Soldier suit for a child aspiring to serve could not have been more pleasing.

I rejected Gene's hand and hugged him, pulling his strong, large torso tightly to me, rubbing my left hand on his back. Tears filled my eyes.

"Thank you, Dr. Brown," he said.

"Thank you, Gene," I replied.

"You became our leader today, taking those painful first steps we all must take when we honestly address our frailties," I said.

"God Bless you, Gene."

Looking around the room I observed the members of the group hugging each other, quietly chatting.

"Are you coming to Buffalo Wild Wings with us for lunch, Michael," inquired Quincy.

Quincy is affectionately nick-named by the group, utilizing the first letter of a very long and difficult to pronounce Puerto Rican last name.

"I sure am," replied Michael, "and I am bringing Gene with me."

Buffalo Wild Wings had been comprehensively investigated months earlier by Tommy Kennedy, a former forward sniper, and BWW was found to be "safe." It had become a favorite lunch destination for the group.

I am unaware of any other restaurant nearby that had passed the safety test.

Two years ago, the Department of Behavioral Health moved out of its temporary quarters in a trailer unit into our present location on the third floor of an attractive brick building.

Unknown to our staff, Tommy made a number of independent recognizance missions into our new headquarters, looking for escape routes and areas vulnerable to enemy attacks.

His role of group hero soared even higher when he reported that he had toured the building from the basement to its roof, inspected hallways, rooms, outside and inside features of construction and deemed the building safe.

Carrying two clip-boards, I walked alone down the long hall way to my office. One clip-board was used as a sign-in roster. The other bore the notes I hastily recorded during the Tuesday Morning Group.

This is the same hall way envisioned as a safe haven by Michael only an hour earlier.

Unless a Soldier needs something from me after the group session ends, I like to sit quietly alone in my office, reflecting on the group discussion.

I try to understand the truth and honesty revealed by the Tuesday Morning Group.

What are these Soldiers teaching me? What can I learn from them that will prepare me to help other Soldiers?

The non-judgmental attachment, mutual respect, and positive regard that characterize this group are healing and precious.

Dear reader, I don't know whether you have ever had an emotional, cognitive, and spiritual encounter you wanted to savor, appreciate, and treasure.

I'm talking about an experience so uniquely genuine and real that you never wanted to forget it.

I'm talking about a sudden consciousness that burst into your awareness as a profound realization that there is no place in the world you would rather be right now than where you are.

This is precisely the feeling and the thought I had with the Tuesday Morning Post-Deployment Group.

For most of us, having such a transcendent, transforming experience on one occasion alone would be abundantly ample. However, the phenomenon I labor to describe is not at all too infrequent as a valuable reward that comes from the privilege of caring for Soldiers.

It is not something I seek. It occurs unexpectedly. It is like meeting Dottie for the first time, winning a football game that looked lost 2 minutes earlier, or getting a second chance to study medicine.

It is an occurrence that arises when I am being permitted to enter into the suffering of Soldiers.

It happens when some of their suffering is lessening.

It happens when a cherished understanding is being born.

It happens when their unsurpassed sense of peaceful safety of coming home is, at last, realized and is shared, even if it is fleeting at first.

Tuesday Morning Group Meets again

"Where do I fit in?"

SGM (Sergeant Major) Hall is soon to retire after 25 years as a Soldier. He has risen from obscurity to prominent senior military leadership, overcoming obstacles all too familiar to minorities.

He is a man of medium frame, muscular, prone to smile, generally quiet and self-conscious.

He spoke in philosophic terms to his fellow group members, all refined by combat.

"I wrestle with a question.

Where do I fit in?

We always want to feel like we have some worth.

I saw a bumper sticker. It reminded me of myself, 'Going from Hero to Zero.'

I plan my day by the weather report.

I know there is a storm heading this way today by noon.

I have to be home by noon before the thunder starts.

I can't stand the sound of thunder.

It sounds too much like Mortar attacks.

My personal security vehicle was hit by Mortars in Iraq.

My men were injured and killed by Mortars.

They were my security team.
It was like in slow motion.
I called for help.
I couldn't get anyone on the radio.
It was so real...so terrible.
I had chosen each of my men personally.
I knew them well.
I knew their families.

None of them would have been in combat except by my special request.

I had a feeling of horrendous responsibility.

Thunder...loud thunder brings it all back."

The group, attentive and understanding, remained silent.

Undeniably, in Sergeant Major Hall's voice, there was strong but unexpressed anger.

SFC Morgan, picking up on the unexpressed anger, said, "I want nothing to do with the Army. When I get out, I will leave it all behind me.

I will not go to my retirement ceremony. The only reason I would have gone was to please my mother.

My mother is dead now.

I am not going."

Last week when confessing to the group that his friend Todd died in his hands because he had "not done enough," Gene wept in his hands, hiding his face in shame.

Today, Gene was feeling better. He opposed the 2 previous speakers.

Gene said, "I've been retired five years, gone from job to job, made good money, but I'd give anything to have my old Army office back. I'd give anything for it now."

"I don't fit in any more"

SGM Hall said, "I went back to the pond where I fished as a child.

A lady came out and asked me what I thought I was doing.

I told her who I was.

I told her that I fished there as a child.

'You can fish here today but don't come back.

The only reason I'm letting you fish here today is because I know your father,' she said.

I went to another fishing hole in my home county.

Same thing.

The man said, 'You can fish here today because I know your brother. Don't come back.'

I don't fit in any more."

Michael: "In the Army you had rank, recognition, and what you said meant something.

Now you are retired and you are a nobody.

Add that to PTSD and it equals zero."

I could sense the combined feelings of rejection and anger in the group, both justified, painful emotions.

"Gentlemen," I said, "this is the heart of the matter. If these fishing-hole-owners knew SGM Hall's father and brother, they knew the SGM had served his country in war and spent most of his life in the Army.

What does that tell you about our country?" I asked.

"Are Americans only giving lip-service to how much they support the troops?" I asked.

"If the answer is mostly in the affirmative, I believe it is because our country does not know what you are sharing with me about the psychological cost of 21st Century War.

Every person who reads <u>Sacred Ground</u> will attend your Tuesday Morning Group sessions, hear your stories and respect you just as I do."

No one said it out loud, but they all said to themselves, "I'm from Missouri, Dr. Brown. You will have to show me that what you say will happen."

Quincy broke the silence, "I miss the Army.

I was medically retired after I was injured."

CWO (Chief Warrant Officer) Donald Winston is a retired Soldier. He is a tall, out-spoken man, now in his late 50's. He visits the group less frequently because he moved to another state. The Chief said, "I live at the beach now.

I meet somebody and they want to know where I live and what I do.

I do nothing much.

I used to be in the Army

I was in the Army forty years.

All my friends now are people who used to be in the Army or had had trauma in their life.

I miss the Army. Most of all, I miss the group."

More on the loss of the sense of self

One of the major losses from the trauma of combating terrorists in Iraq and Afghanistan is the loss of the pre-traumatic self, the person before combat deployment. It was the major topic in another Tuesday Morning Group session.

That group therapy session is reported below largely in the words of our Soldiers.

"Who am I now after combat?

My personhood is most difficult to describe.

It is the essential part of me by which others I love and trust know me.

They tell me I have changed. I infer that the change is undesirable.

In contrast to those who best know 'me,' the me that I know, the me that went to sleep last night and woke up this morning, is fundamentally the same me.

I have undergone some changes, but I am far less aware of myself as a changed person.

Am I happy or pleased with myself?

I am absolutely displeased with myself.

I am too occupied with perceived dangers around me to have the luxury of considering my nature, my being, myself."

Crime scene investigations have demonstrated the importance of DNA in identification of suspects.

Some would argue that the changes observed in Soldiers returning from battling terrorism in Iraq and Afghanistan is of the magnitude of an alteration of DNA, a psychological mutation, a potentially lasting adverse effect.

I do not hold this view.

My experience with these brave Soldiers convinces me that they have been refined in the hottest furnaces.

In Biblical terms, like refined gold, the dross has been destroyed. Like shining pure gold, their value to our nation, to their family, and to themselves is unequalled.

SFC Gene Irving said, "Power is what is lost.

When I lost a Soldier as a medic, I lost some of the power of my self-confidence.

These Soldiers retiring are losing power, too.

Soldiers come into the Army from everywhere and are made into one. When they reach E-5 (Sergeant) and above, they are given power for the first time in their life.

As a medic, I saw death, lots of death. Talk about death, this is real. I knew him so well, Todd.

Like I said earlier, the Army takes photographs before a Soldier is deployed. It is the last thing we did before we got on the plane.

The photographs are used by the Army for identification if you are killed.

We are lined up for the photo-id.

We stand in front of the American flag for the photograph.

It is just the torso.

These photographs are also used at the Memorial Service."

MSG Eddie Olsen (just arrived): "I had the worst panic attack of my life."

Eddie, chronically anxious, socially awkward, divorced and devoted to his 2 children, indifferent to the group's attention to other matters, goes around the room shaking hands with each fellow group member.

"It happened just all of a sudden, at the VA.

I had tunnel vision.

It was like looking down on yourself.

Who is watching me?

I couldn't sit still and fill out the survey.

I must have made 50 to 100 movements in my chair in the lobby."

"What were you afraid of at the VA?" I asked calmly.

Gene said, "The anxiety comes from being judged."

SFC Cecil Upton, a large, masculine dark skinned Soldier with a deep voice, said, "I am a conversationalist and I don't know what to say."

Gene observed, "Our integrity is being questioned.

I don't want to tell my story again.

Being judged by strangers in a new group makes us all anxious.

We went through a stage of hiding symptoms.

A stage of wearing shades.

The age of the provider makes a difference.

The provider doesn't listen at the VA.

They are trying to prove what it wasn't.

Being judged causes anger."

The consensus of the Tuesday Morning Group today is simply stated:

"Our expectations are not being met at the VA now. We are told on TV they want to take care of us but we are not getting the help we need."

"Why are you anxious when you go shopping?" I asked.

Eddie: "Crowds are not safe.

Seeing a Middle Eastern person in the store infuriates me."

Gene: "In the past, before combat, if a woman looked at me, I would think she likes me.

Now, after deployment, I think she is wondering what's wrong with me.

In public, our awareness is increased."

Eddie: "I hate driving now, but I used to love to drive.

I acted strange in the car because someone had left a large white trash bag on the road.

My son, just an eight-year-old kid, said, 'Why are you acting strange, Daddy?'"

Gene: "Before deployment I was afraid of dying; but now that I am back, I afraid of living."

Theme: "I am different"

Looking around the group, I said, "How are you different and how do you experience that you are different?"

SSG Barry Vinson said, "Family members look at me different now."

There was 100% agreement among the Wednesday Morning Group regarding these statements:

"We are all in the military or we have recently retired.

A lot of people look at us different because of some of the things we might have done or seen done during deployment.

They wonder why we are not talking to them.

Men are worse than women in the way they look at us.

They don't know how to talk to us.

They are scared of us.

There is a problem with people who know I have been there (combat).

They treat me different.

They don't want to set me off.

Our situation puts a lot of pressure on family members."

SFC Rob Lacey said, "We got spit on coming back home at Langley.

It may be part of that group that pickets military funerals, the ones the Supreme Court said it was okay for them to do it.

It is a small group, but it seems like they are everywhere.

I blame the media. They were nice in the beginning because they wanted to be embedded with us, but now they only print negative things about the military."

SSG Allen Burch, easily annoyed, a married Soldier soon to medically retire with both physical and psychological issues said, "I kind of like it because people leave me the Hell alone."

SGT Harry Robertson, a thin, blond-headed medic with kind blue eyes, said, "But my wife wants me to do stuff with her.

When I don't want to do it, she calls me 'sick.'

My daughter tells her not to do it.

I am not really sick.

Home is a whole different situation.

I make my own decisions at home.

If I want to be left alone I am left alone.

In the military, I do not have that luxury."

SGT Howard Stewart, a stern, annoyed, anxious Soldier with an unchanging frown, said, "If you go out to eat, people notice your legs moving and that you are scanning."

Harry said, "Shopping can be a problem.

It has to be done, but I can't go shopping if it is busy; I get anxious.

We went out to eat. There was a long line inside and the parking lot was full.

I had to leave.

I had to get out of there fast.

My wife didn't like what I did.

My wife gets upset with me."

Allen: "Little things bother me a lot.

We have a new broom, but my wife uses the old broom. It looks like it was used to sweep rocks.

It drives me crazy every time she uses the old broom."

"That's an easy one, Allen," I said. "You can do the sweeping in your house."

"I hate it when people stare at me and don't speak."

SGT Billy Dawson said, "The Police hate us.

I couldn't sleep so I got up and drove around to relax.

I don't know this area.

I was in town and got lost in one-way streets.

A cop stopped me.

'What are you doing here at 2am?'
I am just riding around.
'You are a liar,' the cop said.
'Give me your operator's permit and registration card!'
He was getting madder with me.
Another cop drove up and said, 'He's military. Let him go.'"

Rob said, "You were on a mission…looking for an escape route."

MSG Keith Johnson said, "Racial thing. Hatred or heritage? The colors in the American flag don't run.

It is ignorance.

Living off the grid may be the best answer for all of us. A simple life. No cell phone or TV or computer.

War is easy. Coming home is Hell."

The Post-traumatic Self

The post-traumatic self replaces the pre-traumatic self in varying degrees, depending upon the severity of the PTSD symptoms.

"Roll call is so sad because part of you is gone.

A piece of me is dead."

To what degree is the posttraumatized self formed by deaths in combat? I wondered.

To what degree is the post-traumatized self influenced by strong but unsuccessful, even heroic efforts to be unaffected by death?

"My grandfather died two weeks ago.

I attended the wake and the funeral.

It was like I was on alert.

I was busy watching other people.

I refused to look at grandfather's body at the family viewing.

I did not look at him during the funeral.

I was just trying to cope.

I was emotionally detached.

It is needed for me to become emotionally detached."

Jose's Grandmother died.

"I went to the funeral, but I didn't bawl like other family members.

She was buried on top of my dad. Just a piece of plywood separates them.

I didn't cry.

I didn't get down like that.

My dad's picture was on the tomb stone.

I cried later… in the shower… alone."

SFC Albert North, 38-year-old, quiet, thoughtful Soldier who no longer has a sense of trust, said, "My mother died in 2004, the day I got back from Iraq.

It was terrible. No one had let me know she was sick.

'We didn't want to burden you because you were away in war,' they said.

At the funeral, it was like I wasn't coherent.

My body was there.

People talked to me, but I was expressionless.

I tried to avoid people.

I was really sweating.

I didn't know what feelings to have.

I just wanted it to be over.

I tried to keep my mind off of it.

Emotional detachment is needed as a Soldier.

You can't show your emotions. It is seen as weakness.

We have to put our feelings to the side.

You still have to go to work every morning.

We are told, 'Be a Soldier and take care of your troops.'

I even take my gun to church.

It ain't real safe anywhere."

The Paradox of the Post-traumatic Self

The post-traumatic self embodies a painful, self-centered, self-interested, nearly emotionless, incomplete being.

The post-traumatic self feels whole only in the presence of Soldiers whose newly formed lives were also created in the furnace of combat trauma, unique to fighting terrorism. No war is free of trauma.

Puzzling to me, however, even after years of treating these brave Soldiers, is the unanimity of their opinion regarding the post-traumatic self, "I like it."

To comprehend the post-traumatic self, it is necessary to examine its essential components separately.

No Soldier enjoys the re-experiencing symptoms of the trauma.

These symptoms may be as real and as disturbing as the actual, original trauma.

The effort and the energy required in blocking the recollection and re-experiencing of these dreadful thoughts is exhausting, emotionally and physically.

No Soldier enjoys the isolation that results from nearly constant attempts to avoid situations reminding them of the combat trauma.

Soldiers don't like feeling numb, the price they pay for avoiding feelings they cannot contain.

Traumatized Soldiers also accept emotional numbness because they fear that the expression of their feelings may be too overwhelming for others to accept.

No Soldier likes the embarrassment following his or her exaggerated startle response.

No Soldier likes their intolerance of "stupidity" or "injustice" orbiting them into anger that too often becomes near-rage.

Traumatized Soldiers would readily rid themselves of sleepless nights and nights wrecked by nightmares.

What, in God's name, about the post-traumatic self might our Soldiers find likeable? This important question is addressed below.

Another Wednesday Morning Post-Deployment Group

What I like about PTSD

The negative components of PTSD, already well known and perhaps too often emphasized, were not listed as a part of this pedagogical exercise. I was pleased and surprised by the following list of the positive aspects of combat-induced PTSD proposed by Soldiers with combat-induced PTSD.

"What I like about PTSD is being fully alert. It is a good feeling. It lets you know you are alive."

"I am more compassionate."

"I am more thankful."

"My sense of smell is better at night. In the dark I can smell anything."

"We are hyper alert to some things, but not in all areas of life."

"I am feeling alive."

"I have more understanding of the suffering of others."

"I have increased feelings of love."

"I have increased feelings of loyalty."

"I more fully appreciate the feelings of attachment."

"I believe I have keener perception."

"I have a stronger sense of trust, once another is found trustworthy."

"I now have a strong sense of the value and importance of my family."

"I have a sharpened sense of awareness that another person cares for me."

"I have a stronger sense of the need to protect those I care for and those who care for me."

Early in my training as a psychiatrist, I was taught to expect and to look for one main reason or explanation when a patient presents a long list of reasons or explanations.

The rationale will be developed in this manuscript but for now let me tell you why many Soldiers "like" having PTSD. **Soldiers like having combat-induced PTSD because they believe and behave as if they will be prepared to protect and defend us when the enemy attacks us here at home!**

Dream Interpretation Group

Ken, 27 years Active Duty, Mortuary Affairs, reported a dream about the group.

He turned to Harry, a younger Soldier, and said, "You were in my dream. I think I dreamt about you because we are in related fields (Mortuary Affairs and Combat Medic)."

Harry said nothing.

Looking serious, Harry turned to me and stared as if to ask, "What do you make of this, Dr. Brown?"

"I agreed with Ken. Both medics and mortuary affairs have the highest prevalence of PTSD," I said.

Addressing Ken, I said "Another reason for dreaming of Harry, Ken, is your wish that your son, a Soldier in Special Operations, was also in a group like this where he could get encouragement and warmth and support."

"You are correct, Sir. I have three sons in the Army, all in Special Ops, and I want the best for them all."

Harry, only one week remaining before he medically retires from the Army because of PTSD and Depression and returns to his wife and children in a faraway state, said he also dreamed about the group.

"But it was like a court room, not the group therapy room. A jury was asking difficult questions. They were wearing funny clothes and strange, square-shaped hats. It was like we were on trial."

Associations by the group to Harry's dream led to the conclusion that "funny clothes and hats" most likely symbolize graduation gowns.

Months ago, Harry asked me about our form of psychotherapy for PTSD.

"Is it just trial and error?"

I reminded him of his question, suggesting that the dream was not about the group being on trial, but rather the therapist and his treatment may still be on trial in Harry's mind.

He did not reply.

He changed the subject, and said, "I'm going home next week and my wife does not understand what's wrong with me."

Harry was again bringing up a subject of importance to him.

We are told in our psychiatric training about the uselessness of taking notes during treatment sessions. "If it is important to the patient, they will remind you. You don't have to remind the patient."

"My wife tells the children I am sick. I do not feel sick. I don't believe I am sick. I tell her not to tell our children that I am sick.

My daughter even told her, 'Dad is not sick.'"

I suggested to the group that expecting one's family or one's friends or one's military unit to understand PTSD is unreasonable.

No one yet really understands PTSD.

It is more prudent to ask others to try to accept PTSD, not to try to understand it.

The implication for psychotherapy of PTSD is the need to emphasize these and related positive attributes achieved at the expense of combat. It may well be the foundation upon which a more stable, stronger, enduring sense of self can be achieved.

The attachments or strong positive bonds formed in combat between Soldiers, "battle bonds," hold the secrets needed to be studied to restore the new version of the former "self."

Awareness of the above positive attributes of PTSD may require a "readiness" that is unique for each Soldier in the same way a child may be said to be ready to learn to read.

Many of the positive attributes listed above, in fact, came from a Soldier who was severely injured by an IED in Iraq.

He went through a divorce and was arrested several times for assault.

After six years of psychiatric treatment, he is now an honor student pursuing a business degree in college.

He is a loving father, and a volunteer coach for Little League soccer and football.

MAJ Kelly, on the other hand, dealing with severe recurrent depression and PTSD, two years into treatment, made the following statements.

"I came back hateful and not close to my family. I don't let people get close to me.

I just feel numb.

My father died and I didn't process it.
I fear closeness. I see it as a lot of extra baggage.
The last time I let people in, they died.
It causes bad dreams of people getting killed and lots of painful emotions.
I want to get close…but more than wanting closeness, I fear it."

Post-traumatic Self Relationship

"I told my new wife that I have problems.
Some days I'll be mad and don't even know why I'm mad, but don't you get angry. Understand you have done nothing wrong. Try not to feel bad.
I've been learning (in church) to be humble and to have self-control.
I feel drained after I get upset.
My wife says to remind myself that there are no bullets flying and nobody is dying. Yesterday is gone. You have today. Try not to be paranoid.
I have the love of and for my brothers (group) and love is stronger than death."
Michael commented on being alone.
"The wife and son went away for the weekend.
I thought I'd loved to be alone, but when I was alone I could not stand it.
I couldn't get myself together.
The dog was there, but I put him in the garage.
I couldn't find anything on the TV.
I was afraid.
The thought behind the fear was, 'I can't be alone.'
There was a battle within.
I felt like I'd cry if someone said anything to me like, 'You'll be okay.'
If I phoned my wife, she could tell in my voice that I was not doing well.

I can't identify the feeling.
I'm so sad.
I felt like a woman in menopause.
I am afraid of crying.
I was afraid that I'd go into a deep depression if I let myself cry."

Another Wednesday Morning Group

"I can't live with my wife."

"This is the most important day of the week for me.

I live from Wednesday to Wednesday. I just feel I can drop my guard here…just be myself…there is no other place where I feel more like myself than in this group."

After each Soldier reported in, their present life issues, problems and accomplishments reviewed, a knock on the door startled Allen.

Allen was seated immediately next to the door, Group Therapy Room One's only entrance or exit.

The other Soldiers formed a semi-circle in their chairs in the large room.

Directly opposite from the door was a wall of bronze colored metal framed windows.

The window blinds were partially closed, keeping out the intense mid-summer heat.

Waiting for no response to the door knock, Lawrence entered.

Lawrence is a 50 year old Soldier, recently medically retired for chronic depression and combat-induced psychiatric problems.

Lawrence was dressed in dark blue knee length shorts and a dark, but slightly lighter shade of blue, T-shirt.

A grim expression emphasized his sharply angular face.

He walked without a purpose into Group Room One.

A multi-colored wash cloth covered the top of his head.

He silently went to each group member, shook his fellow group member's hand, including mine, picked up the sign-in roster attached to a dark brown clip board, printed his name and social security number, and quietly took a seat.

By this time, the multi-colored wash cloth was grasped in his right hand.

He periodically mopped the sweat off his face, brow, and hairless, shining scalp. Oddly, Lawrence nearly always comes late to each group session. This time he arrived after the session was half over. This may explain why he always knocks before coming into the room.

He looked sad, bogged down with worry, and nearly paralyzed by indecision over returning to his wife and high-school-aged son.

"I know now that I cannot live with anyone. I just need to be alone.

My sister has been with me for the past 3 weeks and she bickers and wants to argue all the time.

I can't take it.

I promised my son that I would come home, but I can't.

I can't live with my wife."

A feeling of helplessness spread throughout the group.

No superficial encouragement would help Lawrence.

A modern Ansel Adams could photograph Lawrence as the epitome of despairing, dreadful suffering.

"I took my blood pressure the other day and it was 289 over 198."

I gasped and said, "Lawrence, are you taking blood pressure medication?"

He replied in the affirmative.

"You must see your medical provider today, Lawrence. Are you aware of the negative consequences of such a very high blood pressure?"

He dropped his head.

Staring at the floor, again he replied in the affirmative.

"How do you feel about the possible severe negative consequences of dangerously high blood pressure?" I asked.

"Do you really want me to tell you, Dr. Brown?

I am afraid you will put me in the hospital again if I tell you the truth.

To tell you the truth, I welcome it!"

Ken: "If you die, not from your own hand, you would welcome it?"

Lawrence: "Yes."

Shawn: "Lawrence, I know you read the Bible and pray. Are you a doer of the Word or just a hearer of the Word?"

Lawrence: "I know I am not living by the Word.

Sex is my problem.

I love sex.

Since I was 5 or 6 a little girl pulled up her skirt and I put my… you know…in there and it felt good and I have been hooked on sex ever since then."

Shawn: "We all have that problem, but I have found that by reading the Bible, sitting on the front row of my church every Sunday morning, right in front of the preacher, really helps me.

Look, I could tell you some of the things I've done that are so bad you could not believe me, but God is helping me deal with lust.

I went to a restaurant yesterday and the friendly waitress wanted my phone number, but I did not give it to her because I know where that leads. Sin leads to death."

Rob: "Lawrence, we really care about you.

Think about your son if you died.

Think about all the bad that could come from something happening to you.

I told you about the woman in Germany that I was involved with, but it ended and I am better off for it ending. I believe in God and I believe God can help you if you let him."

Harry: "Your son is a grown man.

You don't have to go back for his sake.

Soon, he will be gone, out on his own.

Come to Michigan with me. You can get a house for $75,000 with 10-15 acres."

Ken: "Something has been missing for the past 2-3 weeks.

We don't end with prayer because the Chaplain is not here...but we don't need the Chaplain...we can pray."

The meeting was over. The men stood up in a circle.

Lawrence prayed sincerely to his "Lord, God," a salutation he enunciated reverently and repeatedly.

Tranquility and love flowed abundantly into the hearts of all of these brave Soldiers...and into the heart of its leader for whom Lawrence most sincerely prayed.

"Lord, God, from the time of his birth you called Dr. Brown to this work. Thank you and bless him."

The Soldier needing help, I pondered, is praying for the person trying to give the help. I was humbled by the sheer honest sincerity of the Soldier, and strengthened by it, though undeserving, I felt.

I saw Lawrence later in the day.

His countenance was lifted from the depths that nearly drowned him in the morning.

With complete assurance, Lawrence said, "God spoke to me today through those men. I heard God when they spoke to me."

Dream Interpretation Group

"Nobody sent me anything in the desert"

Albert reported dreams of "dead relatives...I don't know why I am dreaming of dead relatives...people dead for years...and it bothers me," he said, sadly, while adjusting his cap, and repeatedly removing and replacing his much blackened sun glasses.

"I don't like funerals. I don't go to funerals. Two of my aunts died and I did not go to their funerals. I don't want people to see me break down and cry.

I don't want to be around people...people living or dead.

People ask 20,000 questions.

My father knows me and he forgives me because he understands me.

People will act like they care and say, 'Oh, it is so good to see you. I am so happy you came home safe.' But they don't really care.

Nobody sent me anything in the desert."

At this moment his voice betrayed him. Tell-tale tears, those awkward messengers from the depths of the universally recognized aching heart.

With both hands, he covered his face, already partially hidden by the pulled down brim of his NY Yankees baseball cap and by his black sun glasses.

His chest heaved.

He apologized quietly for unsuccessfully fighting the perceived enemy, his own tears.

An image rushes into my mind of a little child who has been beaten in the old fashioned way that parents disciplined their children years ago, striking the small frame painfully with a belt, shouting angrily.

"If you don't stop crying, I will beat you with all my might, so help me God."

Whimpering, the child begs for forgiveness and for mercy, its whole body trembling, unable, of course, to silence every single tear, now too numerous to measure, too plentiful to stop.

"Albert," I said, "thank you for sharing your tears with us.

Your tears are a gift more valuable than gold.

I see you today as having a breakthrough, not a breakdown.

The label we put on things is very important in helping us understand ourselves and others.

When our labels are accurate, then we come closer to understanding the truth of our situation.

It is difficult for men to cry in front of others.

It must be very difficult for Soldiers to cry in front of other Soldiers, even in a psychotherapy group like ours, but it is very important to be courageous enough to cry.

You were hurt by the hypocrisy of your family and friends who tried to act like they cared for you, but did not care enough to remember you with even simple expressions of concern while you went to war to protect them.

It must be a horrible feeling of disloyalty. I wonder if you connect your dreams of deceased family members with the hurt that you feel today.

I believe you have quoted your father, a man you respect and love, who said, 'don't show me sympathy after I am dead; show me that you care while I am alive.'

The family that sent you nothing in the desert was not listening to your father's wise and sincere counsel. Their inaction caused you pain.

I can imagine that you often went to mail call in Iraq. You were keeping hope alive that your family would remember you.

Dad after day, week after week, month after month, a year and more passes, but no letter or favor from home finds its way to you.

It's okay to cry; it is even better than okay to cry: it is healthy, natural, and one of the most normal things you can do.

Later, I will tell you about the saddest day of my life and my own inclination not to cry. It happened on June 28, 1971. It was the day of my mother's death."

Dream Interpretation Group

"I want you to know that I kept my promise"

As is often the case, the group session began with a review of each Soldier's most pressing issues and most pleasant experiences of the past week.

The main purpose of the Dream Interpretation Group is to discuss dreams as a method of uncovering the truth of the dreamer's situation.

The fruitful associations of combat Soldiers to the dreams of fellow group members are often astonishing.

Their associations become framework with which important thoughts are brought into awareness where cognition can do its work.

Harry said earlier, "I can't talk about my combat traumas, but I can talk about my dreams."

Harry's dreams, unsurprisingly, as expected, are about his combat traumas.

Sharing dreams is also a form of intimacy, enabling attachment between members of the group.

My cell phone rang. I asked the group to excuse me to answer the call.

All my patients have my cell phone number.

My patients reliably know I can be reached by them nearly any time.

My patients are not ordinarily perturbed when my phone rings, knowing it is most likely a fellow Soldier in distress.

Tommy Edwards was calling. He is a former member of the Dream Interpretation Group, who retired three months earlier after 20 years of brave, honorable service.

"Dr. Brown, this is Tommy.

"My mother died at 7:50 PM last night in Macon, Georgia, where she was visiting her sister."

"Tommy, may I put you on my speaker so your former group members can also communicate with you?"

The speaker was permitted. In fact, Tommy was calling specifically to communicate with the group, knowing the time the Dream Interpretation Group meets.

Tommy continued.

"Dr. Brown, I want you to know that I kept my promise.

I am very sad that my mother died and died so unexpectedly of a heart attack, but I am so pleased that I kept my promise to her."

"This is Harry, Tommy."

"Harry, are you still there? I thought you would be back home in Michigan by now."

"No, you know how it is sometimes with the Army, but I want to say how sorry I am about your mother."

"Thank you, Harry."

"This is Q, Tommy, I am sorry for your loss. My mother's death has been the worst thing in my life."

"Tommy, this is MAJ Kelly, I too am very sorry, but don't avoid grieving for her like I did for my dad. I was just numb. I felt nothing. I just forced myself to get through it. I will have to grieve for my dad sometime in the future."

"Thank all of you," Tommy said.

"You helped me so much to get through the toughest decision I ever had to make in my life: should I ask my mother to move out of the home I promised she could live in the rest of her life?

I kept my promise, the promise I made 20 years ago to my mother, the promise she could spend the rest of her life in the house I purchased for her.

The group remembers, I'm sure, that my new wife wanted my mother to move out. It put me in a terrible position.

I struggled for a long time about the right thing to do. It was hard to make my wife and my mother happy.

I even repaired the house myself, inside and out, even in the hot weather.

My new wife and I moved into the house with my mother.

We all three lived together.

I am so pleased that I kept my promise to my mother."

Tommy spoke with a voice of self-confidence, a voice of strength and purity we had not heard from him before now.

He did what he knew in his heart was the right thing to do.

He kept his promise.

"Now I am making all the arrangements. She will be buried in her family plot in Macon."

"Tommy, if you can do it, I hope you will speak at your mother's funeral," I said.

"Tell those gathered for her service how much your mother meant to you.

Tell them how much you meant to her.

Tell them that you made a promise to your mother 20 years ago.

Tell them you were a very young Soldier when you made the promise.

Tell them your mother was in a vulnerable position in her life when you made your promise.

Tell them you returned from 20 years in the Army and from many combat missions as a Soldier.

Tell them you kept your promise to your mother.

Remind them how wonderful it feels to keep a promise, over many years, to someone you love."

13

THE UNIVERSITY

"Give this young man a chance"

AT THE RISK of redundancy, I focus the reader's attention once again on my relationship with the University.

People, institutions, and circumstances change. It is an unchanging understanding, however, that when one speaks of "the" University one is speaking of, without exception, the University of Virginia.

My admission to the College of Arts and Sciences, University of Virginia, must be counted as one of the major miracles of my life. I revisit it here in greater detail.

I did not have the grades the admission office would require. I did not have the athletic ability that invited letters of interest from college football coaches. I did not have the money for tuition or lodging. I could not afford the cost of living for a student in Charlottesville in January 1950.

I cannot rationally explain why the University would give this young man a chance.

Kitty Garnett, about whom I reflected in Chapter Eleven, it now seems to me, must have masterfully orchestrated each of my steps to the Rotunda.

I search for the words of tribute she so richly deserves. Not finding them, I puzzle, dumbfounded, over my unawareness of the magnitude and persistence her work on my behalf must have demanded.

Lacking most of the important pieces to this remarkable puzzle, known only by Kitty Garnett now many years deceased, I resort to my reminiscence of this important opportunity and privilege to study at the University.

I was 18 years old and had never been to Charlottesville. Technically, I had been "through" Charlottesville via the Chesapeake and Ohio Railroad, chaperoning youngsters en route to Camp Greenbrier.

I remember Charlottesville in those summer days as a hot, humid town, so hot I got the 8 or 10 boys from the train station platform onto the air conditioned train as quickly as possible.

If one could see the University from the train, I was not aware of it.

I saw the University for the first time when I arrived on that cold January day in 1950. I arrived hoping I would be given a chance to matriculate.

There were no visits to colleges, unlike the way most high school juniors and seniors today go about selecting "the best place to study." At least, in my case, it did not occur. I had traveled little and was comfortable in my small world.

I spent the first and second decades of my life in Lambert's Point, a neighborhood of blue-collar, low income families, in Norfolk, Virginia.

I walked to nearby Burrows Memorial Baptist Church where both my religious and most of my social life occurred. I walked to the James Madison Community Center located in the basement of James Madison Grammar School where my interests in athletic participation began. I rode my Western Flyer to Maury High School where my academic interests were encouraged.

I enjoyed a close relationship with my family and with three caring friends, Bobby Clyburn, George Munden, and Baxter van Pelt. We did just about everything together. We all sang in the church choir, played on the same teams sponsored by the Norfolk Recreation Department, and we all attended the same schools from elementary to high school.

It was idyllic. It was difficult to leave. Even to attend "The" University.

As first mentioned in Chapter Eleven, it was arranged that I would be offered a ride to the University by Nicholas G. Wilson, III, Kitty Garnett's nephew, an upper classman at Virginia.

He was to arrive at my house on a Sunday afternoon in mid-January, one day before the beginning of the second semester, which for me, of course, would be my first semester.

I lived in a neighborhood that Nicholas Wilson, III, is unlikely to have ever previously had a reason to visit.

Oddly, I don't recall that I was embarrassed or ashamed of my home at the time. Probably I was too caught up in the adventure itself.

However, now, looking back, I shudder over how I must have appeared to Nicholas and to the other Virginia students also traveling with him in his car.

I was not in their social class. I did not know their code of conduct or even their dress code. It must have been instantly clear to them that I would not fit in on the grounds of the University of Virginia.

It was many weeks later before I discovered that I was a fish out of water in Mr. Jefferson's Academical Village. For example, I had failed to observe that Virginia gentlemen wore blue blazers, conservative striped neck-ties, and khaki pants, not pink bow-ties, light green zoot suits with pegged pants.

As I said earlier, my mother called the family into the living room before my ride arrived. It was time to pray for me. We got on our knees. My mother prayed loudly, sincerely, and faithfully.

I believe the Lord had no reluctance in answering her tearful but bold petitions. The ritual had been established shortly after my mother became a Christian when I was a young teenager. No important event went unprayed for, nor with less sincerity or less faith.

I once shared with a friend at work the story of my mother's love of God and her love to pray. Later my friend referred to her as a "prayer warrior," a term aptly capturing her faith.

The prayer warrior's prayers were made for me so often that I became a well-known name in her church years before I ever paid her church a visit.

My mother scraped up a small amount of cash and placed it in my coat pocket.

She also gave me an aluminum suit case filled with food.

I was to use the aluminum suit case to mail home my dirty laundry to her each week. She washed and ironed the laundry and mailed it back, always enclosing something good to eat and a note of encouragement scribbled in her uneducated hand writing.

Three years later, one of my college friends commented that my room always smelled like apples, a reminder of my mother's thoughtful, nourishing little weekly gifts.

Mr. A. B. Bristow was my principal of Maury High School. He was a quiet man, but one sensed his power and authority from his unsmiling face and his efficient, conservative use of words.

A man of medium build, Mr. Bristow always dressed in a gray suit with a smart neck tie, and vest. His neatly coiffed ample head of hair was decidedly graying, not only above his ears, but it was beginning its perceptible march throughout his mane.

His thin and rimless eyeglasses had a gold nose-piece and stems.

I had only two encounters with Mr. Bristow during my 3.5 years at Maury.

I shook his hand at graduation. A month before graduation, I went to Mr. Bristow's office to ask for a favor.

Despite some unmistakable popularity, I was and I still remain a shy person.

I am at this moment remembering the crowded hall ways and crowded stairwells at Maury High School when students changed classes, a carefully timed procedure controlled by the "first and second bell."

One day while climbing up the steps at a rather slow pace established by the crowd of fellow students, I was approached by a younger student. I did not know the student.

Kindly and sincerely, the fellow student said, "So you are Bobby Brown! How did you become so popular?"

I replied quickly that I did not know that I was "so popular." I never sought popularity. I just tried to do my best at whatever I did. The second bell rang.

It was not easy to go into Mr. Bristow's office.

I had spent some of my early childhood as a beggar. Had Charles Dickens lived in my generation, he would have had much to write about the character I depicted.

As a young lad, I was a thin boy with uncombed and uncut hair, brown and curly, with brown eyes. Most of the time, my face was unwashed.

I wore knickers with drooping socks. My several old and unkempt sweaters were conspicuous for their gaping holes. The holes were variable in size, not only in the elbows, but also in the front.

This must not be understood to reflect discredit upon my mother. As my sister Edith reminded me, "we were poor but proud." I was always clean and tidily dressed each morning when I left home. My mother had no knowledge of my begging occupation.

My mother also did not know that I frequented Tayloe's Garage at the corner of Hampton Boulevard and 47th Street, Norfolk, Virginia. Tayloe's Garage was located less than 25 yards from the house in which I resided from birth to age 10.

Circumstances required my family to be industrious. My brother Randolph transformed empty tin cans into beautiful flowers for sale. Ingeniously, tin snips reduced the can into many one-fourth inch strips of tin made into flower stems by folding their ends around colorful crepe-paper "flowers." Randolph's artistic talent flourished in early artificial flower arrangements.

On good days, I found clean appearing Collier's or Life magazines in trash cans to sell door-to-door at reduced prices. On very good days, I sold the magazine to its original owner whose trash can I scavenged.

On very hot days, I was retained to swat flies in Tayloe's Garage office. The flies were lulled into the sauna-like small, hot "office" space. The job description demanded dexterity and extremely rapid reflexes ordinarily found only among National League baseball all-stars.

If the flies I killed were retained and counted, I was paid handsomely but less than the minimum wage.

Regrettably, on days of low batting scores, the less than 10-year-old Dickensian kid resorted to begging.

I was in pursuit of five pennies, the price of a Pepsi Cola.

Sizing up people approaching the little food and drink counter attached to Tayloe's Garage, I asked, barely above a whisper, "Sir, do you have a penny to spare?"

Truly, not many people had extra pennies during the great depression.

Most of the people just walked on without acknowledging the little beggar.

As I walked into the office of the principal of Maury High School, I felt I had receded into my little beggar role again.

One can only imagine the feeling. It has to do with asking for something that is not my right to have, to expect rejection, and to be covered in shame of the most despicable type.

To my most unexpected disbelief, Mr. Bristow warmly welcomed me into his office, smiling broadly, pointing to a chair, motioning to me with his hand to be seated.

It was my first and last visit to his office.

Located in an eye-catching place on the wall immediately behind Mr. Bristow's desk, was his degree from the University of Virginia.

The deep red seal in the lower left hand corner of the attractively framed document is what first caught my eye: Master of Arts

Degree in English, University of Virginia. Upon close examination, the red seal read "University of Virginia, 1819."

"Of course I will write you a letter of recommendation to the University of Virginia, Bobby.

George Ferguson is the Dean of the College of Arts and Sciences at the University. He is a good man. I've known him many years.

Return this afternoon for the letter. Give the letter directly to Dean Ferguson when you get to Charlottesville.

Tell Dean Ferguson I send him my best wishes.

I believe you will do well there if they give you a chance. I will follow your career with interest."

We shook hands warmly.

Mr. Bristow's words, "If they give you a chance" stuck in my mind as I left his office. It put me on notice that the matter of being accepted by the University was by no means settled.

Nicholas G. Wilson, III, found a place for my luggage in the trunk of his car. The only passenger seat left for me was in the right rear. As I mentioned earlier, it was not a good seat for a person prone to motion sickness. Thankfully, I did not have to throw-up during the long trek to Charlottesville.

As mentioned in my chapter about Kitty Garnett, I was taken to 504 Rugby Road, Charlottesville, Virginia, the "football house." Many of the University's football team members resided in the "football house."

Coaches took turns monitoring the "study hall," a euphemism for repeated episodes of very loud shouting, "Hold down the noise!"

Bus Male, a former star athlete at the University and valued member of the Athletic Department's coaching staff, came right over in response to my phone call, greeted me, took me to the second floor and assigned me to an Army cot located in the left side of the room near the window.

I was the fourth man assigned to the room. I was also allocated a small desk with a goose-neck lamp.

My presence added to an already crowded room of moderate size. I heard no complaints

Bus Male, the Virginia coach for whom I worked at Camp Greenbrier, was the only person in the whole new world of academia that I knew that January Sunday night in Charlottesville.

The Show

I was shocked but amused by the Football House 2nd floor ritual that occurred promptly every night about 10 PM. The players rushed into my room, switched off the lights, fought for the best viewing positions, the window nearest my bed, and waited impatiently for "the show" to begin.

A vacant lot separated the Football House from the next house. A window in the neighbor's house was converted into a stage upon which a shapely woman thoughtfully undressed to the unheard cheers and shouting from the football players.

"Is Barney there yet," the players loudly wondered.

"Give him time," someone shouted. "He'll be there unless he's immovable at the Virginian."

Apparently, an essential feature of the ritual was the antics of one of the well-known athletes.

Perhaps Barney was near-sighted or uncomfortable in crowds such as the one invading my bedroom.

Nonetheless, it was his preference to climb the shrubbery adjacent to the wall of the bare woman's window, peer in forthrightly, and heroically bear the envy of the entire team.

Meeting Dean Ferguson

My first day in Charlottesville was a cold, rainy one. Mr. Bristow's unopened letter to Dean George Ferguson was kept dry inside my coat pocket, but I had no umbrella for the half-mile walk down Rugby Road to the Rotunda in the rain.

It was registration day for the second semester.

Registration was held on the stage of Old Cabell Hall, a building at the opposite end of the Lawn from the Rotunda.

No one could register for classes who had not been accepted as a bona fide student by the University.

Dean Ferguson's office was in the east end of the basement of the Rotunda.

The Dean's office was an elongated, somewhat narrow, room. The walls were lined with books and the floor was nearly full of handsome wooden desks and long tables.

If the Dean had a secretary, I do not remember seeing her.

When I slowly opened his door, the Dean was standing, bent over papers on one of the tables.

He had the appearance of a gentleman of distinction, tall and fit, erect in a navy blue suit with vest and striped tie.

His hair was as white as snow. His eyes, soft gray, peering through delicate eyeglasses, acknowledged my presence. He did not speak.

"Dean Ferguson, I am Bobby Brown from Norfolk. I want to study at the University of Virginia."

The Dean did not respond.

I walked toward the Dean, removed Mr. Bristow's letter from my coat pocket, and passed it to the Dean.

"Sir, this is a letter from Mr. A. B. Bristow, my principal at Maury High School. He told me to give you his best regards."

The Dean opened the letter slowly. He read it slowly. He placed the letter on the table slowly. He walked slowly to a filing cabinet and slowly removed a document.

"Sit down, Mr. Brown.

This is your application for admission. It is the document I just removed from my files.

Frankly, I did not know what to do with the document.

You do not have a strong academic record. You had a good last semester, but it was an extra semester.

We like to see a student's grades improve over time. Your grades got better, but there is inconsistency in your performance.

What makes it an even more difficult decision for the admission office is your wish to enter our pre-med program, one of the most academically demanding major areas of study at the University."

"Dean Ferguson, everything you said is true," I replied respectfully.

"Students are judged by their grades. I did not know how to study until I was tutored at Camp Greenbrier last summer and was permitted to take Chemistry One and Two at Maury High School last semester.

All I want is the chance to study at the University. I want to prove that I can become a good student and a good physician."

The Dean read Mr. Bristow's letter again.

The Dean's eyes sparkled.

"Mr. Brown," speaking articulately in a deep tone and with seriousness, the Dean said, "Over the years, Maury High School has sent some very good students to the University. Maury is a good school. A. B. Bristow is a man whose opinion I respect.

Welcome to the University of Virginia, Mr. Brown, as a first year student in the College of Arts and Sciences.

If you give me your Charlottesville address, I will mail you an official letter of acceptance."

I successfully resisted my impulse to hug or even kiss the Dean on the cheek.

I could not have been happier or more thankful.

When I reached the door to leave, the Dean called me back.

"Mr. Brown, if I find a DuPont Scholarship to take care of your tuition this year, will you vigorously object?"

"Dean Ferguson," my eyes filling with tears of gratitude, I replied, "thank you…I vigorously thank you."

I walked with a purpose.

I could not have been aware of it, and I know it sounds preposterous, but I was falling in love with the University of Virginia.

As these pages will reveal, my love affair with the University had its precious as well as its perilous moments.

At times, thankfully infrequent and for only brief periods, the University, I perceived, did not return my love.

I continued down the brick sidewalks in front of the East Lawn, famous original Jeffersonian buildings housing students and faculty.

When I reached Cabell Hall to officially register for classes, it was still raining, but in my heart the sun was shining, even bursting; my steps were lighter.

The first steps of a very long journey, one that has yet to end, were begun.

The University of Virginia was a small school in January 1950, fewer than 3000 students, about one-seventh the size it is today.

Registration was largely informal.

Faculty advisors were available, but it was generally understood that a Virginia gentleman neither needed nor took advice of any kind very well.

Mistakenly, as mentioned earlier, I registered for an advanced Philosophy course taught by the renowned University Professor William Weedon who used Alfred North Whitehead as a primary text.

The second mistake, also mentioned earlier, was registering for Parasitology, an advanced course in Biology.

I had never previously taken a Philosophy course. Alfred North Whitehead knew me as well as I knew him. We were total strangers to each other. Sadly, it was the same kind of relationship we enjoyed at the end of the course as well as at its beginning.

The Parasitology course was taught by Professor Bruce Reynolds. Regrettably then, maybe humorous now, some of my naive questions embarrassed him into patent blushing.

The course I most wanted to take, Chemistry, was denied to me because it was mandatory to have previously taken the first semester Chemistry before one was permitted to take the second semester of Chemistry at the University.

John Coleman, a gentleman and scholar, taught my English class. It was all about learning how to write effectively. He had great wit, missing no opportunity to be prickly or make caustically cutting comments. It was done in good taste.

Our small class admired and respected Professor Coleman.

It was my good fortune, many years after my English class, to know him as a dear friend until he finally retired.

American History rounded out my course load. I can visualize the professor's face. It was rounded and healthy. The class was large. The course required more reading in 4 months than I had done in my whole life up to that time.

If my memory is correct, I came home with two D's, Philosophy and Parasitology, a C in History and a B in English.

I had been given a chance to study at the University, but was it justified?

Of all the people who wanted me to succeed, I was the most disappointed.

"I was a lab prep assistant at the University"

Ed Weise was my best friend in college. I keep his 1953 photograph on my desk today.

I first met Ed when I moved from the University Football House on Rugby Road into the Baptist Student Center on Main Street, now called University Drive, in 1950. Ed and his older brother, Reinold, resided, along with 5 other University students, in the 2-story white shingled structure standing adjacent to the University Baptist Church. The building was razed years ago for a church parking lot.

Ed was the serious brother. Reinold was the prankster. Their father was a German physician who practiced medicine in Jacksonville, Florida. Ed was tall and quiet. Reinold was short and talkative. Ed stood at 6 feet with dark hair and hazel eyes. Reinold and Montgomery Clift, a Hollywood actor, could have been twins with the same acting coach.

I studied German for 3 years at the University, but the Weise brothers taught me the German language that I still value and occasionally use to impress others.

Ed and I took many of the same classes, studied together, and later were lab partners in Anatomy at the University.

We were lab assistants in the Biology Department during our 4th year at the University. I was also the "Lab Prep Assistant."

The "Lab Prep Assistant" prepared materials, from frogs to media culture, needed for the biology lab courses.

It was a beautiful warm and sunny early spring Saturday afternoon when I went to the Miller Building, then the home of the Biology Department, to check the list of materials needed for the early Monday morning labs.

It was a short list. I needed to prepare culture media, a concoction of several substances on which bacteria thrived when streaked on its thin layer congealed in a Petri dish. The same principle is employed in a "throat culture" to see if the patient has "Strep Throat."

The ingredients and instructions for my task were typed out cook-book style on a 3 by 5 inch card. Everything needed was available, including the Bunsen Burners to heat up the batches needed by students in the Monday morning lab.

The Bunsen Burners were attached by small black rubber tubes to the gas nozzles strategically placed around a large table in the center of the prep room on the Miller Building second floor.

I've tried to never let a beautiful day pass without breathing its fresh air, basking in its delight.

The lab preparation was the only remaining obstacle keeping me indoors.

With a light heartedness, I set about completing the detailed lab prep task and soon found myself walking speedily to Scott Stadium where I stretched out on one of its bleachers, inhaling the Charlottesville day.

Hours later, I walked back to the Baptist Student Center where I learned that Ed Weise had been searching for me.

I went to Ed's room.

Ed, already serious by nature, was even more serious appearing.

"You are really something, Bobby Brown. Do you know that? You are really something." Ed was not mean, but he could not have been sterner. He could have been an irritated Police Officer arresting me for a serious traffic violation.

Ed's brother, Reinold, looked up from his desk across the room. He smiled in an anticipation of something woeful at which he could yet again burst in laughter over my absurdity.

"You could have burned down the Miller Building, Bobby Brown. It's a good thing you broke the rules and left the windows open."

I had no idea what he was about to complain.

"Black smoke was billowing out of the 2nd floor windows in the Biology Building. I raced in and turned off the Bunsen Burners. The media was boiled out all over the table.

I could hardly breathe.

It was as dark in there as the middle of the night…but it was the middle of the afternoon.

I doused everything with water. I even had to climb up on the table and stomp out the flames.

I was ready to pull the fire alarm, but the flames started to die down. In another minute, the Miller Building would have been ashes."

Reinold could not stop laughing. "And Brown's career would have been ashes, too. Ed, why are you always rescuing him?"

Ed smiled.

Ed kept my secret.

Together, Ed and I went back to the Miller Building. We finished the clean-up. The culture media was prepared properly. The Monday morning labs carried out their business as usual.

I am told that Professor Runk asked around about the "unusual odor" in the Miller Building on Monday morning. No one identified the peculiar aroma to his satisfaction.

Had Professor Runk asked me about the "unusual odor," I was bound by the University's Honor System to reply honestly. Fortunately, he never brought the matter to my attention.

"Never Grow Old"

During college, Ed Weise, John Buchanan, later to become a member of the US Congress from the grand state of Alabama, Jim Small, and I, formed a quartet.

We enjoyed singing more than our audiences enjoyed listening. There was one exception.

We were asked to sing at the "homecoming" of a small, rural church, 10 miles south of Charlottesville.

"Never Grow Old," an old gospel hymn, touched their hearts to such an extent we were literally restrained from ceasing the singing of it.

Clapping hands signified their merriment, louder than the country church piano.

From their hearts, they kept us singing "Never Grow Old" as if it were a promise and a guarantee that aging would come to an end if we did not stop singing. Sing we did.

To say we really got into the song and into the spirit of the occasion would be a British understatement.

No corner of the tiny old country church was unreached by our lyrical enchantment. I think we got to the point that we could not stop singing even if we wanted to stop. It is a most pleasing memory.

"You can take the man out of the University, but can you take the University out of the man?"

I came to the University in 1950. I was invited to stay by Dean George Ferguson. My name was on the List of Distinguished Students when I was awarded a BA in Biology in 1953.

In 1954, I was invited to leave the University by Assistant Dean Oscar Thorup. The University's School of Medicine, based on a transcript needing more Oxygen and marred by excessive immaturity, recommended heavy doses of growth hormone or its equivalent. It was a kind of "don't call us and we won't call you" departure.

I returned to the University in 1958. I was invited to stay by Dean Ralph Cherry.

I moved to Atlanta in 1959 with a University MEd Degree in Educational Psychology in hand.

I returned to the University in 1961. Two years later, the University awarded me its PhD.

I refused to leave the University until it awarded me its MD in 1967.

I helped the University meet its quota for interns for the 1967 – 1968 requirements.

My last really generous gesture towards the University occurred in 1968 when I accepted its munificent offer of a three-year residency in Psychiatry.

During my psychiatric residency, I published two professional articles and won the William James Research Prize.

The author sincerely hopes that his humor will not be sacrificed by his reckless use of immodesty.

Teaching in the Curry School of the University

While I was in medical school, I taught in the University Summer Session each summer after earning my PhD in Education. In the afternoons, I also administered psychological tests for Dr. Burke Smith, Chief of Psychology, School of Medicine, to patients who were admitted to the Davis Wards, the Psychiatric Inpatient Service.

We lived across the street from the University Hospital. This made it convenient to have lunch with Dottie and the children.

I sensed we were happy, working toward a long pursued goal.

Happily, I was able to dart home to watch "Hogan's Heroes" on TV with Dottie and our children, only to return to the lab for further study into the night with fellow classmates.

I could tell the Summer Session classes were going well when uniformed University employees garbed in white, painting the open windows outside the class room, would stop and listen intently to my lecture, even if some of my students found comfort in meaningful naps.

These were happy summers.

Teaching Mental Health at the University

Fourteen University students gathered in the Tumor Clinic of the University Hospital in 1968 at 7 PM. This was my first class of Mental Health scholars. The class met for 3 hours on Wednesday nights each semester.

The Tumor Clinic was strategically selected because it was located less than 100 feet from the ER (Emergency Room). I was a first-year psychiatry resident. Like all hospital residents, I carried a "Beeper" attached to my belt. If called, I could readily reach the ER.

The Mental Health students understood my situation, accepted it, and may have even liked being instructed by someone fully engaged in mental health issues.

For the next several years, I taught Mental Health in the Medical School Auditorium. It was located even closer to the ER. The auditorium accommodated the ever-increasing number of students enrolling in this elective University course.

Let me be straight and on the level with you about my Mental Health class at the University. I believe in intellectual and moral virtue. It may have taken a Sherlock Holmes of the mind to uncover Mental Health's intellectual and moral virtue.

In good taste, even with charm, certainly with good humor, I was often greeted on the grounds of the University by small groups of students chanting, in cadence with my walking pace, "Gut, Gut, Gut!"

A Gut Course at the University at my time was "an easy A." Other courses earning this epithet included "The American Circus," and "Cinema 101," among others.

I admit that Mental Health raised the eyebrows of the various and sundry deans of the College of Arts and Sciences with whom, on more than one occasion, I was invited to meet and address their concerns about my course.

Administrative concern peaked when the enrollment of University students in Mental Health reached 800.

First, no classroom at the University could accommodate a class of 800 students.

Unlike the University administrative staff's perception, I saw limited classroom space was too easy. I rented the University Baptist Church, located 100 yards from the University grounds, and used its sanctuary for my "large class," a term later used by some derisively.

In the spring of 1977, each Mental Health class was monitored by a professor from the University. Each proctor submitted an evaluation to the dean.

In general, by and large, the proctor's comments were favorable, but they unanimously recommended that Dr. Brown bring his Mental Health class back to the grounds of the University and its enrollment strictly limited to 500 students each semester.

I received a phone call from London the following semester. "Bob, this is Bob Pate. I'm one of the professors who monitored your class last semester. How are you today?

"I am spending a year in England at Oxford University. We are having the annual European Counseling Conference in Oxfordshire in November, and Kenneth Cooper has had to cancel at the last minute. Could you come and talk about your interests in physical exercise and mental health?"

Dottie and I went. We had an enjoyable time. We stayed at the White Horse Royal Hotel in Chipping Norton. I joined the Darts' Team at the Bunch of Grapes public house.

I visited the Department of Psychiatry at Oxford and met its chief. We even purchased books at Blackwell's Book Sellers and experienced the special charm of Oxford's historic colleges.

My interest in the relationship between aerobic exercise and mental health was later described in Time Magazine in July 1978 in an article entitled, "Jogging for the Mind." It was preceded by an article written for <u>Physician and Sports Medicine</u> entitled "The Prescription of Exercise for Depression," in the same year.

The students' chant about my "Gut Course" referred to a non-demanding academic course. I always smiled when privileged to hear it because I was thinking about the other gut, the one too often protruding from one's abdomen.

"Life style diseases" was a newly emerging term when I was a medical student. Autopsies of young men killed in motor vehicular accidents provided the evidence of the ravages of a life style too rich in fats and sweets and too little physical exercise.

Today, after 40 years of clinical practice as a psychiatrist, I have never treated a physically fit depressed person.

I moved physical exercise out of my life when I moved myself out of the Football House at the University in 1950. I was physically active as a counselor at Camp Greenbrier during the summers of 1949-1953; however, my life style until 1954 qualified for the "before" photograph in an advertisement showing the health benefits of exercise in a "before and after" poster.

In 1964, on a rigorously regular schedule, I started following the Royal Canadian Physical Fitness Manual. I rediscovered the sense of well-being I had known as an athlete. I knew this perception was too real to be merely or substantially "in my mind" or psychological.

The discovery led me on a search for the causes of the sense of well-being from achieving physical fitness. Fred Goodwin, NIMH, encouraged my research. He offered to study urine samples before and after jogging.

Research reported a 7-fold increase in endorphins in young women who exercised on stationary bicycles. Other studies, however, showed that endorphin-blocking injections did not lessen the "runner's high." Thus it was not endorphins causing the increased sense of well-being.

I reasoned that the hyperthermia of exercise (increases core body temperatures up to 104 degrees, an observation I presented as a poster at an international meeting in Philadelphia on Treatment Resistant Depression), accounted for the positive mood effects of exercise. A Japanese scientist communicated his finding to me: as core body temperature increases, the circulation, and likely the metabolism, in the brain optimally increases.

It also seemed reasonable that college students needed to adopt a healthy life style before it was too late.

I offered academic credit for physical exercise. Yes, you understand correctly. My Mental Health course was soon dubbed, "Run with Bob."

I needed TAs (Teaching Assistants) to realize the full benefits of the unique Mental Health curriculum. The number of TAs soon rose to 26. It became a class within the class. The "Head TA" became a coveted position, not for its small stipend, but for its major leadership opportunities.

The large class was divided into small sections, each with its own TA. The TA sections met after each lecture to discuss it relevance.

I met with the Head TA and all the TAs every Wednesday night one hour before class. This enabled me to get to know each TA. It formed the basis of my letters of recommendations for TAs planning to attend graduate school.

Through my weekly interaction with the TAs, I got to know the members of the class.

In addition to a mid-term and final objective examination, Mental Health students were offered several electives from which to choose. The elective comprised one-third of their final grade.

The "Exercise Elective" was the most popular elective. It required a First Day and Last Day at the University track, 30 minutes of aerobic exercise at least 3 times weekly. The exercise required the University's honor pledge.

Students were encouraged to get an exercise partner, a fellow classmate, to keep up the motivation to the commitment to exercise.

I believe approximately 30,000 University students enrolled in Mental Health during its survival from 1968 to 2003.

The University formerly conducted "exit interviews." Students were asked to recall some of their best experiences during their tenure. Mental Health received favorable remarks in the "exit interviews."

Well after I gave academic credit for exercise in Mental Health at the University, Dr. Fred Gage of the Salk Institute discovered that exercise remarkably increases the release of brain BDNF (Brain Derived Neurotropic Factor).

BDNF increases neurogenesis and synaptogenesis. It causes brain cells to regenerate. It causes optimization of the synapses or connections between brain cells. Depression and other forms of stress kill brain cells.

If I had said that a brain cell could grow after its death, I would have been laughed out of medical school in the 1960s.

BDNF does for depression many more times better what antidepressant medication attempts to do for depression.

I will not ask for a formal apology, at this time, from the deans of the College of Arts and Sciences who wished to tar and feather me for my pedagogical twists and turns in my "Gut Course."

Mr. Jefferson himself, advocating exercise and learning, would have immediately seen how their combination in the classroom of the mind would have been a strong point of agreement between him and John Adams.

When it comes to grading a "Gut Course"

Most teachers will confess that grading is the most challenging aspect of teaching. This was true for me when I taught at the Norfolk Academy, at the Blue Ridge School where I was also the Principal, at the Curry School, and at the Medical School at the University.

Mental Health received its fair as well as its unfair criticism from its students.

Student evaluations, the world's least reliable assessment of teacher effectiveness, may turn up with graffiti like the following: "Your exams are too picky, Dr. Brown." "I feel like I learned more than your tests allow me to demonstrate." "I thought this was reputed to be an easy course but I spent more time on Mental Health than all my other courses combined."

I wondered how honest students could be in making their own self-assessments. Early in the history of Mental Health at the

University, when we met in the Medical School Auditorium, 188 students were enrolled.

I created unintended but obvious anxiety among my students when I asked them to submit their own mid-term grade to me. "Give yourself a letter grade from A to F. Justify your grade with written documentation telling me how you arrived at your most accurate self-assessment."

The results were pleasing. The grades ranged from D to A. In every case, a reasonable explanation justified the grade submitted by each student.

Two weeks before the final exam, I made the same offer. Can you guess the results?

One hundred eighty-eight students in Mental Health submitted 188 A's.

The Kent State University Shootings

On Monday May 4, 1970, 4 Kent State University students were shot and killed by the Ohio National Guard. Nine others were wounded, one with a permanent paralysis. Some of the students were shot after protesting the Vietnam War. Others were watching the protest or walking past the protest.

It was an unthinkable tragedy.

It occurred during a period of marked unrest in America. Our nation was divided over the Vietnam War.

The outcry over the shootings was widespread. It is said that 4 million students protested the shootings and many colleges closed in protest.

Most of the protesters of America's escalating role in Vietnam were college students. To my knowledge, University of Virginia students were seldom visibly involved in public demonstrations opposing the war.

The final exam in Mental Health was scheduled for Wednesday night, May 6, 1970, two days after the shootings.

The Dean of the Curry School sent word that course examinations following the Kent State University catastrophe would be left to the discretion of the faculty. I understood that no reasonable alternative would be unacceptable. Exams could be given as scheduled, rescheduled, or postponed until further notice.

During the Spring Semester 1970, I taught Mental Health in Classroom C-2 in the Old Medical School building. About half the 100 students in Mental Health were enrolled in the School of Nursing. The remainder of the students was typical fun-loving Virginia students from the College of Arts and Sciences.

The reader must not conclude that nursing students at the University were opposed to fun or in any way were less fun-loving than their cohorts in the College of Arts and Sciences. Moreover, as will be disclosed below, one might conclude that University nursing students were more fit.

The Exercise Elective was not yet in place, I had no Teaching Assistants, and Mental Health's prognosis was indeterminable in 1970. Standing in front of the Mental Health students Wednesday night at the University on May 6, 1970, I reviewed the Dean's examination options.

These were upper classmen (a permissible term in 1970), the majority of whom were graduating in 2 weeks. I sensed some sadness and anxiety, but these resilient young men and women were not somber.

"We want to take the exam now, Sir, as scheduled."

I turned to the green board directly behind me. With yellow chalk, in large letters, I wrote, 310 Carrsbrook Drive, Charlottesville.

With the seriousness of an English Public School Headmaster, I said, "For your examination, you will be graded on how successfully you can throw a party at my house," underlining my address on the green board.

"The party begins one hour from now." With that, I hurriedly left the class room, answering no questions.

On the phone, I said, "Dottie, we are having a party in one hour. Get ready to enjoy it. You will have no other job."

In the 4 decades that followed the Mental Health Final Examination party, I have enjoyed no party more. It was a party to remember. Nothing that makes a college party great was missing, including the Police, called by annoyed neighbors who were uninvited, complaining about the "noise," also known as music.

In every way, it was a wholesome party. No alcohol was served and the fun and games were fun and games. For example, "Tug of War" separated the men from the nurses.

The front yard of my residence was far from level. The thick rope used in the contest, I was informed, was on loan from Memorial Gym.

After much debate, it was considered fair by all the contestants that the winners of the "Tug of War" would earn an A+, the losers an A as their final exam grade.

Picture the strain, pain, and sweat required to pull a thick rope with all one's might in a "do or die" contest that was sustained for what seemed like "hours." Picture the rope burns in the red palms of these motivated scholars.

The nursing students won. Their opponents complained, "They were pulling us downhill, Sir. That is not fair!"

The nursing students agreed to a "re-examination." Their opponents could not complain this time. The nursing students pulled them uphill as successfully as downhill.

There were good feelings all around. A good party was enjoyed by all, except for my neighbors.

At the time of this written recollection, the Mental Health students who were graded on their ability to celebrate life at the time of the 1970 Kent State Shootings must be 65 years old. I hope they retained their recognized ability to create cheerfulness that conquers sadness.

I hope they have continued to find ways to struggle to win at the "Tug of War" of life.

"The University gave this young man a chance"

Lou Gehrig, the former captain of the New York Yankees baseball team, put it best in his farewell speech on July 4, 1939. "Yet today I consider myself to be the luckiest man on the face of the earth."

When I arrived on its "grounds" in January 1950, 18 years old, the University was an oasis for me in the middle of the dry, parched desert.

If I were from West Virginia, I would sing the University was "almost heaven."

I was unprepared to appreciate its architectural genius that historically stood watch over its "lawn." I was even less prepared to appreciate its architectural genius that came from the heart of its founder, Thomas Jefferson.

In 1819, its founder explained that he desired an idealized "father – son" relationship between the University faculty and their students. Jefferson was a child when his own father died.

In a strange way, the University as an institution is referred to in the feminine gender. It is "strange" only in the sense that I add the University to the list of the strongest influences on my life. They are primarily also of the feminine gender.

My mother, my wife, my substitute teacher Kitty Garnett, and my choral director, Sena B. Wood are women of strong character. In addition to its academic excellence, the University is best known for its Honor System or strong character.

I first knew the University as a striving student whose good professors were tolerant of my lack of knowledge.

Failure was my master teacher. It taught me humility. It taught me how to study. It taught me to count my blessings.

Failure taught me to value opportunity.

Failure taught me to never give up.

Failure taught me to be thankful for a second chance.

I am reminded of an old joke, the one about a man asking his psychiatrist, "Doctor, is it possible for a man to fall in love with an elephant?"

The psychiatrist replies, "No, it is not possible for a man to fall in love with an elephant."

The saddened patient asks, "Then what am I going to do with this big engagement ring?"

Dear reader, is it possible for a man to fall in love with the University?

14

War on Temperament

"It bothers me that I am not in control of my feelings"

SSG (Staff Sergeant) Cecil Upton is a large, masculine Soldier whose huge triceps delineate his light grey Detroit Tigers T-shirt. He has a large, deep bass voice, the kind best suited for singing "Old Man River."

Cecil is not singing today. Something important is on his mind. He looks perplexed, unsettled.

His skin is dark, matching his piercing dark eyes. His shaved head is shiny. His biceps bulge even with minor gestures made by his hands used when speaking, as if he is giving directions.

Cecil is 38, married for the second time with adult and teenage children in a blended family. He is devoted to his wife and children.

He is one of 9 children. Cecil grew up on the streets of a large city. He enlisted in the Army at 17 with the written consent of his mother, with whom he maintained a very close bond until her recent death.

"I can't sleep," Cecil told the Tuesday Morning Group.

"Things make me cry. I don't know why. Before combat, things would make me feel sad, but I wouldn't cry about it."

"I'm either mad quicker or sad quicker."

"Yesterday, we had a mother bird in our attic. I heard her up there at an earlier time but it didn't bother me."

"I'm more sensitive to animals since Iraq."

There was a general agreement among the Tuesday Morning Group members that they too now find their interest in animals is much more serious. It did not surprise me, but the extent of these combat Soldiers' concern for animals was unknown to me.

"I watch Animal Kingdom on TV when I can," one Soldier reported. Others acknowledged similar fondness for the program.

Cecil continued. "My wife was in the heating and air conditioning business before she took a job at a local medium-security prison.

My wife said it was unsanitary to have a bird in our attic. She wanted it removed.

My son went up and found the mother bird's nest in the attic. It was made of scraps of candy wrappers and just about anything she could find. Three eggs were in the nest.

After we saw the bird fly out of the vent in the attic, my son stuffed some rags into the vent so the mother bird could not return to the attic.

He used some purple plastic gloves, the kind used to clean the commode, to bring the nest downstairs.

I watched the mother bird try over and over to get back into the vent.

It was raining yesterday. I placed the nest under the tree for the mother bird. I tried to keep it dry.

I could see the mother bird up in the branches of a nearby tree, but she wouldn't come near the nest.

I got angry with my wife…but I didn't tell her. I thought she let those (soon-to-be) birds starve to death.

I took my wife's lunch to her at work. She's on the night shift.

On my way to the prison where she works, I thought of saying to my wife, 'What if I didn't feed you?'

This happened yesterday. I could not sleep at all last night.

I got up at 0230. I went outside to check on the nest.

We have a cat that prowls around the yard at night. What if the cat got the eggs?

I wasn't man enough to tell my wife what I really thought. Those eggs would have hatched in a few weeks. The mother bird would have taken them out. She would teach them to fly.

I cried alone.

My whole day is messed up because the mother bird can't get back inside the attic."

"What bothered you the most about this situation, Cecil?" I asked.

"I don't know. The mother bird seemed so helpless. She tried over and over to get back through the vent.

We saw so much helplessness when we deployed. Mud houses…substandard living…kids barefooted…kids begging for everything…starving…kids fighting over the MRE (Meals Ready to Eat) that we threw to them from our vehicles."

"We saw a lot of helplessness over there," said Hank, a quiet, sensitive, deep-thinking fellow group member.

"I don't think it was the helplessness of the mother bird that affected Cecil," said Hank.

"It was the problem between Cecil and his wife.

She didn't understand how Cecil wanted her understanding more than he wanted to help the bird.

Cecil felt she should have known how sensitive he was to the situation.

It hurt Cecil deeply that she did not understand his feelings."

Cecil's unashamed tears confirmed Hank's discernment. His burden was lighter.

He was understood. Cecil was immediately comforted.

Now he knows why some things make him cry. He is learning why some things make him angry.

Like most Soldiers who battled terrorists and now battle PTSD, Cecil is painfully sensitive to death, even the death of three unborn baby birds. The session ended on this melancholy note.

"All my buddies were hurt real bad"

Peter is a tall, stocky 27 year old married Soldier, the father of 2 young children to whom he is devoted.

Despite his strong physical features, Peter is a kind, gentle person whose articulate speech is soft and mellifluous.

He has completed two years of college, having studied at the University of the Virgin Islands and at Rutgers University. Currently, he is enrolled at Central Texas College.

Two of Peter's 6 years in the Army have been spent in Iraq, first from November 2008-December 2009, during the surge, and from November 2010 to December 2011.

Peter has an unblemished military record, carries a Secret Clearance, and has received a number of military awards.

His name was on the promotion list until he was charged with a felony on 8 May 2012, less than 6 months after returning home from his last deployment.

Peter's MOS (Military Occupational Specialty) is 92 Bravo, "All Wheel Mechanic." Every Soldier, despite their MOS, is a rifleman, expected to respond unhesitatingly when called upon in combat to fight as a well-trained warrior.

During his first week in Iraq, December 2008, Peter was a gunner in an MRAP (Mine Resistant Ambush Protected Armored Vehicle).

The vehicle was traveling fast on a mud-covered road, responding to an explosion, when they encountered small arms enemy fire.

A member of the MRAP crew shouted "Roll-Over!"

Peter, positioned in a gun turret at the top of the MRAP, was returning enemy fire when his vest was yanked down by a fellow crew member. He was half-way down the turret when the MRAP rolled over.

"I was banged up pretty bad and confused for a while. We were all shaken up but okay. We got out of the MRAP, reacted to the enemy fire, and moved out."

The rollover was traumatic, but it paled in comparison to the "thing that really messed me up," Peter said.

"I was on duty at the gate that first week in Iraq in 2008. I was supposed to be in the convoy, but my seat in the truck was assigned to a civilian who had to be taken to the next location.

All my friends were in the truck.

I was closing the gate immediately after the truck went out.

An explosion knocked me down. It felt like I was struck in my back. In a panic, I thought, where is my weapon? I was freaking scared.

Two grenades had hit the truck just outside the gate. The explosion was gigantic. It blew off the leg of my best friend and hit the civilian who was in my seat.

I ran to the truck to help the wounded. I put a tourniquet on my friend's leg. He was begging me not to leave him.

I helped remove the civilian. A big man, he was already dead, but we rushed him to the medics.

Another friend was injured badly. It looked like his face was peeled off. It looked like his eye protection glasses were holding his face on. He is the friend I told you about in the Spiritual Domain Group. He is the one that committed suicide on Ash Wednesday this year. I had just spoken to him a week before his death.

After the explosion at the gate, I couldn't sleep for days.

I wet the bed.

I didn't want to go for help. It was too embarrassing."

Peter kept functioning.

He learned that his fear and his mood were better when he was "on the offensive in combat."

"I was assigned to a Sniper Unit. We kicked in doors.

We were given a bolo ("Be on the Look-out") list. It had detailed descriptions of people we wanted. It may say the Iraqi man we wanted had a mole on his left ear lobe and a scar on his left elbow, for example.

We could even take his finger prints and see if they matched the ones we had on an apparatus we took inside the house with us.

I was the 'Snatch Guy.' I walked in behind the Soldier with the gun. If we got the right man, I would snatch him, zip-tie his hands behind him, place a pillow case over his head, and put him in the truck.

I carried pillow cases in the left lower leg pocket of my ACU (Army Combat Uniform).

I was really pumped up.

About 12 of us would storm in.

The building would be surrounded on the outside by our armored trucks. A number of our vehicles would also be circling the perimeter.

It was dangerous.

We would watch out for women in the huts who wore a suicide vest.

If it were a high value target, we went in with knives only.

I was with a PSD (Personal Security Detachment). We rode with a CSM (Command Sergeant Major) and the BN (Battalion) Commanding Officer, a LTC (Lieutenant Colonel).

We had to have good shooting scores from the range to belong to the PSD.

We slept in a stinking, unsanitary mud-house. Mice would snip at my ears when I tried to sleep.

I stay in touch with my friends. Four have committed suicide and 3 were killed later when they deployed to Afghanistan."

Peter stays in touch with his friends from combat. Peter does not stay in touch with his feelings.

The loss of Peter's friends, the closest friends of his life time, is reported objectively, but the losses are too unbearable if given access to his sentiments.

"She almost knocked over me and my bike on Interstate 95 in rush-hour traffic"

Peter did not imagine that chasing, at a high rate of speed, a driver who struck his motorcycle while she was texting, would end as it did for him.

Redeployment combat anger is widespread. It is a potentially dangerous symptom for which meaningful answers too often evade us.

Dangerousness is one of the most feared consequences of combat-induced anger.

Road-rage is a common symptom of PTSD. In Iraq and Afghanistan, most of the violence our Soldiers encountered took place in vehicular convoys on roads and highways. It is natural to anticipate danger while driving on our roads at home once the combat deployment has ended.

The woman driver nearly knocked Peter and his bike down into the paths of speeding cars and large tractor-trailer 16-wheeler trucks.

When Peter's motorcycle was struck by the other driver's car, it "wobbled a little."

His fear of crashing to the ground triggered his exaggerated startle response, one of his PTSD symptoms. His emotions wobbled more than a little.

The rapidity of Peter's startle response was "faster than a speeding bullet." Like all human reflexes, it is often outside voluntary regulation.

Peter's startle response significantly contributed to his combat readiness. It was life-saving when kicking in doors in Iraq. It helped make him a good "Snatch Guy."

The traffic was congested on Interstate 95 during the busy rush hour.

When apprehended at the gun point of a police officer, Peter was forced to lie face down in the dirt on the side of the Interstate.

Peter was shamefully cuffed, a knee painfully thrust in his back, and wrestled into the confined space of the back seat of a police cruiser, but not before a second police officer also put his knee into the back of our prostrated Soldier, still lying face down in the roadside dirt. The snatcher was being snatched!

He was transported to the police station, where his clothes were removed and replaced by prison orange.

He was finger-printed. He was locked up in a claustrophobically small cell furnished only with a commode and two bunk beds.

Without bail, Peter would have spent months in jail awaiting a trial that has been repeatedly rescheduled for 24 months.

Peter lost the liberty and the freedom for which he was bravely fighting in Iraq less than 30 days earlier.

A moment of thoughtlessness, never to be retracted, only regretted, led to an uninterrupted series of painful consequences that will prove inevitably to be costly in cash and suffering.

Peter was charged with "Felony Eluding Police," in addition to many lesser crimes, while unaware of being the subject of a pursuit by two police cars.

PTSD is rarely an excusing condition in criminal courts. Combat-induced PTSD, however, is often a complex, challenging, and pervasive mental disorder, complicated to explain to a court.

Combat-induced PTSD related criminal and civil litigation is best and most fairly judged in "PTSD Courts," similar to "Drug Courts," not in our circuit courts, already strained with heavy dockets.

The author implores communities to divert Soldiers and Veterans, suffering from combat-induced PTSD, who face legal charges, to special courts that are fully informed about the psychological consequences of our 21st Century War. Peter's session ended on a note of uncertainty.

"It made me so mad I could have choked the Hell out of my sons"

SSG Allen Turner, called "Turner" by his fellow Soldiers, is a quiet man. He has distinctive, unique facial features, a combination of Asian and Puerto Rican heritage, that form a pleasant expression.

He has the body build of a physically fit, athletic person, standing 6 feet tall, weighing 200 pounds with a very low percent body fat.

Turner returned from 4 combat deployments physically intact, having suffered no apparent injuries.

"He came home with more anger after each deployment," his wife observed. She was frightened by his behavior when he was angry. Fortunately, Turned never "lost his temper" with his wife or his two young sons.

Turner had several close calls with his temper in public, according to his wife. In each case, he did not act out on his anger.

Recently two young men, windows down, music blasting, drove their car recklessly into the filing station on post, cutting off Turner, stealing the parking space that he was approaching cautiously in his car.

Even though the rowdy young men were themselves at fault, they shouted obscenities at Turner.

Turner got out of his car with his weapon, a Louisville Slugger baseball bat, held down by his side.

He approached the young men calmly, saying, "I understand you wish to speak to me?"

Seeing his weapon, the young men apologized profusely, removed their car from the space Turner, and witnesses, readily agreed was appropriately his parking space.

No one was injured or threatened.

In another recent traffic situation, an irate driver cut off Turner's car and stopped in front of him, blocking Turner's movement in traffic. Quick thinking led Turner's wife to hastily exit their car and race to the offending driver.

"Sir," Turner's wife pled, "my husband has just returned from Afghanistan. Please don't upset him. He may be dangerous."

Good sense immediately returned to the offending driver. He sped away to safety.

No one was injured or threatened.

Imagine the burden borne by Turner's loving, clear-thinking wife.

"This is how I try to handle my anger," Turner explained to me, "First, find the trigger.

Next, I assess the environment; where am I at the time?

Then take a step back...back up...count to 10 slowly to calm myself.

And then I dismiss myself. In my mind, I shout "Dismissed!"

I have to dismiss myself or I may hurt somebody."

I listened attentively. He needed to talk. I needed to listen.

"It was embarrassing"

"I need to tell you the story of the painful part of taking my children for school orientation," Turner said.

"My children got up late, did not have breakfast, and we left the house together rushing to attend school orientation, the first day of school.

The teacher had a table with cookies and juice.

My sixth grade sons piled their paper plates high with cookies; I mean they really stacked them up...even to the point of falling off the plates.

It was embarrassing.

The teachers and the social worker were thinking that we don't feed them at home.

It made me so mad I could have choked the hell out of my sons...so hard their eyeballs would pop out.

I had wanted to talk with the teachers, but not after this happened.

When we got back home, I sat my sons down at the table and told them how angry I was at them. I didn't speak to them for the rest of the day.

Yes, my temper is different after combat. Little things bother me. I am easily irritated.

Now I watch everything. I watch people.

I don't like to sit with my back to the door.

I am not playful any more."

"What would have happened," I asked, "if you expressed your anger at school during orientation?"

"The Police would have been called. There would have been an altercation. No doubt about it.

Either I would have been hurt or the police would have been hurt.

I know how to take a gun away from a person if the man with the gun got close enough to me."

"You handled it by going home, saying nothing to the teachers. Can you think of another way of handling it?" I asked

"There is no other way to handle it once my anger takes over. I must leave."

"Can you think of a way to keep your anger from taking over?" I asked.

"There is no way to keep my anger down once it is triggered.

I guess I could have fed them at home or gotten them up earlier so that breakfast could have been prepared.

I just don't know."

"Was it the cookies they took, or was it something else that made you mad?"

"It was the greedy way they piled up the cookies on their plate... for certain...that's what made me mad enough to want to choke them."

"You said the teachers and the social worker were also involved."

"Yes, they considered me to be a poor parent, one that must not feed my children at home."

"Did they tell you that?" I asked

"No."

"How did you know they were thinking that you are a bad parent?"

"That's what anybody would think when children behave like that."

"What is the evidence they thought you were a bad parent?"

"It was written on their face, a disgusted look.

They may have snickered under their breath. I just knew what they thought about me after my kids grabbed the cookies."

"Was this the first time the teachers and social worker ever saw sixth grade boys grab a lot of cookies?"

"I don't know."

"How could you find out?"

"I could have asked them, I guess."

"What do you think would have been their answer?"

"I really don't know."

"That is correct. Nobody knows what another person is thinking unless they ask him or her.

Would you be willing to role-play the school orientation situation with me to see if you may be prepared to deal with the situation in a different way, in a way that will decrease the chances of getting angry?

Let's imagine it is school orientation day. Your sons have just grabbed the cookies and returned to their seat. I will be the teacher and you will be yourself. I will speak first.

'Good morning, SSG Turner, I am Ms. Smith. I am pleased to be your sons' teacher this year.

Let me also say that it is an honor to have the sons of a Soldier like you in my class.

Thank you for serving our country.

How are you this morning?'

"I am not good, Ms. Smith. I am so embarrassed. My sons grabbed those cookies like they are neglected at home. What do you think about that?"

"Boys will be boys, SSG Turner.

It never crossed my mind they are neglected at home.

I just wish all the boys in my class had a father like you who cared enough to attend School Orientation with them.

It is such a wonderful thing to see fathers come to school events with their sons. Thank you."

"Thank you, Ms. Smith, for those remarks, but are you being honest with me about those cookies they took?"

"If boys did not grab cookies, no matter how much they eat at home, SSG Turner, I don't believe the sun would rise in the morning.

My memories of the cookies will fade quickly, but my memory of a Soldier who is the father of two of my students will encourage me to teach the very best I can for the whole school year."

Role Playing ended.

SSG Turner appeared relieved, almost smiling, and surely less tense.

"I never looked at it like that before…that is a whole new way to look at things.

It was not what my sons did, but what I thought the teachers and the social worker thought of me that angered me.

It's a whole new way of thinking. I know it's going to take a long time to change my thinking."

Turner, staring into space, thinking out loud, said, "People in the US don't know what the war was like.

Everything is chaotic over there…under attack all the time… can't sleep. Kids starve over there.

Once an area is bombed, they block all communication for 1-2 weeks.

If there are fatalities, then we cannot communicate with anyone back home for weeks.

It changes the way we think when we return home.

Combat changes the way we look at everything.

Now anything, no matter how small or meaningless, can make us irritable and angry.

My wife doesn't know that she irritates me at times, how she talks when I'm watching TV or how she will say, 'You are not listening.'

We celebrate our 14th wedding anniversary this weekend." Turner is changing the way he thinks.

"I was on the Recovery Team in Iraq. I don't like to think about it…but I can't stop"

SFC Bobby Davis sat in front of me in my office. His round face is friendly, but his eyes did not return my gaze. He was making a "threat assessment," almost constantly visually checking the safety of my small office.

This 36-year-old married man, father of 3 children ages 8-14, was visibly tense, rapidly moving his left leg up and down.

He is overweight, a common side effect of his antidepressant medication. He stands 6 feet and weighs over 225 pounds, based on my estimation.

There is an unexpected gentleness in his demeanor and in his speech.

SFC Bobby Davis is frightened by his intrusive thoughts of combat, thoughts that need to be examined in therapy. Regrettably, he spends considerable time and effort trying to avoid his haunting thoughts.

He let me know at the beginning of the session that he chooses to remain non-self disclosing.

"I like group therapy," he said, "as long as we don't talk about combat.

When we talk about combat in group, it comes into my mind when I drive home on the weekends. I have a 3-hour drive. My mind fills up with combat memories. It upsets me, Dr. Brown.

I know that's what we need to be talking about but," looking away, "it can ruin my whole weekend."

My office has been untidy recently. Our Department of Behavioral Health is preparing for the Joint Commission Accreditation inspection. Stacks of files were piled on my desk, filing cabinet, and even on the floor.

"Bobby," I said, "Soldiers tell me that it helps to discuss their painful combat memories. When you get the troubling thoughts out of the depths of your mind, you can try to make sense of what happened."

He nodded in agreement.

I continued. "If I put these files under my rug, I would trip over them all day. I don't want you to trip over the bad memories you have tried to place under the rug of your mind."

At first, he did not reply. If one could visualize the complexity of the brain struggling whether to talk about frightening subjects, I would be observing it now.

SFC Davis, convinced I could contain his emotional reaction, as well as my own, sighed audibly and began to speak.

"I was on the Recovery Team in Iraq. I don't like to think about it," said SFC Davis.

"The things I've seen in Iraq!

I saw Iraqi dead bodies.

I saw the aftermath of American Soldiers killed or severely injured in combat."

His choice of the word "aftermath," I was to learn later, had a significant meaning. It was an interesting choice because he was in my office to talk about his "aftermath" of combatting terror.

"If one of our vehicles is hit on the road, the job of the Recovery Team is go out and bring that vehicle back in.

The unit would take care of the killed or injured Soldiers.

The convoy commander would MedEvac the injured Soldiers out by helicopter.

The convoy commander would also radio Mortuary Affairs to deal with the remains of the dead.

The unit would remove sensitive items from the vehicle, like radios.

The convoy would keep moving.

The unit would contact us by radio. They would give us the map coordinates to locate the messed up vehicle.

Our job as 91 Bravos (Mechanics) was to pick up the messed up vehicle and bring it back to the FOB (Forward Operating Base).

The vehicles were mangled by explosions.

Too often the mangled vehicles had things I did not want to see or smell.

I saw blood, lots of blood, brain matter, and guts. It was splattered inside the mangled vehicle.

When the Recovery Team went out to get the vehicle, it was at risk of being attacked by the insurgents.

We had to set up a perimeter around the vehicle. We had to be on guard for safety.

The enemy would often try to hit us when we went out on a recovery mission.

One day on; the next day off. That was my job for 12 months in Iraq.

We would bring the vehicles back to a holding area. We would see if we could fix them. If it was too costly to fix them, the messed up vehicles were used for parts.

We had to spray out the blood.

We tucked the vehicles away, behind barbed wire. We did not want American Soldiers to see what we had to see in our recovery mission.

If they were real bad, we covered the vehicles with a tarp.

At the time, I didn't think it had any effect on me. I didn't dwell on it or think about it. I was hard-core then. My only thought was to get home.

Now it bothers me a lot to think about it.

"We grew up like brothers"

My cousin was deployed to Iraq at the same time.

My thoughts get mixed up.

I have disturbing dreams now that I am home.

In my dreams, I see the messed up vehicles and, for some reason, I start to think it was my cousin's blood that I sprayed out of the vehicle.

I know it's not true.

My cousin was killed by a sniper while he was walking beside his Bradley (tank).

He was not even inside a vehicle.

In Iraq, he was 4 hours away from me by helicopter.

Is that how he looked when somebody came to pick him up? I wondered.

How was he?

I was not told where in his body he was hit by the sniper. A sniper bullet can leave a big exit hole.

I tried to get more information, but they wouldn't let me get it.

I tried to bring his body back home, but they wouldn't let me.

We grew up like brothers. He was 5 years younger than me.

We were e-mailing each other over there. I last contacted him about a month before he was killed.

It doesn't make sense."

SFC Bobby Davis could have been arguing like a prosecuting attorney in a felony trial, mercilessly pounding the weak defense.

The veins in his thick neck became visibly distended. I could hear both anger and fear in his voice.

The case was being tried in his mind.

He was the prosecutor, the defense, the judge, and the jury.

No verdict had been reached in a trial that could become interminable.

He abruptly stopped talking.

His expressive eyes, watchers of the most unholy, imparted discouragement, sadness, and confusion.

I cleared the courtroom.

I wanted to prevent further contempt.

We both sat in silence.

Finally, I spoke. "How do you feel now, Bobby?" I asked.

"I'm okay right now, in here with you. I always feel good when I'm here in the clinic, either in the group or with you.

I just don't know how I will feel later. That's what always bothers me."

"Bobby, do you have my cell phone number?"

"I remember you gave it to me on the back of your professional card, but I don't know where it is now. I lose things, even my car keys.

Can you give it to me again?"

I gave him my cell phone number, praised him for sharing some of his difficult memories with me, and reassured him of my determination to help him.

"Bobby," I said, "when I first saw you months ago, you had a different problem. Do you remember?"

"Yes, I was abusing alcohol. It took away my bad dreams."

"I told you I could not really tell the effects of combat on you until you stopped drinking."

"I went to ASAP (Army Substance Abuse Program). I didn't really want to go to ASAP. I know you strongly recommended it.

I completely stopped drinking months ago."

"I can't tell you how proud I am of you, Bobby. You are winning that battle. You can win this one, too.

Based on your nightmares, your need to avoid things that remind you of your combat trauma, and the symptoms you talk about in group, I believe you have PTSD."

"That's not good, is it, Dr. Brown?"

"PTSD is not something we can say is good or bad. It is a disorder that we can treat," I told Bobby.

"My wife told me that PTSD is bad because it keeps you from getting a good job."

I explained that federal law prohibits an employer from asking a veteran whether he or she has received psychiatric treatment, except for violence.

The patient appeared clinically stable. I will see him in weekly Post-Deployment Group Therapy in 5 days.

I reminded him to call me between sessions whenever he needed to talk.

I said, "We are going to make sense of your dream."

SFC Bobby Davis smiled.

We shook hands and parted.

"I can't walk through the parking lot"

SSG (Staff Sergeant) Kurt Vest is best described as aloof. I can't say whether repeated exposure to blasts in Iraq explains his reserved, indifferent, detached, and unfriendly comportment.

This forty-one year old married man has good eye-contact, but poor communication skills. He also has some hearing loss from combat.

He does not ask others to accommodate for his hearing loss. He just does not appear to understand or even to process what is being said to him.

This introverted Soldier is tall and thin. He has a military bearing, always neatly dressed in his ACU (Army Combat Uniform).

SSG Vest, in a recent Wednesday Morning Post-Deployment Group Therapy session, spontaneously spoke. The group became quiet and attentive. This novel change for SSG Vest, speaking unexpectedly, was not anticipated.

"I can't walk in the parking lot. I don't understand why. It's not only the clinic parking lot down stairs," pointing to the third story window below which is our large parking lot. "It's any parking lot."

"Tell us more, SSG Vest," I said.

"I don't think it had anything to do with it, but I saw a terrible accident in Iraq.

I was in a large convoy in Iraq. I mean it was really long. I can't tell you how many vehicles were in the convoy.

I saw a car coming from the opposite direction. He was driving real fast. I guess he was looking for an intersection to cut across our convoy without having to wait to the end of the convoy.

He was speeding when he suddenly made a 90 degree turn right in front of my truck.

His car flipped 7 times. His passenger was thrown out of the car.

The car landed on him.

People tried CPR, but I knew he was dead."

"Would you say, SSG Vest, that that car was out of control?" I asked.

My question remained unanswered.

SSG Vest continued.

"I was the Soldier who reviewed all the road accidents in our sector of Iraq.

I saw pictures of the accidents.

I wish I had not seen all that...all those photographs of all the motor vehicle accidents."

"Do you see any connection," I asked SSG Vest, "between the car out of control that flipped 7 times, all those pictures of road accidents, and your fear of walking in parking lots?"

Unconvincingly, SSG Vest replied.

"I just don't know. I guess."

"I believe the Iraqi experiences you just described are logically connected to your parking lot problem back home.

Your response to what you saw in Iraq is extreme," I said. "See if you can modulate your response, work towards the mean, 'the golden mean,' best described by Aristotle."

I was hoping to introduce Aristotle's ethics. I wanted the group to consider their PTSD symptoms as understandable but extreme responses to combat trauma.

This was not going to happen.

Almost in unison, the group reacted strongly, "What we saw in combat was extreme. We need extreme responses. It's only a matter of time before terrorists will strike America again. They will strike again and again. They will strike big time."

Everyone described their conduct in parking lots. Amazingly, it was even more extreme than SSG Vest's need to walk around the outside of the parking lot, not to walk through it to enter our building.

There was solidarity in the group.

"I drive around every parking lot before I enter it," said one group member. "If it is crowded, I will look for another store."

"My wife complains," said another Soldier. "She always asks why I park so far away from the store."

"I drop my wife off at the commissary here on post. I find a parking space as far away as I can."

Another Soldier said, "The best I ever felt in the commissary was when I found that you, (pointing to a fellow group member), "were in there, too. Every so often, I'd check an aisle to make sure you were still there."

"Help me understand," I appealed to the group.

"The worst things happened in congested areas in Iraq. Congested areas are chosen by terrorists.

The terrorists chose the Boston Marathon because it was known to be a congested area.

It is impossible to perform threat assessments in congested areas.

It is too easy for the terrorists to be undetected in crowds of people.

We are trained to look for anything that doesn't look right. How can anyone tell if something doesn't look right in a congested area?

We are thinking security all the time.

Some areas on this post are not safe. Anyone with a driver's license can drive through the gate and be cleared by the security officer.

Some of our buildings on this post have outside security. They have physical barriers that prevent VBID (Vehicle Borne Improvised Explosive Device) from driving close up, close enough to the building to blow it up.

But the CDC building (Child Development Center) where our kids spend the day has no external security.

At Fort Hood, we had pop-up barriers that can be engaged immediately as needed."

"When I first came here 9 years ago to treat PTSD," I told the group, "I misunderstood that you wanted to keep some of your PTSD symptoms.

Today, you are teaching me which symptoms you want to keep. You told me why you want to keep them.

Now I understand why you are 'thinking security all the time.'

You want to remain vigilant. You want to detect danger. You want to avoid danger. You want to be fully prepared to meet and defeat terrorism in our country.

You want to retain these highly honed skills, sharpened by the horrific experience of defeating terrorists in Iraq and in

Afghanistan, because you love your family, you love each other, and you love our nation.

I want to thank you. I want to honor you. I want to return your love. I want to tell your story with you so that our nation will thank, honor, and love you as I do and as I know they will when the truth of fighting terrorism is revealed."

"Our Rules of Engagement hurt us a lot"

MAJ Rhett Williams is a perfectionist. His grim expression connotes his disappointment with himself.

A small, physically fit, trim man in his early forties, he emits sadness.

"I've been deployed 4 times. We had no rules of engagement when the war started in Iraq in 2003. We went in to win.

With each deployment, I've watched the tightening of the Rules of Engagement.

Now our Rules of Engagement hurt us a lot. We can't even engage the enemy unless we can document that our military response is defensive, that they attacked us first.

Often it is too late to respond when the enemy initiates the fight.

Our Rules of engagement hurt our Soldiers emotionally.

You can see it on their face at the Memorial Service.

The expression on their face tells us what they are thinking. They are saying, 'We could have done more to stop the killing of our buddy we remember in this ceremony today.'

I question myself. Did I do enough to help my Soldiers?

Did I lack the courage to stand up to my commander when I thought he was wrong?

My commander was a good man, but he had a flaw that was toxic.

He liked to go outside the wire 'to check on the troops.'

Every day, the commander went outside the wire. It was totally unnecessary for his rank and his responsibility. It was dangerous to himself and to his PST (Personal Security Team).

His PST included 7 Soldiers and two vehicles.

Eight Soldiers died needlessly when the commander and his PST were directly hit by enemy fire.

I have a very disturbing recurrent dream about the commander. He is telling me that he admires some of my traits and dislikes others. We are on top of a tall building. We both fall off. I see him hit the ground. I wake up startled.

When I visit friends and family now, I get asked more questions. They ask, 'What happened in Iraq? '

I don't answer because I only think of the negative things that happened in Iraq."

"I'm not happy with the person I am"

Six Soldiers attended the Tuesday Morning Group today. Attendance varies from week to week from 5 or 6 to 11 Soldiers.

Once a Soldier has served in combat, he or she is and always will be a Soldier in my book.

In today's group there are Soldiers in various stages of active duty. Two have been medically retired. One will soon retire after 30 years in the Army. The rest remain on active duty.

Clinical depression is no stranger to this group. It was their constant struggle with depression that was talked about today.

"My depression lingers all the time. It gets worse when the news gets worse.

Any news about death makes me feel more depressed," said MSG Michael Yoder.

Michael arrived late today. He wore a black baseball cap with the brim pulled down so low that it covered his face when he looked down. He looked down a lot today.

Michael has a medium build, dark eyes, fair complexion, and a completely bald head always covered by a cap. His superior intelligence is apparent in his articulate speech.

Clinical psychologists would describe Michael as a quiet, withdrawn introvert.

Michael joined the Tuesday Morning Group 5 years ago, the same year he retired. Housebound by Major Depression and Chronic PTSD, Michael has been unemployed since leaving active duty.

He is dedicated to his 13-year-old son whom he loves. Michael is loyal to his wife of 20 years whom he loves and respects.

The group sits in chairs arranged in a semi-circle that begins at the door to my left and ends at the wall of windows to the right. I sit in front of the group. Michael sits in the chair to my far right.

Upon entering the group room today, Michael stopped in front of each fellow group member to shake hands. Unlike his usual custom, he did not shake hands with me today, an incident to which I will return.

Michael continued.

"I lost my whole weekend because I was depressed. It comes with anger. I got mad because the sun came up. I wanted it dark.

I'm talking about severe depression. It's been worse recently.

I could easily lie in bed all day. I don't want to take a shower.

I withdraw and wallow in my own misery."

Quincy said, "I don't want to be big any more. I'm tired of being heavy."

Quincy is morbidly obese. It makes him depressed.

He was severely injured when he was blown out of a truck in Iraq. Unable to exercise, taking medication for pain, and poorly controlled Diabetes contributed to his present seriously unhealthy weight.

Michael said, "I don't feel like doing anything.

I'm not happy with the person I am. I don't socialize. I don't relate.

I isolate myself because it keeps me from being hurt. I also don't trust.

But we are not meant to be alone. We need affection from others."

CSM (Command Sergeant Major) Paul York is new to the group. He recently spent 28 days in a nearby psychiatric hospital for depression and PTSD. He is a naturalized American citizen whose past 3 decades has been spent in the Army.

Paul is a quiet, small man whose education has been British and whose ethnic background has been Asian.

Paul said, "We are all wounded. As Soldiers, we always had someone to our left, to our right, and in the front and back of us.

I am also very sensitive to death. What happened in the Boston marathon bombing this month really saddened me.

The world is not a safe place.

We've got a lot of work to do in America."

CWO (Chief Warrant Officer) Edward Zimmerman just returned to the group after 6 weeks in a partial hospitalization treatment center. Edward suffers from depression and PTSD.

Edward said, "The thing that happened in Boston took me right back to Iraq.

I've seen it. I've seen people running everywhere for help after an explosion.

Crowds of people! Congested areas!

It was the exact same scene as in Boston.

Pushing through clouds of smoke…you can't see in front of you.

It took me back to my zone."

Michael spoke again. "There are reminders of death everywhere.

On the road the other day, a man threw his cigarette butt out of his car window. The cigarette landed on my windshield. Sparks went everywhere.

It took me back to Iraq. Immediately, I was in my zone. I was in tears.

Everybody here is still feeling the same way. I am tired of taking medication. I know I can't stop abruptly.

I think we all go through phases of medication-taking.

At first we are embarrassed that others will see it.

Then we start to depend on the medication.

Then we are still depressed.

We get sick and tired of it.

We are still depressed.

This is why I want to be quiet and not communicate in public."

Tom Kennedy had been distracting himself on his cell phone up to this point. He said, "Our mood depends on our plan or mission.

I don't want to be bothered when I go out.

I don't want to answer questions.

When I go anywhere, it is as if I am on a military mission.

If my mission is ruined, it makes me depressed.

When I go out to eat, I'm on a mission.

I don't want somebody to come up to my table and chat. I want to complete my mission and get back to the FOB (Forward Operating Base).

I don't want to share my story with strangers.

I don't want to hear their complaints about life.

When I go out to a place, I want to go in and get out.

I don't want people at my table."

I looked around the group. The jury had reached a unanimous verdict. The six group members were in agreement.

"It seems you all want the same thing. What is that?" I asked.

The answer was immediate.

The answer was one word.

The answer was "peace."

"Before we end our group session today," I announced, "I wonder if Michael will tell the group why he did not greet me with his usual friendly handshake."

Michael smiled and said, "Dr. Brown, I'm glad that my handshake is important to you. It means a lot to me. I'm sorry, very sorry. I have so many unpleasant things on my mind that it honestly slipped my mind."

Michael jumped out of his chair, shook my hand tightly, and hugged me warmly.

Like my Soldiers, I too am on a mission. When my routine or expectation is ruined, it upsets me as well.

Being greeted by Michael at the beginning of each Tuesday Morning Group is an important part of my mission.

15

Picking Up the Pieces

"In a word, I was not pleased with myself"

IT WAS EMOTIONALLY wrenchingly painful to tuck away my lifetime dream to become a physician, but it was, for the most part, an unspoken aching.

I was immensely happily married, a very proud and most loving father, and my employment as a Boys Work Secretary for the Norfolk Central YMCA was fulfilling in many ways, some of which I described earlier.

But at the same time, sometimes inexplicably more torturing than at other times, the agony and anguish of failing out of medical school haunted me.

Perhaps it is not difficult to understand now, but the heartache throbbed most when I sat in church. I had then as I have now the deeply held belief that God's will and plan encompassed my becoming a physician despite all its improbable, implausible, and incongruous likelihood.

In a word, I was not pleased with myself.

I took evening courses taught by good professors through the University of Virginia's Extension Division in Norfolk.

The Norfolk Public Health Department

I left my employment in good standing at the YMCA after one year and worked as a Bacteriologist for the City of Norfolk's Public Health Department, applying my degree in Biology, hoping to increase my chances for a second crack at medical school.

Mr. Farmer, a competent and caring Director of Laboratories, was a good man for whom to work. Harry Snyder was my supervisor. He was a remarkable man: a faithful husband, caring father, Hebrew scholar, and gifted Bacteriologist.

At his invitation, I studied Hebrew under Harry at the Temple on Granby Street; however, I learned little Hebrew, but soon learned to love kosher food, often having lunch with Harry in a Hebrew Delicatessen on Church Street.

Mr. Randolph, an equally gifted Bacteriologist at the lab, took me on field trips where we tested milk. The names, but not the kind faces, have faded from my memory over time, but it was an intellectually stimulating work force, all willingly sharing unselfishly their wisdom and knowledge.

The Norfolk Academy

In 1956, after a year as a Bacteriologist for the Norfolk Public Health Department, I joined the faculty at the Norfolk Academy, a major favorable change in the direction of my life.

Mr. Farmer, Chief of Laboratory, Norfolk Public Health Department, unhappily accepted my resignation on the grounds that much effort went into my training with the reasonable expectation that I would continue working in the laboratory over a period of years. On many occasions, however, we had discussed my ambition to return to medical school.

Unlike Mr. Farmer, I saw a teaching and coaching job at the Norfolk Academy as more likely enhancing an opportunity to return to medical school. The Norfolk Academy was an all-boys school at that time, located at Ward's Corner in Norfolk. It traces its heritage from 1755.

James B. Massey, the Head Master, a fearless leader, guided the school into an enviable academic institution of unmatched supremacy.

Kitty Garnett and her husband, Theodore, who also taught at the Academy, helped me land the job. I enjoyed no employment and benefited from no position more than my tenure at the Academy.

Nothing comes close to the Academy as an idyllic life: teaching attentive, intellectually curious, well behaved boys (Lower School) and young men (Upper School) in the morning and early afternoon and then coaching the same young men in the afternoon on the athletic fields.

The class room building, the gym and dressing room, and the athletic fields were all conveniently adjacent to each other.

Each day began with a chapel service held in the gym. Mr. Massey was reared in the Presbyterian persuasion, son of an acclaimed professor of Religious Studies at Hampden-Sydney College, the best kept secret in higher education.

Theologians might describe the morning chapel services at the Norfolk Academy as "short, sweet, and deep." A short prayer preceded the concise reading of a brief Biblical passage, followed by the singing of a hymn whose lyrics were nearly always related to naval-inspired composers.

The closing prayer and announcements, along with the entire chapel service, took no more than a quarter of an hour, but its lingering elevation of the human spirit, an incredible way to begin one's day for student and Master (teacher) alike, is one of my fondest memories of those promising days lighting the footpath of the twenty-five year old man I was in 1956.

Joe Massey

Joe Massey, next to the youngest of the Massey children, was a gregarious, friendly, out-spoken, happy young man who was not more than six or seven years old when we first met, a uniquely likeable person, one that leaves a pleasant lasting memory, warmly welcomed like a beautiful spring day.

The Headmaster's house was situated near the gym. As one of the Headmaster's sons, Joe pretty much had the run of the place, but none were frequented more often by Joe than the gym and athletic fields.

I believe Joe loved sports as much as I did. He soon became my shadow in the afternoons, my favorite time of day. That is when I donned my coaching gear from my locker in the gym dressing room. I jogged out to the field to coach the junior varsity football team, walked into the gym to coach wrestling, or assisted with basketball or baseball.

Interestingly in retrospect, having paid little attention to it at the time because it seemed so natural and insignificant to me, but Joe kept some of his athletic gear locked up in my locker in the Norfolk Academy gym.

It was often no more than a small football or an old beat up baseball glove or ball.

Every afternoon, Joe and I met at my locker to retrieve our respective gear.

One of Joe's frequent questions, originating from a quizzical and unquenchable thirst for information and knowledge, revealed to me the value Joe and I had invested in our friendship.

Out of the blue, Joe sincerely inquired, "Mr. Brown, are you one of my dad's boys?"

I answered in the negative, Joe's countenance changed immediately. He looked down at the floor, attempting to hide his disappointment.

"I thought you were one of my dad's boys," his voice communicating sadness.

How perceptive Joe was even at such a young age. In many ways, I was more immature and less sophisticated than most of Joe's dad's teachers, more naïve, more anxious to play than to work.

"Joe," I said, "I'm one of your dad's teachers, but can we still be friends?"

Joe, beaming one of the world's biggest smiles, let me know it need not change our friendship. He continued to stow his gear in my locker until I left the Academy to become Principal of Blue Ridge School in 1958.

Many good memories come into my mind from the Norfolk Academy.

First and foremost, J.B. Massey was like a good father to the faculty, a firm parent to the boys, and a virtuous leader to us all.

I can't imagine that the school could pay him for what he was truly worth.

I recall standing behind Mr. Massey, at a church service, as he knelt prayerfully on his knees for a Communion Service; large holes of various depths revealed that his shoes were well worn. Only a thin layer of brown leather hid his socks from view.

Even if he knew the poor condition of his shoes, I do not think Mr. Massey would have been shamed or embarrassed by them.

Subjects more important than worn out shoes occupied the scholarly mind of the Headmaster.

Two of his ideas came to fruition merely as a result of saying them in my presence, "We need a wrestling team," and later, "We need a summer day camp."

The First Norfolk Academy Wrestling Team

Robert W. Herzog, Senior Master and Director of Athletics, Norfolk Academy, sent Charlie Cumiskey, Bill Harvie, and me to a one-day wrestling workshop at a nearby tidewater school on a cold winter Saturday.

Wearing suitable clothing for the occasion, we got on our hands and knees, not to pray, a better idea, but to be preyed upon by larger, better, and stronger wrestlers who, in the pretext of instruction, easily and often physically humiliated us.

The long car ride back to Norfolk after the wrestling workshop was solemn and mostly silent. It was decided I would be the newly appointed Norfolk Academy Wrestling Coach, the first wrestling coach in its long history.

I could find no acceptable, masculine way to decline the honor. I was soon to learn how regrettable the appointment could become.

Billy Martin, Granby High School Wrestling Coach at that time, is a legend in secondary school wrestling coaching history. The "Granby Roll," a specific technique used world-wide in high school and college wrestling, came from the celebrated Billy Martin. A true prince of a man of medium build, sandy colored hair, blue eyes, who was a friendly and humble person.

Our first wrestling match, as one might guess, was against Granby High School.

Fortunately, the match was poorly publicized and it was only attended by a small crowd.

The speed with which each of my wrestlers was pinned by the incredibly superior Granby team was record-setting.

Billy Martin warmly shook my hand as the match ended and said, "You have some fine young wrestlers. I know they have a bright future."

Years later I learned that Billy Martin was telling the truth, not just trying to cheer me up. One of my wrestlers that night against Granby was a youngster named Bill Miller.

Bill Miller made it to the top in wrestling and became a successful wrestling coach himself. Others may have done equally as well, but I confess I did not long follow wrestling after I moved on to Blue Ridge School.

The Norfolk Academy Summer Day Camp

The Norfolk Academy Summer Day Camp was born June 1957, two months after the birth of our second child, David Milton Brown, his middle name honoring his maternal grandfather.

David is our second blue-eyed, blond-headed son, DNA transcripts from their mother.

From his beginning, David, a lover of animals, art, and adventure, has been self-reliant, and independent.

When David lived in the country, he owned more cats than anyone could count. He was a prize-winning photographer early on, and he got his pilot's license before he got his automobile operator's permit.

I watched his first parachute jump. He was a mere teenager. I was a frightened observing father, having failed to talk him out of jumping, but his joyous shouts upon landing safely on the grass at the Orange, Virginia, airfield were unforgettable.

David has resided in New Zealand for the past fifteen years, first teaching high school photography and then on to the practice of law, first in Balclutha, a small town south of Dunedin, and then in Dunedin, his favorite New Zealand City, where he has lived for seven years.

When Dottie and I visited David in 2010 in Dunedin, South Island, New Zealand, we were warmly welcomed by some of the friendliest people in the world.

The School of Law, Otago University, Dunedin, is led by the laudable Dean R. M. Henaghan, truly a scholar, a gentleman, and an altogether most pleasant person.

Rex Adair, Professor of Law and Religion at the Otago Law School, became a fast friend.

I cannot tell you whether the Norfolk Academy Summer Day Camp survived after I left for Blue Ridge School. I can only tell you about its beginning.

Mac MacConochie, one of the Academy's most respected teachers, Bill Harvie, a new teacher like me, Allen Tyler, a popular teacher of French, and I formed the Day Camp staff.

We operated out of two sites, Virginia Beach and the Norfolk Academy.

Each day I drove the large yellow school bus from school to the beach, parking it in my driveway at home each night.

Our son, Bobby, our first child, then only three years of age, happily greeted me at the door at the end of each day's work at the Day Camp. His large blue eyes were filled with a special love, unique between father and son.

Bobby honored me by following closely as a child in my every footstep. As an adult, Bobby followed my professional footsteps, readily surpassing my psychiatric and forensic accomplishments.

It would be an understatement to say that 3-year-old Bobby was impressed with the school bus. In fact, when asked the familiar question, "What would you like to be when you grow up, Bobby," unhesitatingly and with the immediacy of an enthusiast he would reply, "I want to be a bus!"

As I recall, we conducted two sessions of the Summer Day Camp, soon learned that our enterprise was proving popular, and, perhaps most important of all, everyone had a happy and safe summer.

We had every conventional game and sport one could imagine at the Academy Day Camp.

A healthy lunch was followed by the telling of ghost stories.

A pleasant round-trip bus ride to Sea Shore State Park on the Chesapeake Bay for swimming and running on the beach was the day's main feature. Sadly, in just a couple of years, Sea Shore State Park closed its gates to fight integration.

The boys came mostly from the Lower School of the Norfolk Academy. They were at an age where ghost stories fell on receptive ears and fertile imagination.

Long before the present television and movie craze and obsession with vampires, I had a rich resource of similar tales.

I had been frightened out of my wits by my mother's endless telling of stories from an invisible world where strange things without rational explanations permanently thrived.

Self-anointed vampire expert, I soon had recognition and popularity I never deserved nor ever dreamed would be my fate that hot summer in Norfolk.

Suspending my sense of reality, I straightforwardly told preposterous accounts of the life and work of vampires struggling at night for ways and means to replenish their dwindling supply of life-giving red blood cells, rich in hemoglobin and iron.

Students sitting at the feet of Plato or Aristotle could not have been more attentive, more rapt, or more admiring and impressed than the young students gathered in the shade under a tree.

The Academy Day Campers, sitting inches from my feet, absorbed every fabrication and misrepresentation that was formed by my uninstructed tongue about the life and limb of vampires.

Hands shot up as polite forms of interruptions, all asking what in their inquisitive minds was the critical question, "Mr. Brown, how can I become a vampire?"

Without intending it, I had made vampires heroic, if not pathetic figures.

There is only one way, I assured the students, to become a vampire, replying half-heartedly, unable to think on the spot of a better answer.

"To become a vampire," I announced, "you must go to vampire school."

To my surprise, my answer did not end the discussion.

"How can we go to vampire school, Mr. Brown?" they replied in unison.

"Look guys, rest hour is over," I announced. "We have to move on to another activity. Can't you see I am in a hurry," I pleaded.

"We don't want to go to another activity. Tell us how to go to vampire school!"

Okay, I thought to myself; these are bright kids. They are turning the tables on me. The joke is on me, I thought.

Walking away, almost as an afterthought, I simply said, "If you want to attend vampire school, bring a note from home. It must be signed by one of your parents."

First thing the next morning, a ten year old boy walked up to me and placed a note in my hand.

What is this, I wondered. I unfolded the note and read, "Johnny has my permission to attend Vampire School." It was signed by his mother.

The Extension Division

The Extension Division of the University of Virginia was staffed by competent and caring people at its Center in Norfolk in the 1950s. I do not believe a year passed since I left medical school without my taking at least one evening course.

In order to fulfill the requirements for a master's degree, however, a year of course work in residence at the University of Virginia in Charlottesville must be completed.

Now the father of two fine young sons, I was happily married, and well settled into a good life as a master and coach at the Norfolk Academy. These good circumstances made leaving the Norfolk Academy for the foothills of Virginia less appealing to anyone other than me.

I was working on a plan to return to medical school, but it was a scheme whose only visible indicators were all on the negative side, letters of discouragement from the Dean of Admissions.

If there is going to be a second chance to attend medical school, it must be granted by the school where the academic failure occurred. No other medical school willingly takes on the problems of one of its sister schools.

The Blue Ridge School

In the late 1950s, Blue Ridge School, an Episcopal co-educational Boarding School, grades one through twelve, originally a "mountain mission school," geographically close to Charlottesville, urgently needed a principal.

Rev. Loving, the Headmaster of Blue Ridge School, was ill. The school was struggling financially.

If I agreed to come to the school almost immediately as its principal, it was understood that time would be made available to complete my master's degree in educational psychology at the University of Virginia.

Remaining my friend after leaving him and the Norfolk Academy at mid-year for Blue Ridge, J.B. Massey proved to be a steadfast colleague.

Independent school administrators in Virginia and the southern region are a tightknit group. Dr. William Presley, Headmaster of Westminster School in Atlanta, contacted Mr. Massey at the Norfolk Academy.

Dr. Presley asked Mr. Massey to help him find a suitable candidate to run Hillside Cottages, a respected home for children from broken but mendable families.

Mr. Massey, of course, had no way of knowing when he called me after one year at Blue Ridge, about the Atlanta position, that a major hurricane would strike the center of the Blue Ridge campus, destroy vast amounts of property, and usher in entirely new objectives for the school, transforming it into the fine boy's school it became and remains today.

I was a teacher and principal at Blue Ridge at the same time I was a full-time student at the University, commuting almost daily to Charlottesville.

Mr. Loving was devoted to Blue Ridge. As an Episcopal Priest, he had spent much of his career at Blue Ridge. He was a thoughtful, caring, and strong-willed person who always treated me with kindness and respect.

The teachers were dedicated. The children came from diverse backgrounds. I enjoyed teaching them.

Bobby, David, Dottie, and I lived in the principal's house, a stone structure next to the chapel. We regularly entertained students and faculty in our home.

A "mountain woman" and her young daughter occasionally helped Dottie with the housework. We soon learned, however, that mountain people do not wish to become "beholden."

The mountain behind our house was tall, steep, and rugged. We were surprised by a knock at our front door at the end of a hot, humid summer day during which the mountain woman, an industrious and laborious worker who spoke less often than a deaf mute, had worked with Dottie at our house.

"Here are your two Cokes, Mam," said the sweating and nearly breathless mountain woman, passing two Coca Colas to Dottie.

"No," said Dottie, "I gave you and your daughter those to drink with your lunch today. I did not expect you to replace them…they were a gift from me to you."

Shaking her head and speaking firmly, the mountain woman said. "No, mam, take them…I can't be beholden," and she quickly marched off the front stoop and soon found her path back up to the top of the mountain.

Virgil Scott Ward

Virgil Scott Ward, PhD, Professor of Education, Curry School of Education, University of Virginia, became my academic advisor when I returned to the Charlottesville area by way of Blue Ridge School.

I underestimated the power of his intellect at our first meetings. I could not have known at that time that his influence upon my future would be transforming. Dr. Ward gave me a new perspective. He gave to me abundantly. All that he gave to me was given selflessly, a comment I will attempt to clarify later.

He was a tall man, standing about six feet, but his bushy white hair, failing to stay slicked back with repetitive combing, added inches to his image.

Three of Dr. Ward's features stood out: dark eye glass frames with lenses not unlike the thickness of the bottom of a Coca Cola bottle; command of the English language most resembling the learned guests on a British radio talk show; and an uncanny knack of attracting and welcoming criticism and debate.

He was reared as an orphan in South Carolina, served in the Army, and earned his PhD at the University of North Carolina.

He became a leading authority on education of gifted students. Although he never acknowledged it, owing to his extremely private nature, he was likely a gifted child himself whose education was unsuitable, if not distractingly disrupting.

His entire academic career was dedicated to teaching about the distinct characteristics of gifted children and creating guidelines for teachers of the gifted. It is therefore puzzling that Dr. Ward took an interest in me and my aspirations to return to medical school and to practice medicine.

It is not a disguised form of modesty to admit that I am not and never was considered by myself or by my teachers to be gifted. I did not express to Dr. Ward, or to anyone else, that I had an interest in the education of the gifted.

Mine was an entirely selfish motive, if not an obsession, to get back into medical school. Dr. Ward understood.

In August 1958, while Principal of Blue Ridge School, I earned a Master's of Education Degree, specializing in Educational Psychology, under the tutelage of Dr. Ward.

Our third child, Nancy Elizabeth, was born while we lived at Blue Ridge School.

It is exactly twenty-six miles from Blue Ridge School to the University of Virginia Hospital.

"Gunsmoke," one of my all-time favorite TV shows, was playing. Yes, Dottie thought she was having labor pains, but could she not be mistaken, or, at least, could she not wait until Matt Dillon shot the bad guy?

These admittedly important if not critical topics were addressed, during the commercials, of course, and not during the show itself. Trying not to be insensitive or indifferent to Dottie's feelings, I believe I even started the car and moved it, engine still running, to the front of the house.

It turned out that we were both correct: she was in labor and she could wait until the show ended, justice prevailing.

We made it safely, thankfully, to the hospital. Nancy Elizabeth's big beautiful eyes, for the first time in her life, no sooner than two hours after we were greeted at the delivery room, opened with tears flowing, warmly welcomed by all that she beheld.

Thanks to Encore Westerns, I still enjoy Matt Dillon, Doc Adams, Miss Kitty, and Chester Good every night. Sadly, I watch the show alone at night in my rented house near the military facility where I treat Soldiers. My dear Dottie tells me she also watches Gunsmoke in Charlottesville at the same time

While relishing Gunsmoke, I also relish the nutritious dinners prepared for my week away from home by Dottie, always lovingly devoted.

Blue Ridge School opened in 1903 as a "mountain mission school," a credit to the Episcopal Church who recognized early the need to take education, both religious and secular, to the children who lived high up in the steeply rugged Blue Ridge Mountains of Virginia.

At its beginning, Episcopal priests on horseback carried the Word of God and the instruction of man to these all but forgotten children.

On Sundays, the priest took his message to at least three small remote churches; soon these priests were called "circuit riders."

The children who lived near enough walked to the Blue Ridge School. Those who lived far from the school represented the majority of its student body. They were housed at the school during the academic year.

Dedicated men and women were recruited to live and teach at the school.

Testimonies of the children educated at Blue Ridge School, emotionally moving, describe how they became enlightened by the school. Without it, their lives were doomed to the poverty and illiteracy of common mountain folk. These students were ethnically diverse. They lived many miles from electricity and other common place conveniences.

Over time, progress reached even the peaks of the tallest mountains of Appalachia. Few people continued to reside there. This forced Blue Ridge School and the Episcopal Church to reexamine its mission. The process was slow. Change came with difficulty.

The vacuum was filled by other children in need, children from other geographical areas of Virginia.

When I arrived five and a half decades after its origin, Blue Ridge School's student body had few if any "mountain children." Instead, many of the children, boys and girls from age 6 to 20, came from welfare departments who happily placed their wards in the safety of the geographically isolated school.

Some of the teachers were retirees from various professions; others were young and motivated by genuine devotion to helping these rather unique students, many with great unrealized potential.

Tucked away in the foot-hills of the Blue Ridge Mountains, the Blue Ridge School formed a warm and protective environment.

It is a rather special place with its own Post Office, beautiful stone chapel, exquisite mountain stone Battle House nearly adjoining the chapel, adequate dormitories, fine dining hall where three healthy meals are served daily, a good gym, a stone school house, a stable with horses, and spacious athletic fields.

Reverend Loving, Superintendent and Episcopal Priest, dedicated his life to the school during some of its most financially challenging times. He was physically exhausted, confined to his bed when I arrived.

Reverend Loving's failing health was the main reason my arrival could not wait till the end of the academic session at the Norfolk Academy. It was a trying situation for everyone involved.

Mr. Massey deserves the credit for bearing the burden on his end and permitting me, without malice, to leave with our friendship intact.

I was twenty-three years old when academic failure barred my continuation in medical school at the University.

I had left Charlottesville in 1954 in a rented truck, moving back to Norfolk, Virginia, nearly all my hopes of returning to the University dashed, largely replaced by self-loathing and disappointment greater than any I had ever known.

I was twenty-seven when I became Principal of Blue Ridge School, the same time I returned to the grounds of the University, an applicant for a Master's Degree in Education.

Thomas Jefferson's "academical village" fostered and rekindled my hopes through the strong authentic support I received in 1959 from Dean Ralph Cherry and Virgil S. Ward, my mentor whose friendship I came to cherish.

The contrast between the way I left the University as a medical school failure and the way I was welcomed back to the University as a graduate student in the Curry School is of the degree one comes to expect between night and day.

No professor in medical school was more demanding or more intellectually honest than Virgil Ward in the Curry School. This quiet, socially avoidant scholar was not known for his friendliness. In fact, he was argumentative, a stickler for even minuscule facts, and reserved his respect for those who succeeded in debating him, not put off by his intellectual ruthlessness.

I arrived as Principal of Blue Ridge School in January 1958. Accommodated by evening and summer classes, I was permitted to teach and administer at Blue Ridge simultaneously.

I received my Master's Degree in Education in August 1958.

Hillside Cottages

Mr. Massey, my former Headmaster, Norfolk Academy, called in the fall of 1958 and suggested I consider an offer suggested by Dr. Presley, President, Westminster School, Atlanta, to become director of a children's home, "the oldest charity in Atlanta…started by a group of Atlanta women for orphans and mothers with children… all victims of the Civil War and originally known as the Home for the Friendless."

"Bobby," Mr. Massey said, "the future of the Blue Ridge School is uncertain. I know you want to be a teacher and more than a teacher, Bobby. Look into this position in Atlanta. I have a lot of respect for Dr. Presley. Based on what I told him about you, he is convinced that you are the man they are looking for in Atlanta."

Mr. Loving's health had returned. Several of the teachers were readily capable of replacing me.

Dottie and I talked seriously about the Atlanta option.

On a Friday, I took the night train from the old train station in Charlottesville to Atlanta.

I rode in a Pullman train car, hardly slept, arrived rather disheveled at the Peachtree train station about seven AM, took a taxi to Hillside Cottages, and waited, quietly walking around the middle income neighborhood, killing time until I met the Women's Board of Directors.

Hillside was an attractive collection of four brick "cottages," all neatly landscaped, a more recently constructed attractive brick office complex, and all were nestled on a gently upward sloping hill with tall, mature pine trees.

Mamie Ruth Bartlett, President, Women's Board of Directors, Hillside Cottages, joined by several members of the Personnel Committee, welcomed me to Hillside.

It was a bright, clear Georgia fall day. These sophisticated, educated, and seriously dedicated women treated Hillside and its wards with affection and firm executive responsibility resembling the seriousness with which one takes the oath of office.

They were rightfully proud of its history, and its changed but ongoing mission to care for children from "broken but mendable families." They wanted an executive director who shared their perception of its mission.

In 1959, each cottage housed sixteen school age children, was staffed by a house mother and dietitian, and had its own pediatrician who volunteered his services as needed.

The Kiwanis Club of Atlanta had built and maintained an in-ground swimming pool. The assistant director, Ms. Waggoner, a Licensed Clinical Social Worker, worked with community agencies in arranging for admissions and discharge planning.

The children attended nearby public schools, and most children came from single parent families who were able to have their children return home for weekends.

"Going home for good," an electrifying pronouncement that brought broad smiles of joy to everyone, was the ultimate goal of Hillside Cottages for all of its children.

The position was offered to me and I accepted, got back on the Saturday night train, slept as peacefully as rail travel permits, arrived in Charlottesville early Sunday morning, and drove the twenty-six miles to Blue Ridge School.

I was 27 when I became Executive Director of Hillside Cottages, Atlanta, Georgia.

Dottie shared my excitement. The Board of Directors wanted to fill the position immediately, but understood that I must delay my departure from Blue Ridge School until the end of the fall semester.

It was a beautiful 1959 January day. Our station wagon was packed with all that we could carry, when Dottie, Bobby, David, Nancy, and I drove out of the winding country roads of Greene County, Virginia, onto US 29 South to Atlanta, an all-night, nearly non-stop trip.

Bobby was 4, David 2, and Nancy, our "Gunsmoke" baby, was only 3 months old.

A severe, unexpected winter storm accompanied us with sleet and ice, but we arrived in front of the administration building at Hillside Cottages just as dawn's first light danced on the sparkling ice that weighed heavily on the tall pine trees.

In the station wagon, we dozed intermittently until a light shone in the office building, then used by the assistant director as a temporary residence.

Ms. Waggoner, LCSW, a delightful southern woman in her mid-fifties, spotted our car and welcomed us inside and then took us to a nearby hotel.

The hotel was to be our home until the renovation of the old wooden school house, tucked in a wooded area behind one of the brick cottages, was completed.

Initially, there was excitement about living in a hotel, a new experience for our children; however, as the weeks of waiting slowly passed, impatience became annoyance and then frustration hardened itself around us like concrete.

Eating meals, mostly of fast foods, taken into our large hotel room, with all the necessary beds, was an awkward problem, one standing out in my memory.

Finally, the Board permitted us to move into our house before it was completed. Soon thereafter we began to feel at home.

Woody, our German Shepherd family pet, completed our sense of being together. A dog barking in the distance on the dark night when I now recall this important phase of our life, momentarily takes me back to the good feelings and good memories evoked by Woody, now long deceased.

More may be revealed about Woody in these pages, but I am compelled to share one thought about him at this point. The children at Hillside loved Woody, and he was very gentle with them. From the time of our arrival in Atlanta, Woody was my shadow.

He quietly slept under my desk at work, jumped into the Hillside Volkswagen Bus, and on my all too frequent trips to Miss Georgia Ice Cream parlors, I always treated him to the same ice cream cone that I enjoyed. Woody consumed his treat from the sidewalk, leaving no trace that it once served as a dessert serving tray.

Dottie, the children, and I soon felt completely at home at Hillside; however, no work before or since Hillside, the possible exception being my current position as staff psychiatrist to our fine Soldiers who fought for us in Iraq and Afghanistan, had such a strong personal, emotional impact upon me.

Witnessing the children painfully separating from their mothers, the ones requiring psychiatric hospitalization in distant Milledgeville, Georgia, resonated with me in the most inner part of my soul.

It touched a long ago memory when my own mother intuitively knew I could not manage separation from her at five years of age. As described earlier, my mother subjected our entire family to weeks of quarantine, restricted to our small Norfolk house because of my contagious "Yellow Jaundice."

My sadness over the plight of the children at Hillside became depression.

I did not know what had befallen me.

Dottie's wonderful culinary art and skill lost its captivation. My loss of appetite led to significant loss of weight, and I was incredibly anxious.

Looking back from my professional position today, I was clinically depressed and had panic attacks that made me seriously wonder if I was losing my mind.

Two things helped me out of despair.

First, we had joined Druid Hills Baptist Church when we arrived in Atlanta, transferring our membership from our church in Virginia.

Louie D. Newton was the pastor. He was an intellectual giant. He moved from journalism to ministry, never having the benefit of a seminary education.

Louie Newton, a man of contagious love for Jesus Christ of Nazareth, taught a "healthy minded religion," not unlike that advocated by William James in his 1903 <u>Varieties of Religious Experience</u>.

We attended church religiously. Dottie and I sang in the choir. I taught an adult couples class prior to which, in the long history of this wonderful church on Ponce de Leon Avenue, men and women were always taught separately.

Secondly, Dr. Bernard Holland, Chief of Psychiatry, Emory University, volunteered to see one Hillside child a week with me.

Dr. Holland, "Bernie" to his friends, was a friendly, warm, kindhearted, genius with a full head of blonde-white hair.

Dr. Holland healed primarily through caring. His love was palpable. As each child recovered, my emotional burden lifted, thank God, never to really return.

Hillside flourished. It was a happy time in the life of our family, and our family gradually included every child at Hillside.

I was very pleased by a phone call after our first year at Hillside.

The kind voice of a mature woman said she was pleased with the mission of Hillside and wanted to donate the funds for a fifth "cottage." Recall that the "cottage" of Hillside Cottages was a grand brick structure attractively landscaped, housed sixteen children, had its own dining room, and accommodations for a house mother and for a dietitian.

I thanked the caller. I told the kind and generous person I would contact the President of the Board of Directors and promptly return her most welcomed call.

Mammie Ruth Bartlett, President of the Board, firmly advised me to decline the offer.

"Tell the woman we cannot accept her gift unless it includes furniture and complete furnishings for sixteen children."

It was not easy for me to call back the generous lady with the message from the Board; however, I could almost detect a smile in her voice when she agreed to the terms of her gift.

The fifth cottage was built, finely furnished, beautifully landscaped, and sixteen additional children joined our large family.

"Fruitful" describes our two and a half years in Atlanta.

The location of Hillside was in the Morningside neighborhood of Atlanta, and geographically close to Emory University. I was permitted to enroll in Emory's Graduate Department of Psychology, staffed by eminent scholars, several of whom took a personal interest in our work at Hillside.

I was also privileged to serve under General Carl Sutherland as the Assistant Division Chemical Officer for the 80th USAR Infantry Division.

Hillside was also the second consecutive job in which we lived on the premises, the good part of which was being near my family.

If there were a down side to living on the premises, it contributed to periodic and strong feelings "to get away."

In those days, we prayed together as a family. One prayer was for a "safe trip to Miami." Taking turns praying, David, our second son, then still very young, sincerity and seriousness in his voice, prayed for a "safe trip to my Daddy's Ami."

God answered David's prayer. In the words of Pope John Paul II, "Each child is God's irreplaceable gift."

No person is poor who has the love of his or her children. Dottie and I count our children as our greatest blessing.

Dr. Virgil Scott Ward Calls Again

In August 1961, at the Atlanta airport, at his request, I met Virgil S. Ward, my former academic advisor at the University of Virginia.

"To fulfill your destiny," Dr. Ward said, "you must complete your PhD. If you want to come back to Charlottesville, I will be pleased to continue our work together."

Dottie agreed. Like a whirlwind, we made our way back to the place where all my roads lead, not to Rome, but to the University of Virginia whose founder, Thomas Jefferson, influenced by Roman architecture, built one of the most beautiful universities in the world.

Others may observe living in "Old Copely Hill," dilapidating wooden barracks surviving since WW II, or managing on limited income made available through loans, grants, and scholarships, as "hardships." We recall them now as among the happiest days of our long life.

We never felt deprived.

We were working toward a goal, making dreams come true, identical to our neighbors. We never counted the cost, and we never worried about tomorrow's challenges.

We knew who we were. We were students whose income at that time would have qualified for food stamps, had they been available in the early 1960s.

We were happy people filled with hope. We were people willing to work and wait. We were free of envy. We were joyous when a neighbor graduated, got a good job, or passed an important milestone in his or her personal and professional life.

Harold P. Warner, our banker for fifty years, was referred to fondly by our family as "Uncle Hal." He often saw us through troubled waters more hazardous than the Straits of Hormuz.

In those days, all interest paid on loans was tax deductible. For us, that literally meant that many of our loans were interest free in the long run.

Hal Warner believed in our potential. He took many risks. Government backed educational loans evolved long after my formal education ended.

I earned a stipend as a graduate assistant to Dr. Ward. The University charged only $40 monthly for our three-bedroom apartment. Fortunately, in looking back, we lost no sleep over financial worries, knowing that somehow our debts would be paid, and they were paid.

It was not easy on Dottie. Nevertheless, she was more than can be expected of the good wife that she was. She was more than can be expected of the good mother that she was to our three young children.

We pulled together as a team.

The two years between 1961 and 1963 speedily vanished.

My PhD in Education was awarded May 15, 1963.

As the successful completion of my PhD studies appeared to be coming to a happy ending, it was generally understood I would buy a navy blue suit for job interviews.

It would, however, be misleading, if not dishonest, to report, in the unique case of the Browns, that one's wife's perception of a job interview and the husband's perception of the same term were unalike.

They were miles apart.

One party assumed an academic appointment, a job, at last, with regular income and benefits that such a position brings immediately to mind.

The other assumed a second crack at medical school, eight to ten more years as a lowly student, intern, and resident and fellow, with little or no opportunity for income for at least the next four or five years.

Some dreams never die.

Some dreams may become nightmares for others, fortunately not true in this case.

When one's dream is buried deeply in one's heart, there is no rest for the dreamer, none until every possible approach to fulfillment is exhausted.

The New Navy Blue Suit

Clad in the new navy blue suit, I sat nervously in front of Dr. Frank Finger, Chairman, Pre-Medical Evaluation Committee, University of Virginia, and three members of his important team.

"Mr. Brown," Dr. Finger asked, "are you not nearly thirty-two years of age, and will you not be at least forty years of age if and when you complete medical school and post-graduate training?"

It was true, I admitted, but my age had never been a major concern of mine.

"Mr. Brown," he continued, "you have not taken a single course in science since you left medical school a decade ago."

For the past ten years, I was almost never out of a graduate school program, I needlessly reminded the Committee, but my choice of courses was determined by their availability to me, operating under the constraints of full-time employment.

All the good questions raised by Dr. Finger deserved better answers than I could credibly provide.

I was no more than an older student whose desire to study medicine might be perceived by the Pre-Medical Evaluation Committee as commendable. Beyond that, I lacked even the most rudimentary academic accomplishments for medical school.

Furthermore, Dr. Finger may well have said, "Why give a second chance to a man who has already failed once, when so many good students have not been given their first chance?"

I don't believe I ever learned what Dr. Finger's committee finally decided.

Many years later, as I mentioned earlier, I was honored to have a locker at University Hall, University of Virginia, adjacent to Dr. Finger's locker.

Dr. Finger was a prize-winning master athlete, an Octogenarian, a record holder of yet to be surpassed track and field events.

We worked out at noon nearly every day, often including weekends and holidays. Dr. Finger had his own key to University Hall.

We met in this way for many years, discussed many topics and concerns, but the Pre-Medical Evaluation Committee was never mentioned.

Dr. Finger was the most popular guest speaker in my Mental Health class at Virginia. I counted him among my best friends over the past twenty-five years.

Several years ago, Dr. Finger's daughter phoned me with sad news.

"Dad will not be speaking to your class tomorrow night. He died of a stroke today. I found your class presentation written on his calendar."

I was very saddened. At the same time, I was very pleased that Dr. Finger had such a long, productive, and physically active life.

He was a hero for many of us. Each time I introduced Dr. Finger to the five hundred Mental Health students at Virginia, I always sang the first stanza and part of the chorus of "You are the Wind Beneath my Wings." The round of applause, of course, was for Dr. Finger, not the vocalist.

Everyone who applies to medical school knows the importance of grades, particularly grades in science courses, letters of recommendation, and MCAT scores.

For my application, there were no recent grades in the sciences and no MCAT scores. Letters of recommendations would have to mean more for me than for my competitors for one of the seventy-five seats in the medical school class of 1967.

Dr. Morris McKean, Professor of Anatomy, remembered me favorably from the class of 1957. He agreed to write a letter on my behalf.

Dr. William Sandusky, Professor of Surgery, was Chairman of the Admissions Committee. He was an excellent surgeon and enjoyed the reputation as a man of integrity.

Years after the fact, I learned from Dr. Sandusky that Dr. Virgil S. Ward not only wrote a letter on my behalf, but he also met with Dr. Sandusky and "put his reputation on the line for you."

When the letter arrived from the Committee on Admissions to the School of Medicine, University of Virginia, my reaction was not unlike that of Rudy, the character in the movie bearing his name, when his admission letter arrived from Notre Dame.

It was the culmination of a decade of hope, prayer, visits and applications to medical schools here and abroad.

Most important of all, I promised Dottie this would be my last attempt to attend medical school. If I was not accepted this time, I would make a life-altering decision, give up my dream, and close that chapter forever.

I read only the first line of the letter, "It gives me pleasure...." It was fifty-one years ago, or was it yesterday, or earlier today?

A sincere prayer of thanksgiving struggled for the right words. The right words came right from the heart.

"I was given a second chance"

I was given a second chance.

I came to believe in second chances for everyone. I had not given up. Those I respected had not given up on me.

I believe in and try to practice never giving up on others.

Medical school was tough, more difficult than the first time, but I had learned how to study and I had the loving support of Dottie and our children, Bobby 9, David 6, and Nancy, 4 years old.

In many ways, we went to medical school together as a family. We went nowhere without the children.

Our favorite place to eat was the University Cafeteria, sadly no longer at the University Corner. We also enjoyed a chicken salad sandwich on toast at Chancellor's Drug Store.

Regrettably, like the University Cafeteria, Chancellor's and the good people who were employed in these full-of-life businesses exist now only in our memories. They must also live on in the memory of the thousands who, like us, were privileged to find meaningful respite there.

Clinton Addison Brady Brown, our fourth child, the one on whom the remaining family names were liberally bestowed, was born early in my second year of medical school.

Hunter Faulconer, a remarkably kind and generous man, inexpensively rented houses near the University Hospital to medical student families and hospital personnel.

I could leave our back door on Park Place, walk across Jefferson Park Avenue, and enter the main entrance of the hospital in a matter of a few minutes. The reverse trip home was made even more speedily.

Except when I was on call, I could come home for dinner with the family, return to the pathology lab to view microscopic slides, run back to watch a family favorite TV show such as Hogan's Heroes, help put the children to bed. If necessary, I could run back to the lab until all assignments were completed.

Dottie deserves most of the credit, but we raised our children together in the shadow of the University of Virginia School of Medicine and Hospital. I could not have been happier. Happiness infused the family. We had no shortage of problems, what Freud called "the common miseries of life," but ones that were besetting were endured together. We went nowhere without the children.

My identity, or sense of myself as a person, was mostly influenced by the people I loved and by people who loved me. It was also shaped by my hopes and dreams. My successes and my failures changed and guided me.

"...the endless thread that has woven meaning into my life."

A concise review, at this point, may help the reader, as well as the writer, to understand the endless thread that has woven meaning into my life.

My identity was seldom a conscious awareness. It became clearer to me as time and events passed, initially slowly and then seemingly speedily.

From an anxious, dependent elementary school child, I discovered I could run faster than anyone in school. I did not appreciate its importance at the time; it was merely a score teachers were required to record twice a year as we lined up to run fifty yards. Was it the discovery that I could become an athlete?

Ms. Green, my kind and gentle first grade teacher, created a sense of safety. The same was true of Ms. Gray, my third grade teacher. All the teachers at James Madison Grammar School were welcoming.

I was in the fifth grade when WW II started, and in the ninth grade, then a student at Blair Junior High School, when the war ended.

I wore the red badge of the Safety Patrol in the sixth grade. I wore the blue badge of the Captain of the Safety Patrol in the seventh grade, graduating from James Madison with the sense that others saw me as dependable and responsible.

My primary identity in Blair Junior High and Maury High School was that of an athlete, "fleet-footed football star."

Always wanting to be a doctor, I came dangerously close to not making sufficient grades to first enter medical school.

Going to the University of Virginia in JAN 1950 was all about the study of pre-med requirements and getting into medical school. My identity then was that of Bobby Brown from Lamberts Point, the blue collar section of Norfolk, Virginia, who was going to be a doctor.

The first Florence Smith Scholarships, then administered by the Norfolk Foundation, were inaugurated in 1953. The Smith

Scholarships were for medical students. They were and are today generous scholarships.

How I landed one of the first Smith Scholarships 60 years ago continues to baffle me. The memory of it brings with it a deep sense of sadness that the committee awarding the Smith Scholarship envisioned a future for me that I did not fulfill in the usual and customary way.

After an unsuccessful first year of medical school, 1953-1954, there was a dramatic, decade-long identity change in the fundamental, crucial, and foremost way I regarded myself.

I was and I became the person who failed out of medical school.

Words, apart from the hands and heart of a masterful composer, cannot convey the prolonged, persistent misery that befell me.

I had no words for it, but it is known to all who experience grief.

The sense of failure was pervasive and felt impermeable, like a stain that neither fades nor disappears.

Amazingly, I functioned as a husband, father, employee, and later as a graduate student, but those roles could not have been optimally executed.

No success in any other endeavor removed the strong sense of myself as a failure.

Persistent, haunting thoughts, often in the strangest places, during a church service, for example, created a sense of internal restlessness. I believed I could only find relief in the recovery of my identity, my dream to become a physician.

Earlier in these pages, I described the people who immeasurably helped me return to medical school. They helped me regain my lost identity. To these people, and to my dearest wife, I remain forever grateful.

The long road back to medical school, briefly reviewed and summarized in this memoir, perhaps helps the reader understand the incredible, untellable happiness I experienced to be, yet once again, back in medical school, a state of mind, I imagine, like the return of sanity.

Is one's identity more than stored memories and the meaning given to those memories?

Up to this point in my life, I had failed to achieve the first, major step in the career goal of my life, the meaning of which for me was to keep trying.

The most of the difficulty I encountered was impatience that arose from taking the narrow, short-term view, instead of persistently trying and patiently waiting, taking the long view of life, having faith that what is right and true will rule my life if I permit it to happen.

Was hope, the hope of the second chance to study medicine, replaced by the dread of the revisitation of the ghost of academic failure once I restarted medical school?

The answer is yes and no. The academic challenge of medical school is a cake-walk for no one.

Perhaps my fear of failure at that time, learned like a child who touches a hot stove, is most accurately depicted as a background noise. It was never completely quiet in that part of my mind.

I was reassured and encouraged by my perception that my professors and my classmates wanted me to learn and wanted to work with me to assure that learning was taking its rightful place.

Warmth that combined collegiality with some of my professors and acceptance and respect from my classmates surprised and pleased me very much.

Those who know me well will laugh out loud, or sneer, but the following movie scene best describes the unarticulated feeling that most truly described my inner feelings as I walked, for a second opportunity, into the class rooms of the School of Medicine, University of Virginia.

Joseph Carey Merrick, 1862-1890, the "Elephant Man," in a movie bearing his name, was finally cared for in a special section of the London hospital, circa 1880s.

He was astounded by the kindness with which he was treated and could barely speak of his emotion and gratitude above a whisper. I fight back my own tears, no matter how many times the scene comes before me.

Mine was also a spirit of humility and gratitude for a second chance. I can blame no one but myself for losing my first chance to study medicine.

The hopes of a lot of good people rode on my shoulders when I left Lamberts Point and Maury High School, attended the University, 1950-53, got a BA Degree in Biology, and entered medical school in the fall of 1953.

It was the dashing of their hopes that hurt me the most.

My parents and Dottie were all right with it, I thought.

But Sena B. Wood, Director of the 5th Bell Chorus, Maury High, Mrs. Williams, the Chemistry teacher who permitted me to do what no other Maury student was ever allowed to do (take Chemistry One and Chemistry Two at the same time), Kitty Garnett, the substitute teacher at Maury who changed the direction of my life, and my football coaches, Tony Saunders and William Gray, were all disappointed in me.

I felt their unspoken disappointment as sure as I feel the shoes on my feet.

"The pieces of my life were picked up…"

The pieces of my life were picked up by the caring hands of people I carry in my soul today.

My "doctor's bag," the one into which I reach to treat each patient, military or civilian, overflows with their love.

The greatest antidote for fear and failure, undeniably, is love.

16

WAR ON TRUST

"I was in Iraq for 15 months during the surge, 2006-2007"

Trying not to be late for the Traumatic Grief Group, I walked speedily down the long hallway to Group Room One.

CPT William Abram, previously unknown to me, sat opposite the door, with his back to the window, the only occupant in the large room.

CPT Abram is a man of small frame, black hair, dark eyes, and somber facial expression. I guessed his age to be about 27. He frequently put his right hand, formed into a small fist, up to his closed mouth before clearing his throat.

The repetitive clearing of his throat, sadly, was failing to clear his mind of anxious thoughts.

He was neatly dressed in his ACU (Army Combat Uniform). He wore a combat patch on the right sleeve of his uniform. He wore a sad, serious, and worried expression on his thin face.

I extended my hand, welcomed him to the group and explained that my co-therapist, LTC Mac O'Quinn, would soon join us.

"I'm new to Behavioral Health. My therapist referred me to your group. I can't recall her name, but here is her card."

He passed me the small professional card on which was written the time and date of his next appointment. It did not have his therapist's name on the card.

"We're pleased to have you in the group," I said, passing his appointment card back to him. "I hope you will find it helpful. The Soldiers who get the most of our group are the ones who make a commitment to come every week.

The group is small. I expect several others to arrive later."

Several others arrived. The group started.

CPT Abram spoke anxiously. "I was in Taji, Iraq for 15 months during the surge, 2006-2007. Taji is located 20 miles north of Baghdad, in the volatile Sunni Triangle.

It was one of the hottest places in Iraq.

"I want no one to feel sorry for me"

CPT Abram spoke again. "I drove by here a million times since I was stationed here over a year ago. I couldn't come in. I wanted to go back to Iraq.

About a month ago, my wife saw dramatic changes in me. She insisted I come here to see if I could be fixed.

I was afraid I was going crazy.

I suck in crowds.

I jump out of my skin in malls.

My sleep is really messed up.

I am constantly in the alert mode.

Six years ago this week was a rough week."

The group listened attentively. CPT Abram was telling his story. Would the group be able to contain the emotional blast of his trauma?

"I'm not coming here for sympathy. I want no one to feel sorry for me.

I was in a high guard tower with another Lieutenant, just inside the gate in Taji. It was the week before Mother's Day.

The insurgents had cut the bottom out of their vehicles. As they drove along the road in front of the gate at night, they would carefully drop IEDs (Improvised Explosive Devices) through the holes.

I could hear the clink as the IEDs landed. I called it in, not knowing what was causing the clinking sounds.

Security made the road 'Black' (not safe for travel), but one of our vehicles went out of the gate anyway.

The vehicle was carrying 6 Soldiers. It hit one of the IEDs in the road. The blast was loud and deadly.

There was a huge ball of orange, yellow fire.

I could feel the heat all the way up in my guard tower.

The vehicle caught on fire.

The 6 guys burned alive.

There was nothing I could do."

CPT Abrams sighed loudly, staring into the floor.

"Sometimes now, years later, I think I hear them screaming.

The QRF (Quick Response Force) tried to use a garden hose to put out the fire.

I heard rounds fire off inside the burning vehicle.

I was upset for a long time. I thought I was over it.

The obscenity of what I observed was worsened by my horrible feeling of helplessness."

"It was a brutal week"

CPT Abram continued his emotionless reporting of the tragedy. It could have been a weather report.

The group, attentive, said nothing.

"Later the same week, I learned something happened to a buddy.

Peter and I worked in the same building before the war. I admired him, an inspiring man.

He enlisted first. Six months later, I joined up.

I joined the Army because of Peter.

We were both deployed to Iraq at the same time. We were in different FOBs (Forward Operating Base), 4 hours apart by helicopter.

A woman suicide bomber killed Peter on Mother's Day.

I found out late.
I wrote a letter to Peter's parents.
It made me feel extremely human. It could have easily been me. It was a brutal week."

The group expressed its respect silently with knowing nodding, slowly upward and down.

"I have a different view of the world now"

After a long pause, another deep sigh, CPT Abram continued.
"I can't explain what happened next.
I redeployed to Germany.
While I was stationed in Germany, I married a German woman. We lived there 5 years. I had no serious emotional or psychological problems.
This is what I can't explain: I was okay in Germany.
The change came when I got back to the US.
The minute my feet stepped on American soil, the symptoms I have today started.
In Germany, we lived in the beautiful country side. It was very peaceful.
I came back to my hometown from Germany for an R and R party with my college buddies. These were my old fraternity friends.
My buddies sat on one side of the room. I was on the other side.
I was suddenly aware that these people have no idea who I am now.
I have a different view of the world now."
The CPT did not say it. He also has a different view of himself.
"The world is a terrible place.
There are a lot of bad people.
I don't recall my former self.
My sleep is inconsistent. It started in combat, but it got much worse when I got back to the US.
Off and on all night, I get up and check the windows and doors of our house.

I have nightmares.

At times, I can't fall asleep."

If this Soldier looked sad when he arrived for group therapy this morning, he looks sadder now.

The group asked technical questions about the vehicle in which the men were killed, unsuccessfully distracting themselves from their own traumatic grief.

"I don't think my wife understands"

"What is it that troubles your wife, CPT Abram?" I asked. "What worries her about you?"

"My wife is very supportive. We have a very happy marriage. We love each other and we love our little boy."

"It may help the group to help you, CPT Abram, if we knew your wife's actual concerns."

"She says I have lost my sense of humor, that I am too serious… the Boston Marathon bombing has made it worse."

"Does she know about your 'brutal week in Taji'?" I asked.

"I have shared some of it with her, none of the gory details.

I don't think my wife understands.

She has no idea how upset I am as Mother's Day approaches.

My wife doesn't know that I deeply ponder Peter's death on Mother's Day."

After another long pause, staring at the floor, CPT Abram continued his soliloquy.

"How awful it must be for his parents, how Mother's Day will never be the same for them."

"I have nothing that belonged to Peter"

It's been 6 years since Peter's death. CPT Abram still cannot recall his friend with less pain.

CPT Abram has not grieved for Peter.

If the CPT shares his tears of grief with us, will we mistakenly think he is looking for sympathy, I wondered silently.

"CPT Abrams," I asked, "do you have anything that belonged to Peter?"

My question sounded innocent enough.

I was looking for something unique to delayed or pathological grief.

I was looking for a "linking object."

"Linking object" is a psychoanalytic term.

It can refer to almost any object that symbolizes and becomes a substitute for the decedent.

The linking object is more than a sentimental reminder of the person who has died.

The linking object acquires the personhood of the lost person, making the expression of grief unnecessarily delayed or nearly completely avoided.

In a complex, mysterious cognitive distortion, certainly unknowingly, the survivor is spared much of the suffering of the natural grieving process by the linking object.

CPT Abram answered, "I have nothing that belonged to Peter."

Interestingly, this is the reply most commonly offered by those who have not grieved because they, in fact, have a linking object, but seldom readily acknowledge it.

I continued. "You have nothing that belonged to or was connected with Peter, not even a photograph?"

The attention of the group was focused on the dialogue between the CPT and the doctor.

"You said Peter had an inspiring influence on your life," I commented. "Nothing connects you to him now all these years after his tragic death?"

"Nothing.

"Wait," CPT Abram said.

"There is something. I forgot.

I have the black arm band that was worn at his memorial service. It has Peter's name on it and the date of his death, 6 years ago."

"Dr. Brown," asked SGT Jim Breeden, a Soldier who delayed his own grief for two years with alcohol, "do you think it would help if the CPT went to visit Peter's parents?"

"That's an excellent point, Jim," I replied. "In a few minutes, I'd like to know what CPT Abram thinks about it.

First, does the group have any thoughts about the black arm band?"

LTC O'Quinn, co-therapist for the Traumatic Grief Group, after a long period of silence, spoke to the CPT.

"Would you be willing to bring Peter's memorial service black arm band to the group?"

CPT Abram, caught off guard by the question, did not know how to answer LTC O'Quinn.

LTC O'Quinn continued.

"I think all of us in this group have lost someone we loved.

"I lost my mother. I was just trying to remember if I kept something of hers...something I really value. I don't believe I have kept anything."

"LTC O'Quinn," trying to be kind, I said, "maybe we should remind CPT Abram that, in addition to the rule of confidentially, we follow another, equally important rule.

No one in group has to speak should he or she choose not to speak.

Soldiers often tell me they learn more from listening in group than by talking."

LTC O'Quinn, a sensitive, caring man, replied calmly. "I didn't mean to make the CPT uncomfortable.

I was wondering if it might be helpful in the future to bring in the black arm band."

CPT Abram replied.

"I'm afraid I have already taken up too much of the group's time today. I apologize."

The CPT said, "Let me think about the arm band."

With the CPT's decision, I felt the level of tension in the group suddenly subside.

"No one wants to be forgotten"

"We all grieve in our own way," I said, addressing the Traumatic Grief Group.

"It is never easy to grieve.

No one wants to be forgotten.

Let your mind rid itself of the horrifying details of the actual death itself.

Let yourself remember the life of the person you lost, more than the details of their death."

CPT Abram was being understood.

I wanted to see at least one tear bravely march down his cheek.

CPT Abram was being comforted.

Sadly, CPT did not return with the black arm band that was worn at Peter's memorial service. CPT Abram did not return at all.

CPT Abram did not return to his individual therapist.

CPT Abram did not return my phone calls.

I have no way to reach CPT Abram. I must not have reached him during the only treatment session he bravely attended after driving past our building all those times when he could not bring himself to come inside.

It saddens me to know that I failed him, that a Soldier who needs help and came for help left unhelped.

I wonder if CPT Abram ever found a way to meaningfully grieve. There is nothing easy, CPT Abram, about grieving; it is hard work. There is little, however, that is more important than timely and eloquently grieving, CPT Abram.

Freddie wore an unchanging, sad expression on his little face

CPT Bell is a big man who stands only five feet four inches tall. This sandy headed, gray eyed quiet Soldier was reared in New England. To return some day to the family farm in upstate New York and settle down there is his consoling dream

He got his military leadership training in the 82nd Airborne Division, a remarkable military organization of which our nation is very proud.

He led his men in combat in Iraq and Afghanistan, brought his unit home without losses, and won the Bronze Star for bravery in combat.

CPT Bell began his Army career 16 years ago. He worked his way up the ranks from PVT to SSG. Then going from "Green to Gold," he was commissioned 2nd LT after OCS (Officer Candidate School).

He loves his wife and three sons, but his wife no longer returns his love.

CPT Bell believes that he was betrayed by a "good friend."

A painful, protracted divorce left him with joint custody of the boys.

"Dr. Brown, this is my son Freddie," said CPT Bell, recently introducing his son to me at one of his individual psychotherapy sessions for PTSD and depression.

Freddie was adorned in a precisely correct, official-appearing ACU (Army Combat Uniform), tailored to fit the frame of a 7 year old. The two bars signifying CPT stood out on the front of his uniform.

My mind raced back to my own childhood, to my love of the Army uniform. In some strange, surprising way, I did not know children today still knew the meaning of longing to wear the uniform of the US Army!

Dottie was very kind and patient with the children of my patients who came with their parents when I practiced in Charlottesville. The children responded to her like they would to Mrs. Santa Claus.

Dottie always had toys for the children. She also provided paper and pencil for drawings. The children's masterpieces were Scotch taped to her filing cabinets.

"Freddie," I said, "here is some paper and pencils. If you make a drawing, I will place it on my wall. Print your name and date on the bottom of your picture."

CPT Bell and I talked calmly about his interesting work instructing newly commissioned Lieutenants.

Freddie made himself comfortable on the floor, proceeding to draw a self-portrait of a little boy in a Soldier suit.

Freddie shared his father's uniform. He also shared his father's physical traits of sandy hair and gray eyes. It did not take a psychiatrist, however, to observe that Freddie wore an unchanging, sad expression on his little face.

Knowing we were talking in the presence of a sensitive child, controversial topics were not on the agenda today for his father's therapy session.

A large painting of a Williamsburg oak tree hangs on my office wall. It is a Pat Rappolt work of art, capturing the blazing orange, yellow, and brown brilliance of the fall season. On a bench beneath the tree sits a Mennonite middle-aged couple.

The painting has been a conversation piece for the 4 decades it has warmed my heart.

It presents an interesting challenge because it is a painting over another painting. The artist, dissatisfied with yet another painting of Monticello, covered Jefferson's home with the Williamsburg oak painting.

The therapy session ended. Freddie gave me his splendid autographed drawing. I taped it to the end of my file cabinet, in full view as one enters my office.

"Thank you, Freddie," I said sincerely. "Yours is one of the best drawings I have in my collection."

Freddie showed little interest in my compliment.

His sad expression remained unchanged.

To my surprise, Freddie pointed to the large Williamsburg painting.

Freddie asked a question about the painting never before brought to my attention.

I later wondered if his question sprouted out of his dad's combat deployments.

I hope it did not come from domestic discord to which he may have been privy.

I hope it was not influenced by heartless teasing from other children that his dad was in combat.

Freddie, his little, serious, inquisitive, sad face turned upward to me as we stood before the Duke of Gloucester Street painting, asked, "Is that an explosion?"

"If it is an explosion, Freddie," I smiled and said, "it is an explosion of beautiful gold, orange, yellow and brown colors of the tree leaves welcoming the fall season. I agree that it might look like an explosion, Freddie...but it is not the kind that destroys things. It is the kind of explosion that nature gives us to enjoy as the seasons change."

"I always looked for the good in people"

The following week, CPT Bell returned alone for his weekly psychotherapy session. My favorable impression of Freddie was shared.

I was pleased that little Freddie has entered counseling in another state where he resides with his mother and brothers.

CPT Bell spends alternate weekends with his sons. It is more important to him than anything in his life.

"I always looked for the good in people. My mom and dad said that about me.

That is changed now.

I see people negatively. I look for their ulterior motives.

I sense danger in people. Danger is not the right word for it.

People are no longer trustworthy.

I was a very helpful guy. Now I steer away from people.

My character has changed. I'm not as open."

"To what do you attribute these changes in yourself, CPT Bell?" I asked.

The CPT paused. He was mulling it over in his mind, not wanting to be deceitful himself, a trait he has come to despise in others.

"I believe it started with my first combat deployment to Somalia in 1993.

It is impossible to explain the feeling you get when you are shot at by the people you are trying to help.

I got the same feeling in Iraq. The feeling was even worse in Iraq. It is lasting so long.

Basic trust is nearly destroyed when women and children are turned into killers."

A long pause preceded his next statement. Hardly visible, small colorless tears slowly left their gates.

"I was crushed by my wife's betrayal while I was deployed. It removed the last amount of trust I had left.

We have been divorced three years."

Another long pause.

More manly tears.

"I still love her."

I wondered if it is more difficult to mourn the loss of one of the CPT's Soldiers in combat or the loss of the love of a wife he still loves. I did not ask the CPT what I wondered. His session ended sadly.

"I leave 3 lights on at night. My bedroom door is locked"

SFC (Sergeant First Class) Bruce Carson, a tall, gentle, light-skinned African American Soldier, meets the diagnostic criteria for PTSD.

This separated, 41 year old man is in the MEB (Medical Evaluation Board) process awaiting his disability rating.

Today, SFC Carson is wearing civilian clothes. He was recently discharged from a psychiatric hospital.

He also has mTBI (Mild Traumatic Brain Injury) from a Stryker roll-over in combat in Afghanistan.

A Stryker is an armored vehicle that can transport an Infantry squad. It weighs 19 tons.

SFC Carson struck his head during the frightening Stryker roll-over caused by an IED blast.

An IED (improvised Explosive Device) wreaks havoc to the human form, forcefully tearing away any of the precious parts of those nearest its hateful massive force.

The shock waves pierce the bony skull, leaving no evidence of damage to the skull itself.

Deadly laser-like waves of energy are unseen.

The powerful rays of energy damage brain cells.

They disrupt the crucially intricate connections between brain cells.

Concussion, any disruption of awareness from being dazed, confused, or seeing stars to unconsciousness, is the medical term preferable to TBI.

Unfortunately, TBI is the term more commonly used than concussion in the military.

The good news is that mild TBI (mTBI), in 80-85% of the cases, will improve over time.

Unfortunately, there is also bad news at this time about mTBI or mild concussions.

Repeated assaults on the brain dampen the prognosis.

It is agreed that PTSD and mTBI produce similar symptoms.

There may be an 80% overlap of the symptoms of PTSD and mTBI.

As in the case of SFC Bruce Carson, it is challenging to separate the two combat-induced disorders.

He is an articulate, intelligent Soldier.

Recently, he disclosed his symptoms in the Tuesday Afternoon Group.

"Sometimes, when I'm talking, I stop (thinking) in my head but keep talking.

I can't listen well.

I can't read well.

Adderall (psych stimulant medication) helps.

I have to go the "Lost and Found" for my train of thought.

I have trust problems with people and with the world.

I leave 3 lights on at night. My bedroom door is locked."

I looked around the room. Heads were nodding in agreement in this Post-Deployment group of Soldiers.

SFC Carson continued "confessing."

"Every time I talk to someone, it is like an interview. I try to see if something negative comes up.

If a person says, 'I'll be right there' and they come 45 minutes late, I end the relationship.

A person has to prove himself before I make a friend.

There is no more forgiveness in me now.

I'm more cynical, more hypervigilant.

I have little trust in myself. I have back-up plans. I have 'what if' plans.

I lost my self-confidence."

By its silence, the group agreed and identified with SFC Carson.

"I need consistency. The slightest inconsistency drives me up the wall.

I have two vases outside my door, one on either side.

They were moved.

I can't tell you how much that upset me!

I first thought someone stole my charcoal grill. It had been moved.

I got real mad.

I called the Police.

I felt bad the whole day.

I felt assaulted.

Life is messed up!"

Another long pause was accompanied by his facial expression of disgust.

"Later I learned my wife did it. She moved the vases. She moved the charcoal grill."

This Soldier's phenomenally exaggerated emotional reaction to the tiny distances the objects were moved, sadly, is not at all unusual for Soldiers with PTSD.

To have his vases and grill moved at all is threatening.

Any change, no matter how small or insignificant it may appear to others, is treated as a matter of life or death by Soldiers with mild TBI or history of concussion and by Soldiers with PTSD. Just as in combat.

"I feel trapped"

SSG (Staff Sergeant) Arthur Darby, a recovering alcoholic, has one year of sobriety. He is tall and thin, speaks very softly, and he is extremely threat-sensitive.

He has waited a year for his wife to sign their divorce settlement agreement. Sadly, his divorce stems from his wife's undeniable infidelity. He continues to wait for her signature.

SSG Darby is a shy Soldier. Barely audibly, almost apologetically, he spoke to his fellow group members in the Tuesday Afternoon Group.

"One night last week, my pastor invited me to his home for a small social gathering.

I was the last person to arrive.

There was only one seat left. It was the middle of the sofa.

I started sweating.

I can't sit in the middle.

I felt trapped.

I saw another seat.

I headed for the seat, but somebody took it.

I got upset.

I couldn't let it go.

I guess I have claustrophobia."

His fellow group members smiled in agreement, no strangers to the fear of feeling "trapped."

"SSG Darby," I said, "it sounds like you are uncomfortable in social situations, even in the presence of your pastor."

"That's right," he replied.

"When do you feel best?" I asked.

Immediately, he replied, "I feel best when I am around my kids. Sometimes I feel best when I am alone, just being by myself."

SSF Darby's voice trailed off, conveying a sense of futility.

"Sometimes, even a lot of sex doesn't help no more," his final comment of the day.

"I don't feel like a hero"

SFC (Sergeant First Class) Gene Velasquez is the accomplished son of proud Mexican parents. He grew up in Texas, joined the US Army 18 years ago, and has fought for his adopted country in 3 dangerous combat deployments.

Gene is a fair-skinned 41 year old married man of medium build, father of 3 children.

Gene mistakenly believes his proud parents would be ashamed should they learn his carefully guarded secret.

Unfortunately, like many Soldiers, Gene hides his depression. He feels guilty about having PTSD.

"I don't want to worry my parents with my problems.

I have problems because I am weak. My parents still believe that I'm strong."

I stared into his sad eyes.

"When I'm depressed," Gene continued, "my PTSD is worse."

Gene is a Soldier who works in a noisy environment. A sudden, unexpected loud noise startled him recently at work.

"It brought back memories of combat."

I could hear the anxiety in his voice. The muscles in his jaw tightened.

"I don't like to talk about it."

I know it is often helpful for Soldiers to retell the trauma story over and over. At some level of awareness, Soldiers also know it is better to mentally revisit the trauma scene.

Another "trip" to the trauma scene (merely discussing it) is sickening, as perceived by Soldiers with PTSD.

It is both a sentimental journey and a sensory trip.

According to what many Soldiers tell me, it may take more courage to travel back in time to terrible combat memories than to fight the original battle.

A terrible image from my pediatric internship popped into my mind. The little boy, no more than 5 years of age, suffered from prolapse of the rectum.

The rectum, the terminal end of the gastrointestinal tract, is normally internally situated. Its contents are released through the anal sphincter, a muco-cutaneous muscular external orifice.

The prolapsed rectum is an oddity to observe. Six to 10 inches of the intestinal tract protrudes uncomfortably outside the body.

One wants to push the uncomfortable prolapsed organ back inside where it belongs. It cannot be done. It becomes a surgically challenging problem.

Gene's painful combat memories are like a prolapsed organ.

These combat memories hurt. Like many Soldiers with PTSD, he wants to push his memories back inside where they belong.

He pushes strenuously with purposeful distractions.

He pushes with attempts to stay busy "so I won't have time to think."

He pushes with ingenious but failed attempts to avoid reminders of the trauma.

He pushes with willful numbness, pitifully but unsuccessfully, trying to feel nothing.

Gene's combat memories are partially protruding like a prolapsed rectum. Like the prolapsed rectum, these painful memories cannot be pushed back inside.

Gene repeated himself. "I don't like to talk about it."

We are at the pivotal point of the session. I think we shared the same thought: If not now, when?

I knew I had earned Gene's trust through years of treatment.

I knew Gene would reasonably receive from me what he had come to expect.

"There will be no surprises from Dr. Brown. He does what he says. He wants the best for me."

These unspoken agreements carry the weight of sacred trust.

I did not want to weaken his trust.

"Gene," I kindly inquired, "has refusing to talk about your combat traumas been helpful?"

"Not talking about it has not helped," he replied without quibbling.

"Will you try to share those aching memories with me, the ones that came to mind when you were startled at work?"

Gene did not hesitate.

"It is a memory of wounded Soldiers and contractors, mortally wounded, looking up at me, knowing they are not going to make it.

I felt horribly helpless.

It makes me feel like a failure.

All those 'what if' questions…

It is not good.

You can never run away from yourself.

I don't feel like a hero. I feel just the opposite."

"I feel like a whimpering child who has just been whipped…"

Staring into space, he paused, reached for the Kleenex, slowly dried his tears, and continued.

"Some were already dead.

The skull was blown off one person.

Legs were blown off."

He paused again.

"I feel like a whimpering child who has just been whipped, but not hugged afterwards."

"Gene, do you believe you were there to treat and save the wounded?" I asked.

"I've been thinking something like that.

I've been thinking I should have prevented it from happening."

"Are those thoughts logical?" I asked.

"No. They make no sense when I think about it.

I'm not a medic.

I'm a Soldier."

"Were you doing the best you could, Gene?"

"Yes."

The more Gene spoke about the details of the trauma, the results of a road-side bombing, the less depressed and the less tense he felt.

Gene was unbridling painful, horrific memories. It was the only way he could direct his logical, analytical skills on his aching mind.

It was the difference between stumbling around in a dark room and perambulating in the light of day.

An hour earlier, his eyes were sad.

We sat in silence. Together we relished the reward of his courage to face his "whipping."

When we shook hands, I hugged him tightly.

"Thanks, Dr. Brown, I always feel better when I come here."

When Gene left, his eyes were smiling.

"I had a sticky feeling on my hands for days"

CPT Ray Evans is a 35 year old married man. He was rejected by his first wife, who tired of his frequent deployments and short-temper.

He has a fair complexion, a nearly bald head, and blue eyes that communicate indifference.

His most remarkable trait is talkativeness.

His attendance at the Tuesday Afternoon Post-Deployment Psychotherapy Group has been inconsistent. When I confronted him about "poor attendance and poor accountability," he launched an angry, unacceptable defense.

Two years passed before he told the group about the consequences of his combat trauma.

"Every time I close my eyes," said CPT Evans, "I see multiple killings by snipers in Iraq.

Every time I close my eyes, I see the floor of our vehicle covered with blood.

I was sitting at the rear of a Stryker (An Infantry Carrier Vehicle that provides protected transport and supporting armor; it can attain speeds of 60 MPH).

A sniper hit the Soldier next to me in the neck.

I did not know he was hit until he keeled over.

Blood poured out.

Later, I helped clean out the vehicle.

The sight, smell, feel of the blood was unique and lasting.

I was covered with his blood from my hips to my feet.

For days I could smell it.

I had the sticky feeling of blood on my fingers for days after I repeatedly tried to scrub it off."

The group nodded, agreeing and recalling their own experience with the blood of American Soldiers.

He was clinically stable, not appearing emotionally involved in the telling of the trauma.

Again CPT Evans said, "Every time I close my eyes, I see the floor of our vehicle covered with blood."

There is a difference between reporting one's trauma and re-experiencing the trauma in therapy.

It took CPT Evans a year of weekly group therapy to finally tell his trauma story.

His understandable reticence to tell his trauma story may explain his inconsistent attendance.

When CPT Evans is at last prepared to share the reliving of his combat trauma in therapy, he will no longer see "multiple killings by snipers in Iraq" every time he closes his eyes.

When CPT Evans is ready to fully open his eyes to his blood-soaked memories, he will be able to close them in peace, to live more fully.

"I'm proud of what I did in the Army for 22 years. Every day I tried 110%"

MSG (Master Sergeant) Hector DeVala is a 41 year old Puerto Rican. His gigantic Army pride and unmatched energetic motivation is carried on a small frame.

A small, carefully trimmed moustache gives a touch of character to his bony, linear, serious face.

Anxiety twitches his body from his capable hands to his repetitively shifting legs.

His dark, penetrating eyes are signaling SOS messages to me.

If I could read Morse code, I would understand that his NCO (Non-Commissioned Officer) Code is informing me "No fallen Soldier is left behind…unless it is me."

His Morse code continues. "Sir, no matter how pitiful I may appear, please understand one thing.

I am not asking for help, Sir.

Take care of my Soldiers, Sir.

Take care of others, Sir."

"It was my 9th deployment"

MSG DeVala, a Soldier with severe PTSD, has kept no appointments with me for the past 6 months.

"My wife had surgery. It was followed by serious complications. She was in the hospital for 60 days.

Before that, I was sent to Kuwait for a 90 day deployment.

It was my 9th deployment.

I had a couple break-downs over there.

I know I can never deploy again."

"How is your wife now?" I asked.

"When she was hospitalized, I spent a lot of time in the chapel.

I made a promise to God: get Mary out of the hospital in one piece and I will put my family first from now on.

The Army was always first in the past.

Mary had a good week…but I'm in bad shape.

I can't fire a weapon at the range. Each round I fire causes me to sweat profusely.

I still carry the pork chop you recommended. It was my favorite smell. I keep it in a zip lock plastic bag and pull it out of my uniform when I get upset. It helps. (Power of pleasant olfactory memory will often obliterate an unpleasant, unsettling combat odor, a common flashback trigger.)

I see images of organs….

I lost family members when all those kids (young Soldiers) died in my arms.

I prayed for the pain to go away.

I feel depression.

I feel despair.

I'm proud of what I did in the Army for 22 years. Every day I tried 110%."

The small brave Soldier, continued.

"The smell of the pork chops calmed me down. It's like a kid's security blanket.

I don't want to kill myself any more.

I sleep 4 to 5 hours at night.

My nightmares are less frequent now. During my last deployment, I had 6 nightmares every 30 days. Two of the 6 were really bad.

My nightmares are really terrible.

They are often about battle.

I see blood.

I smell blood.

I hear screaming.

They can be actual reenactments of combat trauma. I have 8 specific events that reoccur in my dreams.

Some of my nightmares may be about things that never happened. I dreamed that I put human remains in the back of a trailer with MREs (Meals Ready to Eat). I would never do that when I'm awake.

I can't be around raw meat no more…

The other night, I woke up in my bedroom closet. I was in my underwear. I had on my FLACK vest and my KEVLAR (body armor). My 9 mm pistol was in my hand. I was soaking wet with sweat. I was sitting in a crawling mode.

I got up and took a shower. Washing with soap, I looked down. It looked like blood was coming off of me…"

"I don't trust anybody"

MSG DeVala, looking exhausted, trying to tell me all that had happened since our last session, said, "I don't trust anybody.

I trust you. You don't judge me.

I sound paranoid.

I don't know what a person is going to do.

I drive very slowly, always cautious.

In the supermarket, I look for danger.

People get too close to me in the stores. I don't shop on pay-days...too many people.

When people get close to me in public, my skin breaks out."

"Are you ready to come for treatment?" I asked the SGM.

"Yes, Sir, I am ready for whatever you recommend," he replied.

"Are you prepared to let us work together on your health? Will you cooperate 110 % with therapy, MSG DeVala?"

He nodded affirmatively.

"Will you be as proud to be a brave patient as you were proud to be a brave Soldier for 22 years?"

The MSG, smiling broadly, replied, "I will cooperate 110%."

"Go to Piggly Wiggly and buy me some grits"

"Dr. Brown, this is Gary. Are you with a patient?"

"No, Gary, but I am way behind on my notes. What can I do for you?"

Gary is a competent clinician, a Licensed Clinical Social Worker, with a nose for Soldiers in serious need of psychiatric treatment. He screens the Soldiers who walk into our clinic without an appointment.

The Soldiers Gary screens usually come to our clinic after a long period of hesitating, hoping they can manage their symptoms without help.

Gary decides which Soldiers cannot wait for one of our regular appointments, usually a 2-week wait.

When Gary calls, I know a Soldier is in serious need of help.

Gary's record of making the right decision is unblemished. In the 8 years as our screening clinician, none of Gary's patients committed suicide.

"Can I come down to your office," Gary asked.

In a matter of seconds, Gary quietly knocked at my door, apologized unnecessarily but as usual, stood by my desk and said, "This guy needs help, Dr. Brown. It's PTSD, I think. He tells me he smells something. I don't know what to make of it."

"My first available appointment is day-after-tomorrow, this FRI at 1500, Gary. Is that soon enough?

"I think so, Dr. Brown. If it is not okay with the CPT, may he call you on your cell?"

The details were worked out. I wrote down his name and phone number. I would see him in 48 hours.

"Gary, you said the CPT smelled something?"

"Yeah, he said the whole room where he is staying has a strange smell sometimes. It has something to do with his grandmother. I don't know whether to call it an hallucination."

Gary was in a hurry. "I have 3 walk-ins waiting for me in the lobby," Gary said.

Before Gary raced out, I said, olfactory hallucinations may be important. It may mean the patient has a brain tumor, a temporal lobe tumor. I shared this with Gary because he is often anxious to learn.

"Really?" Gary said.

"Yes, a well-known song writer smelled burning rubber, even reported it to his analyst. He died of an undiagnosed brain tumor."

"The CPT looked good to me. He is not complaining of a headache or anything suggesting a brain tumor, Dr. Brown. He can wait 2 days to see you."

Gary spoke with confidence. I was relieved.

CPT Francis Foster looked like a scholar in his horn-rim eyeglasses, the way he often took them off and on, and the way he spoke in an articulate, soft manner.

This 31 year old Soldier, recently left by his wife with their 2 children, is upset. His wife is not permitting him to speak with his children.

If he were not in uniform, he would not be standing straight. I picture his medium build and height bent over in despair when alone.

His 5 year military career has taken him to 21st Century War in two lengthy, destructive deployments.

This dark man was in a dark mood.

I had to strain to hear him.

"I have changed my entire life to become the person I am not.

I have no social life.

I talk to no one.

I isolate myself.

I've changed the way I used to dress, the way I have my hair cut, the way I travel, the way I read my books.

I have to force myself to go to church. It used to be the center of my life.

Before I was deployed, I didn't drink or smoke.

I smoked my first cigarette after we were first attacked in Iraq.

I started drinking alcohol when we first got back from Iraq

I was brought back home early from Afghanistan.

My 90-year-old-grandmother was dying.

She was the most important person in my life.

My Granny raised me."

"CPT Foster," I asked, "were you with your Granny when she died?"

"No, she tricked me."

"How do you mean, she tricked you?"

"She said, 'Blue, go to Piggly Wiggly and buy me some grits.'

She didn't want me to see her pass."

I could see the tears streaming down his face, but I could not hear him cry.

"She passed on 22 FEB 2012 at 1052.

Granny called me 'Blue' because when I was born I was so black I was blue.

As a kid, I watched Perry Mason on TV with her. I'd slip into her room at 0300 and turn on the TV real low. She would say, 'Turn it up, Blue. I'm not asleep.'

Granny loved me being in the Army. That's how my grandfather took care of his family.

To make my Granny happy, Sir, that's why I joined the Army."
The CPT cried.

"Have you been able to remember your grandmother with less pain?" I asked.

"Her death hurts me even more now."

"Have you kept anything that belonged to your grandmother?" I asked.

"I have the belt she beat me with. I have the trumpet she gave me."

The CPT had not been able to grieve for his loss.

Can anyone grieve on top of grief, I wondered to myself. We haven't discussed his combat losses. He was presenting with some of the symptoms of combat-induced PTSD.

I wanted to help the CPT begin the grieving process.

"CPT Foster," I said, "if your grandmother were seated next to you in that empty chair, what you would say to her today?"

"We would just talk…about the news…things in the world…
I would tell her about me.
She always listened.
I would tell her I'm not happy. I'm always depressed.
I don't know how to be me any more.
I'm not the happy Francis.
I'm not like I used to be."

After a long pause, the CPT said, "Granny was the only person that really listened to me."

The CPT cried.

"She gave me the trumpet. It was her way to keep me off the street."

With tears in my own eyes, I said, "Can you let me listen like your Granny?"

"I can't.
You are not her."

The longest pause of the session ended with the CPT's words.

"I'm crazy.

I talk in my sleep.
I should have left that stuff over there."

"You are not crazy, CPT Foster," I said.

"If you did not talk in your sleep, I'd really be worried about you.

I haven't seen a Soldier yet who has been able to leave 21st Century War over there."

"If I'm not crazy, why do I smell my grandmother's kitchen?"

"I grew up in my grandmother's house.
Since my grandmother passed, I think I smell her kitchen."

Reassuringly, I asked, "What does her kitchen smell like?"

"My grandmother's kitchen smells exactly like it did when I was in her house. I can walk into any room wherever I go and sometimes it smells like Granny's kitchen!
I know it sounds crazy."

"It is not crazy, CPT Foster.
What does your grandmother's kitchen smell like?

"It's a wonderful smell.
I smell okra gumbo.
I smell mustard greens.
I smell turnip greens.
I even smell cornbread."

"You are certainly not crazy. Memory of smells is the most enduring of memories. It is a way for you to feel close to Granny.

We can help you understand the thoughts and feelings that seem crazy to you.

Are you willing to work on the painful, confusing issues?" I asked.

The CPT chose to join the Traumatic Grief Group, the Dream Interpretation Group, and to return to see me individually for Cognitive Behavioral Therapy.

We had a risk/benefit/alternative discussion of Lexapro for depression and PTSD and Amitriptyline 10 to 20 mg as necessary for sleep.

He had lost 15 pounds in the past 3 weeks because he lost his appetite as well as his interest in most things he previously enjoyed.

The CPT's spirit lifted. I could tell it in his voice.

"Have you read <u>Where the Red Fern Grows</u>?" he inquired. It was one of his favorite stories, he said. He gave me a brief synopsis.

Was this suffering Soldier going to begin to trust me like he trusted Granny?

It would be a position of great honor.

It will be my sincerest intention.

The session ended. We stood up. We shook hands.

"I will see you Monday, Blue. Have a good weekend. I will read <u>Where the Red Fern Grows</u>."

The following weekend, my wife and I watched the movie, "Where the Red Fern Grows," a story of a boy's unrelenting pursuit and sacrifice to own a pair of hunting dogs. One of the prize winning dogs is killed by a mountain lion; its mate dies of grief. A red fern, said to be planted only by an angel, grows between the graves of the two dogs.

"Where the Red Fern Grows" will be on the agenda when Blue and I next meet.

I sincerely looked forward to working with Blue. I wanted to help him continue the good work his grandmother started, to celebrate her life… but Blue never returned. He was transferred to another Army Post, too far from us to continue his treatment. Sadly, I never heard from Blue again.

Part Three
The End

It has been difficult to write an ending to <u>Sacred Ground</u>. In a number of ways, the end is the beginning or commencement or inauguration. In the strictest sense, it is the conclusion, but not the end, because I am hopeful that America will begin a new compassionate relationship with its Soldiers.

If the story-teller has been successful, truly reporting what he has heard, then it will be a new chapter in the history of America's demonstration of appreciation for its Soldiers.

Almost daily, right up to the last day the approving committee (Army Office of Public Affairs) agreed to review the manuscript, a Soldier told me a story I wanted to include. The story, important to the Soldier, I knew would be an important story to the reader.

Chapters 17 – 24 of <u>Sacred Ground</u> examine the psychological cost of 21st Century war on relationships, on suffering and on lives burdened by uncertainty.

A prescription is written for the reader on how he or she can help. This is followed by a brief review of the book.

The Story-teller's fulfilling life is described as abundantly blessed by a loving, supportive family and by the unsurpassed joy of serving as a physician to American Soldiers. Our Soldiers do not hesitate to put their lives on the line for our nation whenever and wherever their mission demands. Therefore, we cannot hesitate to commit ourselves to learn about the psychological cost of 21st Century War and commit ourselves to bestow compassion on our Soldiers. They truly are our neighbors.

In nearly every story in <u>Sacred Ground</u> there is reason for our nation and for every Soldier to be hopeful. The cases were not screened. No bad outcomes are told because, thankfully, no bad outcomes have been reported to date. It was disappointing when a Soldier came for help, but did not return owing to military change of assignment or by personal choice. Every Soldier who was "lost to follow-up" was diligently pursued, some successfully, but others, a real cause of concern, remained missing. The doors of my heart and mind remain open to them wherever they are. Delaying treatment never proves beneficial, only and sadly detrimental.

17

THE PIECES IN PLACE

The Class of 1967

THERE WERE FEW architectural changes in the School of Medicine, now called "the Old Medical School," between 1953 and 1963, the decade I spent dreaming of returning to medical school.

I am a "space and place conscious" person. Sitting in the same class room I had occupied ten years earlier felt very good. My fondness for sameness added to my comfort.

Ten years earlier, the last time I observed class room C-2, I stood outside its rear door, peering through its tiny window at the backs of my classmates. A lecture I would have been attending captured their attention. My disappointment worsened when I spotted a classmate occupying the seat I would have filled had I not been sent home.

There were few changes in the faculty as well. The difficult-to-define but very real "medical student culture" remained the same, although, of course, the student body was entirely replaced, but for me.

The "culture" in the first few days of classes was all about choosing lab partners for Anatomy, four students per cadaver, buying a white lab coat, buying textbooks, reviewing class syllabi, noting dates of important examinations, and meeting a diverse group of 75 people who needed to learn to work together in order to compete for grades.

It was an exhilarating time. The enthusiasm of hope was in the air. It was profound.

It was announced that our medical school class would hold its first class meeting in class room C-2. Most of us had no idea what our "class meeting" might have in store, but we gathered as required on a warm 1963 September afternoon in class room C-2.

"We are here to elect class officers," announced a class mate standing in front of the class.

"The floor is open for nominations for class president."

Two students were nominated immediately, and one of them was conducting the meeting.

"Thank you for nominating me," he said sheepishly. "This means that someone else must conduct the meeting."

No one volunteered to conduct the meeting. The long period of silence was embarrassing, so I went to the front of the class and said, "If there are no more nominations, then someone needs to move we close the nominations."

Norman Burak, a lanky, outspoken student from Brooklyn, shouted (read as yelled), "I nominate Bob Brown!"

"Thank you, Norm," I said, "but this is no time for jokes."

"I don't joke about important things like this," he replied.

"If you don't write your name on the black board," (it was actually green; yellow chalk was used), "I will come down there and do it myself!"

The three nominees walked into the hallway, permitting the class to cast their vote, a matter requiring no more than several minutes.

I was elected class president, a big surprise and an honor unsurpassed in my professional career.

Tradition is deeply rooted in the University. The tradition in the 1960s, and perhaps still today, has the class president making remarks on behalf of his or her class upon graduation, to the returning alumni of the School of Medicine.

It was a very special moment for me to give the class president's remarks to, among others, the tenth reunion of the class of which I had once been a member.

"On an island far away from the Cultural Revolution"

My medical school class mates were a fine group of people, easy to work with, even friendly, and very intelligent, but they were unique in several inexplicable ways.

The sense I got from them was their strong feeling of the protection, assured in the Preamble of the US Constitution: the right to be left alone.

The Class of 1967 appreciated the tasteful use of sarcasm that characterized my annual class Christmas letters, each year demanding even more absurd application, until unannounced censorship raised its ugly head, robbing me and my class of the pleasure it once delivered.

I don't know if much that has been written about the 1960s included the life of medical students. In retrospect, being a medical student in the 1960s was like being on an island far away from the Cultural Revolution that spread across the country.

I was unaware of anti-authoritarianism or liberal views of sexual conduct among any of my class mates.

As we approached graduation, however, the war in Vietnam cast its dark shadow over my class, affected post-graduate training decisions, and a number of my class mates went directly from their internship to war, some returning with persisting memories of combat trauma, too early in the history of American psychiatry to be diagnosed with Posttraumatic Stress Disorder, a mental disorder first appearing in the diagnostic manual in 1980.

Our professors were unrivaled. Dr. Robert McGilvery, Chairman, Department of Biochemistry, received a spontaneous standing ovation from our class, and Dr. Slaughter Fitzhugh, Chief,

Department of Ear Nose and Throat, was elected by our class as its Outstanding Professor. Dr. David Smith, Chairman, Department of Pathology, was admired for his kind, gentle, knowledgeable teaching style.

I believe my class considered all our professors in the basic sciences and the clinical sciences to be the very best. Dr. William Thurman, Chief, Department of Pediatrics, had a love of his work that readily attracted many of my class mates to follow him into Pediatrics.

Dr. George Minor

Dr. George Minor, Professor of Surgery, was a gentleman and scholar, whose sincere interest in students suited him ideally for his additional job as Director of Financial Assistance. A tall, slim, stately man with silver colored hair and blue eyes, Dr. Minor carried a famous Virginia name.

Dr. Minor was a bachelor, but he intuitively knew the needs of medical students who were married with children. I was thirty-two years old and Dottie and I had three children ages eight, six, and four in 1963 when my second journey in medical school began.

We had accrued some debt in graduate school and came to medical school with no financial resources, an almost unthinkable fact; looking back on it now, it is difficult to imagine how anyone would knowingly expose his wife and children to such great risk. However, I never considered penury a momentous burden; I had been reared in poverty, had no obsession with wealth, and I had faith that funds would be found and provided.

Dr. Minor and Harold P. Warner, my banker, must have tired of seeing me, though they never showed it or impatience, and a combination of scholarships and bank loans were consistently made available.

The Jenkins Brothers

Two other resources, in addition to the generous assistance provided by Dr. Minor and Harold Warner, played major roles in seeing the Brown family through medical school, The Lincoln Foundation in Norfolk, Virginia, and the Summer Session of the University of Virginia in Charlottesville, Virginia.

I had no heart to go back to the Norfolk Foundation and ask for another Lettie B. Smith Scholarship. For some reason, I struggle with my memory of how I found the Lincoln Foundation, but it may have been the result of a suggestion made by one of the administrators formerly associated with the Norfolk Foundation.

I don't think the Lincoln Foundation was well known in the early 1960s. Two brothers, attorneys, I believe, managed the fund.

Visiting the office of Charles Jenkins and his brother, for me, was like walking into a Charles Dickens novel. The small dimly lit room, in a downtown Norfolk office building, was crowded with large dark mahogany desks and chairs. Its walls from floor to ceiling barely held up all the old books whose large size and gold lettered titles suggested law books.

The Jenkins brothers were physically large, but not rotund, wore gray flannel suits, white shirts, and dark neckties.

I was greeted with kindness and received their undivided attention. I recall no secretarial staff or reception area.

The Jenkins brothers were impressed, I believe, that I was born and reared in the Lamberts Point neighborhood of Norfolk, had played football at Maury High School, graduated from the University of Virginia in 1953, failed out of medical school after my first year, and had not given up my dream nor my pursuit of a medical education for the decade following my exit from medical school.

They took notes, during my interview, on white legal pads with No. 2 yellow lead pencils.

Several days later, I received a brief typed letter awarding me a scholarship, renewable each of my four years in medical school. I tried to visit the Jenkins brothers at least annually and kept them informed about my progress in medical school.

Several years after completing my training, I repaid the Lincoln Foundation the amount they had given me, not out of obligation but as an indication of my gratitude.

Painting Minor Hall

The Summer Session of the University of Virginia hired me as an Assistant Professor of Education to teach each summer I was a medical student. It was a delightful experience for me. The students were serious and mature, anxious to learn. I was needy, becoming more mature, and I loved to teach.

I was indebted to good professors in the Curry School of Education who taught me the love of learning and the love of teaching. Most of the classes I taught were held in Minor Hall.

One summer, Minor Hall, a brick building with considerable white trim, was being repainted.

In the midst of a suspenseful vignette I was describing as an illustration from real life to emphasize a major point in my lecture, I suddenly looked up at the large windows opened wide on the hot day.

The five men painting outside the windows had stopped their work and were more attentive to this part of my lecture than some of my students on the front row. It is a very gratifying memory, the reason I mention it a second time, but in more detail. It may have held a special meaning for me of which I become aware as I write. My father had none of the advantages of education. He never knew the joy of reading or mastered the skill of writing, not even his own signature. The last years of his occupational life were spent painting schools for the Maintenance Department of the Norfolk City Schools. I wonder if he ever took advantage of listening to teachers while painting hall-ways and staircases of the school houses. It is an interesting connection with my father, a rewarding, warm thought. I respected him for his manual dexterity and skillful, though, tremulous hands that repaired all that was broken, from cars to construction.

"He was a tall, handsome, heavy smoking Kentuckian…"

Curiously, several tempting and distracting offers found their way in my path towards the completion of my medical education.

I was blessed to teach in the Summer Session during my years in medical school. Ralph Cherry was Dean of the Curry School of Education and Director of the Summer Session at the University of Virginia at that time.

He was a tall, handsome, heavy smoking Kentuckian with a full head of thick blonde-graying hair whose administrative reins were held by strong, firm, experienced hands. I found Dean Cherry easy to respect and to like.

I had only a few conversations with him in his office. The first one resulted in getting housing in Old Copeley Hill, wooden Army barracks that survived WW II, and admission to the Graduate School of Arts and Sciences to pursue my PhD in Education.

Dean Cherry was known to conduct serious business at the water fountain in Peabody Hall, near but outside his office, in the hall-way.

Many years earlier, William Holmes McGuffey, University of Virginia, wrote the famous McGuffey Reader, the standard text for the teaching of reading in the US for generations.

The McGuffey Reading Clinic at the University of Virginia was well established as an institution for the teaching of reading teachers, named for its famous author of the McGuffey Reader.

An unexpected opening, Director of the McGuffey Reading Clinic, was on Dean Cherry's mind. By happenstance, I approached the water fountain just as Dean Cherry was slaking his thirst.

Looking up, mopping a little of the cold water from his lips, with a serious demeanor the Dean said, "Bob, how would you like to be the next Director of the McGuffey Reading Clinic?"

I knew he was serious.

"Talk to Dottie about it. You don't need to prove anything by completing medical school. I believe you are a natural teacher. You'd love the life of a professor, and you could start taking care of your family right now."

He was being kind and persuasive, two of his natural traits. He did not look like Wallace Beery, the former movie star, one of my favorites, but he had a similar "ah shucks….you know you can do it" approach.

"I'll give you a week, Bob, to think about it."

Dean Cherry turned abruptly and walked away, turning his head from side to side as if to say, I perceived, "why in the world can't Bob Brown obviously see how this is the right option for him right now?"

The McGuffey Reading Clinic proposal came as an absolute surprise.

I did not need a week or even a minute to think it over but, as promised, I discussed it with Dottie; we even put the kids in our car late one afternoon and drove from our apartment on Old Copeley Hill to Rugby Road, an attractive Charlottesville neighborhood, and toured the outside of the McGuffey Reading Clinic. It was located less than 50 yards from the "Football House," 504 Rugby Road.

"It would be nice to come out from under the pressure of medical school," Dottie said, "but it is up to you, Bob," already knowing, I believe, what my answer would be.

We never discussed it a second time, never looked back regretting our choice or ever wondered what our life would have been like if a different choice had been made. I would not be the "new Director."

"Dr. Burke Smith, the calmest person I ever knew…"

Another revenue resource comes to mind. Dr. Burke Smith, the calmest person I ever knew, the Chief of Psychological Services, Department of Psychiatry, a man with snowy white hair and sparkling pale blue eyes, hired me, part-time, to administer psychological tests to patients on Davis 2 and Davis 3, the in-patient psychiatric wards of the University of Virginia Hospital.

Interacting with the patients on the Davis wards helped me feel closer to my goal; discussing the psychological test results with Burke Smith helped form insights into psychological illness I would have received from no other experience at that stage in my career.

We became fast friends. I joined many of his friends at his memorial service nearly fifty years after we met; with humility and respect, I commented on his many contributions including his generous spirit of sharing his knowledge with all who were privileged to know and work with him.

I had been licensed as a psychologist shortly after completing my doctorate degree, and thus my summers in medical school were pleasantly spent teaching in the morning and testing in the afternoons. I was also able to enjoy my family with whom I happily spent the evenings and weekends. We never felt deprived. We felt blessed.

Dr. Tsu, an Unmatched Chinese Pathologist

All of the Pathology faculty members were talented teachers, unselfish in sharing their knowledge with us. One stood out from all the rest.

Dr. Tsu, a Chinese physician, said to have performed autopsies in China under threat of being shot, was a small, gentle genius whose modesty and knowledge of Pathology won the hearts of all of us who sat at his feet to learn.

It was said that Dr. Tsu could not be surpassed in his knowledge of Pathology. For example, I saw him, on more than one occasion, hold up a slide and identify it immediately without the use of a microscope.

One of my playful classmates, determined to fool Dr. Tsu, obtained a microtome (very thin slice required for microscopic study) of a hot dog.

Looking befuddled one day during Pathology Lab, my classmate held the tampered slide high into the air and loudly called Dr. Tsu.

"Sir, can you help me identify this slide? I can't figure it out."

Dr. Tsu quickly walked to the classmates' lab seat, held up the slide, without the benefit of one of our Bausch and Lomb microscopes, calmly announced, "hot dog."

He serenely walked away to assist another classmate, keeping his reputation intact.

"Pot Case Method"

Pathology, a second-year medical school course, was ingeniously taught at the University using the "Pot Case" method.

Small groups of medical students were given a plastic 5-gallon pot containing the internal organs that had been removed, with the consent of the next of kin, during a post-mortem examination, minus the brain (that was reserved for the Neuropathology section of the course).

Our task as medical students was to sift through the materials, all well preserved in pungent smelling formaldehyde. We all wore rubber gloves

By gross examination and microscopic study of slides prepared from the remains, we had to make an accurate diagnosis. We were asked to identify the illnesses and or injuries from which the patient, whose actual bodily organs we respectfully and gently touched and studied, was taken from physical life and entered the entirely unknown state referred to as death.

Pathology instructors, adorned in long white lab coats, moved among us in the lab, consisting of work tables and microscopes, answering questions, and, upon completion of our examination, read to us a summary of the patient's relevant medical history and actual cause of death.

"Three autopsies were being performed at the same time"

An equally intriguing part of Pathology was the requirement to attend autopsies.

Delicate readers, I share this small part of my story for its instructive value, not as a deliberate attempt to be indelicate or unaware of its potential to offend.

Autopsies, however, provide knowledge to advance the prevention and treatment of disease; they may be matchless in these regards.

Physicians who devote their professional careers to the study of Pathology, including the performance of autopsies, are held in high regard.

It is the Pathologist, for example, who informs the Surgeon, patiently waiting in the operating room, whether the tissue biopsy sent to his lab is malignant, whether to proceed with surgery, whether the prognosis is favorable, or, for example, whether to remove the breast.

Three autopsies were being performed at the same time in the University morgue when I entered, as required, attracted and repulsed, to observe my first autopsy.

Permit me here, dear reader, to refrain from describing the vivid details of that day and to simply say that the work proceeded quietly, respectfully, and professionally.

It is unthinkable; however, should family members ever observe an autopsy of a deceased family member, without hesitation, the hushed, systematic, gentle procedure would immediately demonstrate care and respect for the remains he or she once knew as a loved one.

Bright lights above each of the three autopsy tables, in rather stark contrast to the sense of darkness that filled the rest of the large room located in the basement of what is now named the Old Medical School Building, dominated the physical features of the room.

Even after all these years, the picture is indelibly stored in my mind. Stored with the vivid visual images are the feelings associated with all that I saw, heard, and smelled. They are no less permanently deposited.

It was an amazing coincidence that all three patients were young adults.

Their deaths were unrelated except for one remarkable detail. All three of these young adults had dramatically visible evidence of advanced atherosclerosis.

Yellow streaks of fat lined their large arteries. In several critical areas, the fat had already formed hard plaques of calcium deposits.

The Pathologists performing the autopsies, shaking their heads, said, "This is the epidemic that is taking the lives of people. It is sad that this problem starts so early in life!"

None of these young people had died of atherosclerosis; however, it was evident to the Pathologists that it would have contributed to their death had they lived a "normal life span."

"What is causing this epidemic?" I asked.

Slowly shaking his head, the Pathologist said, "It is the result of a sedentary life-style. We are sitting around, eating the wrong foods. We are not being attentive to the need for regular physical activity, sensible eating habits, and the importance of good, restorative sleep."

Unaware of it at the time, these first autopsies became a life-changing event for me. I was thirty-three years old. My mother had already suffered a nonfatal heart attack a year earlier at age 62.

In Chapter Nineteen, I will tell the story of how closely observing three autopsies changed the direction of my life.

"Mr. Brown, are you familiar with this case?"

Dr. William H. Muller, a renowned cardiovascular surgeon, Chairman of the Department of Surgery, School of Medicine, University of Virginia, later to become Vice President of Medical Affairs, made a lasting impression with his tall stature, black hair, remarkably keen mind and the nimble dexterity of his healing surgical hands and his firm demeanor.

It was a widely held belief among the medical students and house officers that Dr. Muller was a man we all wanted to please, a man whose fury is best left leashed.

I was not privy to the origin of the Dr. Muller story, but I never encountered a more kind and gentle surgeon; however, I maintained a high regard for Dr. Muller and maintained a considerable distance from him.

Imagine my emotional shock and surprise when I was called to Dr. Muller's office in the middle of my surgery rotation during my third year of medical school.

His face and the tone of his voice could not have been more serious when I was invited into Dr. Muller's office, a large room cluttered with brightly lit X-ray viewing boxes, open surgical text books, wall-to-ceiling mahogany book cases bulging with ancient and modern books on surgery, and told to take a seat.

I will not attempt to identify my emotions, but the one most near the surface was fear of failure, a fear with a firm foundation.

Dr. Muller moved things around on his desk until he found the medical chart for which he was searching. He passed me the chart, saying, "Mr. Brown, are you familiar with this case?"

I turned each page slowly. The chart described a middle aged woman upon whom Dr. Muller had operated. I felt my heart beating rapidly as I read brief notes I had written in the chart, noting that every day I had changed the dressing that covered a large surgical wound on her abdomen.

"Yes, Sir, Dr. Muller, this is one of your patients. I was the assigned medical student. I changed the surgical dressing every day, just as it was ordered, Sir."

"I called you here today to get one thing straight. Is this my patient, or is this your patient, Mr. Brown?"

"She has been your patient from the day of her admission to the hospital, Dr. Muller.

I do not understand your question, Sir.

She was never my patient," I said, with emphasis on "never" and on "my."

"If that is true, then tell me why she refuses to permit me to operate on her tomorrow until, as she said, 'I talk to my doctor.'"

"I have no idea, Sir," I replied in a state of anxious confusion.

Dr. Muller said, "Do you know what she said when I asked her just who your doctor is?"

"No, Sir, Dr. Muller."

"She said you are her doctor.

She transferred her care over to you, Mr. Brown.
She said you cared about her.
She said you were kind to her.
She will not let me operate until she talks to you.

For goodness sake, Mr. Brown, can you go see your patient and see if she agrees to the necessary surgery?"

My anxiety level did not dissipate until, to my surprise, Dr. Muller stood up, walked around his desk, took my hand, smiled widely and said, "Good work, we need more doctors who care about their patients and treat them with kindness."

Dr. Muller, a remarkable man, must have seen the need and did much to restore my self-confidence.

Later I will mention two major steps in my life that Dr. Muller strongly and positively influenced: access to the Duke Medical School Curriculum, and Pedagogy for Surgical House Staff, a didactic series of lectures to improve the teaching skills of surgical interns and residents at the University of Virginia Hospital.

I was soon to learn that medical school education is primarily about making decisions.

I went to medical school to be a family doctor.

Dr. West, Norfolk Public Health Department, wore a dark suit. To be a recipient of his excellent care, one had to be on public welfare. I was fully qualified.

Dr. West took care of me as a five year old with hepatitis for which my whole family was quarantined, just as these pages earlier described.

Dr. West and his lovely blond-headed, blue-eyed nurse, Ms. Anderson, dressed in the Public Health navy blue uniform, were imprinted role models.

My mother with her natural gift of healing was my principal role model.

Dr. Robert Matthews, my family physician, the one who performed my appendectomy when I was sixteen, was another role model.

All these important and influential people formed a composite model I wanted to follow into family medicine.

The University had no department of family medicine at that time.

Medical students were encouraged to consider primary care, but few institutions offered post-graduate training in primary care.

One year before my medical school graduation, I faced a major dilemma.

Should I take a rotating internship and join a family doctor in Norfolk?

Alternatively, should I abandon the idea of family medicine and choose another specialty such as psychiatry?

I was soon to learn that medical school education is primarily about making decisions.

Fourth Year of Medical School

The fourth and final year of medical school was named "Fourth Year Electives," an ingenious pedagogy permitting medical students an opportunity to create their own curriculum, approved by a mentor, with studies at home or abroad.

It provided a great opportunity to take "electives" or externships, a practice ordinarily reserved for interns. It gave each student a chance to see what it would be like to study and practice in a particular hospital under the influence of renowned medical scholars.

I used my Fourth Year Electives and my rotating internship at the University of Virginia Hospital to arm myself with skills required of a family physician: Pediatrics, Internal Medicine, Surgery, Obstetrics-Gynecology, Dermatology, and Psychiatry

I made several trips to Norfolk, met with family physicians who offered me attractive opportunities to join their practice, even with no medical training beyond an internship.

I did not believe I was adequately trained for the responsibilities I would soon assume as a family doctor.

Dottie and I pored over the decision at our kitchen table, often late into the night, and on our knees at our bedside. A couple of funny things happened on our way to the final decision.

I was ten years older than my class mates in medical school, but I became more youthful in my thinking, often caught up in the enthusiasm of my youthful class mates.

The biggest enthusiasm during the fourth year of medical school was making "internship trips," journeys to potential places of study.

It was the most frequently asked question in the medical school hallways, cafeteria, on the Lawn where medical students sometimes ate their lunch on sunny days.

"Where are you going, Bob, for an internship interview?" Pride and vanity were conveyed in one's reply. The better the hospital were known, the bigger compliment one received from one's interrogating fellow medical student.

"Take that Night Train to Memphis"

"Take that Night Train to Memphis," a country music song, comes to mind because dusk was approaching when I boarded a train in Charlottesville.

Memphis was not my destination.

I was going to New York City on an internship interview trip at an influential hospital.

New York Hospital was clearly out of my league. The interview was only made possible because the interest in medical education reform made me and my PhD in Education more attractive to that end.

I had not met Dr. George Reader, a prominent physician and professor at a prestigious medical school in New York City; however, our communication led me to believe he was welcoming, warm and supportive.

It was by Dr. Reader's invitation that I slowly climbed the steps of the Chesapeake and Ohio train to meet him in New York to discuss an internship and additional graduate training with possible employment to follow.

I was the thirty-five-year-old-father of four children twelve years of age and under. We were a settled family, comfortable, and secure in Charlottesville, our home for the previous six years.

The train moved slowly, but my thoughts, mostly doubts about the wisdom of even considering uprooting my family, sped rapidly through my mind.

I ran through several cars and jumped off the end of the train just before the diesel engine gained much speed, landed safely on my feet, a small, old suitcase in my hand.

An excited feeling of relief befell me.

Dottie was surprised when I walked in our front door of our Park Place rented duplex.

"What are you up to, Brown?" she said smiling, holding her loving arms up to greet me.

"Daddy," Nancy, then nine years old said, "Are we moving to New York like you said?"

After the blessing for dinner, I explained to Nancy, Bobby age twelve, David age 10, and Clinton age 2, with wife Dottie's able assistance, all of us seated around the kitchen table, that someday we would visit New York City, but for now we will continue to live in Charlottesville.

As I recall, after brief objections, the topic of discussion soon changed, and the cancelled internship trip to New York City never came up again. Dr. Reader understood.

Looking back, I believe I got caught up in the excitement of internship "matching," the process by which fourth year medical students rank, in order of preference, their dream list and, in return, the hospitals rank the students in their own order of preference.

On "Match Day" the student learns if he or she "matches." Prestige is at stake for the student as well as for the student's medical school.

Thank God, I came to my senses, admittedly late in the process. The best internship for me was at the University of Virginia, and most fortunately, that is where I was trained.

It was not the first time, but it was the last time, I leapt from a moving train. Curiously, not to be recommended, as mentioned earlier, however, and little known about me, was my habit in adolescence of jumping on Norfolk and Western train cars, freshly emptied of their coal at the Lambert's Point Coal Piers, as they slowly made their way westward.

Holding on for dear life to the steel rail ladder on the side of the coal car as it picked up speed, my exhilaration increased with the train's acceleration. When the train crossed Monticello Avenue, I cautiously let my grip loose, dismounted and then walked the rest of my way to downtown Norfolk.

In the name of a well-known British television show, "Don't Try This at Home," I encourage no one to hop trains. Often, two of my best friends, Baxter and George, about whom more could be written, accompanied me, none of us fully appreciating the hazard and wrongfulness of our act.

I understand that a part of the human brain associated with sound judgment remains incompletely myelinated (an essential thin coating of nerve fibers) during adolescence, a fact that may help explain why otherwise normal appearing adolescents do perfectly stupid and dangerous things.

Rotating Internship

The internship year was arduous.

Some rotations placed me on duty in the hospital every other night.

On my surgery rotation, for example, I reported, three-by-five cards in my shirt pocket each containing my hand-written summary of each patient, to the hospital at 0600.

I met my surgery house staff team in the hospital cafeteria.

We made rounds on all our post-operative patients, addressed their issues such as lab reports, X-rays and medications.

After rounds were completed, we raced to the operating room, scrubbed in, operated through much of the day, and made evening rounds on all patients.

Exhausted by the intensity of the long day's work, I unsuccessfully tried to sleep. A small bed in a small room was provided in the Interns Quarters adjacent to the hospital.

Short nights were shortened by frequent calls back to the operating room for emergency cases.

The identical routine was followed the second day.

After all issues were resolved, I would walk across Jefferson Park Avenue to my wife and four children where I had left them at 0600 two days earlier.

I also worked in the emergency room five months on an every-other-night schedule. I loved my internship. Fellow interns, residents, and attending physicians were inspiring and gifted teachers, all working as a unit to understand the causes of our patients' diseases and injuries and to effectively treat them.

Psychiatric Residency

After the painful decision during my internship to abandon the dream of becoming a family physician, I started searching for psychiatric residencies.

Residency decisions were no less difficult to make than choosing an internship.

Dr. Ian Stevenson, a remarkably intelligent gentleman, was chairman of the Department of Psychiatry at the University of Virginia when my clinical rotation in Psychiatry occurred as a third year medical student.

A mild-mannered man, one of few words, Dr. Stevenson congratulated me on my performance in Psychiatry. He encouraged me to consider Psychiatry for my medical career. His encouragement continued during my externship in Psychiatry as a fourth-year medical student.

I visited Johns Hopkins, Duke, and was also interviewed at Virginia. Johns Hopkins, despite its wonderful reputation, did not feel right. I learned later the feeling was mutual.

Duke was entirely different. One might say it was a kind of love at first sight for all the principal parties.

It happened four and a half decades ago, but it remains a vivid memory.

The Duke Curriculum

Dottie and the children and I drove to Durham, and spent the night in a nearby motel. Early the next morning, I went to be interviewed for a three-year residency in the Department of Psychiatry, Duke University School of Medicine.

I was unprepared for what unfolded that eventful fall day in Durham.

"The Duke Medical School Curriculum," a well-kept secret in the late 1960s, was alleged to likely change the direction of medical education in America once it had been comprehensively studied.

"This must be the way they do things at Duke," I thought to myself when Dr. Busse's kind secretary passed me a sheet of a paper at 0800 with a list of names and times of my interviews. Dean Analyn's name was at the top of the list.

I had not met the Dean of Johns Hopkins School of Medicine when I visited Baltimore a month or two earlier. I had not met the Dean of the University of Virginia, School of Medicine when I was interviewed for a psychiatric residency at Virginia.

It was my first trip to Duke University. Then, as now, it enjoyed an excellent reputation.

Asking directions of several people along its long hall-ways, attempting to follow the specific, brightly colored painted lines on its floors, somehow I made it to the office of Dean Analyn, an articulate, impressive and pleasant gentleman.

"You certainly impressed Harry Muller at Virginia. He and I go back many years. I understand that, in addition to your third year rotation in Surgery, you also took an externship in Surgery and spent some of your internship as a rotation in surgery."

"Harry tells me you have a PhD in Education. Harry and I believe you are well suited to inaugurate our Office of Research in Medical Education.

I know you came to Duke today for an altogether different reason, to be interviewed for one of our residency positions in Psychiatry, but I believe you can do both jobs at the same time.

We would like for you to lead our research on the Duke curriculum as our first Director of Medical Education Research," Dean Analyn said to me.

I could not have been more surprised.

I was speechless.

It was evident this important person had little time for a lengthy discussion.

"At the end of the day, I have an escort to drive you and your family around the Duke campus and some of the nearby residential areas. Once you are employed by Duke, your eligible children may receive a Duke University education tuition-free.

I know you have a busy day planned by our staff. Discuss my offer with your wife and family. It has been a pleasure to meet you, Dr. Brown. Have a great day." With a firm grip, the Dean warmly shook hands.

If I said anything, I don't recall what it was, but somehow I felt out of breath.

Fast forward four decades. My twenty six year old grandson, Rhett, a talented, tall, young man with remarkably fine social skills, recently applied for a job with the banquet service of a national hotel chain.

He came to tell us how the job interview went.

"They offered me the top position," he said, a tone of pride in his voice, his eyes smiling, "but I told them I would rather have the second position because I am not ready yet to be the Director of the Banquet Service.

I told them to give me six months to a year to get my feet on the ground. I really don't know their system…how to order on their kind of computer system."

My son Clinton and I thought it was incredible as we listened to Rhett.

"Why not learn on the job, be your own boss, set your own hours?" we glibly inquired.

It is dawning on me now, though, that Rhett must have been feeling something akin to his Paw Paw's reaction to the offer he received to tackle the Duke Curriculum.

I, too, was hesitant; furthermore, I had not dreamed of applying for the job. I knew Duke had a good psychiatric training program. I wanted to be a well-trained psychiatrist.

The remainder of that eventful day went smoothly.

The Duke Chief of Psychiatry was easily one of the top ten psychiatrists in the country, a leading authority on Geriatric Psychiatry. I met several residents, all pleased with the Duke program.

The Director of the Residency Training Program, cordial, articulate, and well informed, told me that the psychiatry residence call schedule was at least every-other-night, and was piled on top of incredibly busy days.

He wondered how one man could be the Director of Research in Medical Education at Duke and a successful psychiatric resident at the same time.

A professional mind-reader could not have better identified my own thoughts on the subject.

The beautiful day ended with, as promised, a tour of the faculty housing at Duke and attractive residential communities near Duke.

Dottie and the children were excited. I was anxious and apprehensive.

"Matching" rules prohibited promises from either party, but it was understood that I would soon let Dean Analyn know my decision about the offer in medical education research. It was all we talked about on our long ride back to Charlottesville.

It is clear to me now, forty-five years later, that most reasonable men in my circumstances would have unhesitatingly accepted the attractive offer in medical education research at Duke. Most reasonable men would have given up the idea of years of additional training to complete a psychiatric residency, and then start earning a living for my family.

Maybe a man with a passion to study and practice medicine is not reasonable. The validity of my previous sentence is confirmed by my failure to be strongly inclined to accept the offer.

Yes, it was an honor to have a prestigious university consider a person of my limited background for a pioneering position in their uniquely progressive innovations in medical education.

Dr. Harry Muller's unexpected, but most welcomed, confidence in me turned on the light in the office window of the Dean at Duke. The rays of that precious light fell on me. Declining the offer caused some regret. I am sincerely sorry for the disappointment it may have caused a man for whom I still have incalculable respect.

"Bob Brown's Body is not Leaving UVa..."

The psychiatric residency issue was settled rationally.

Our family was, once again, not uprooted.

We stayed happily at the University of Virginia. The training was excellent.

Dr. D. Wilfred Abse, a British trained psychoanalyst, became my mentor; he positively influenced my training as well as my psychiatric practice in Charlottesville. He was a remarkably intelligent and prolific writer.

He had served in the British Army in WW II and psychologically interrogated Rudolph Hess, a prominent Nazi military leader who fled the German Army by parachuting into England during the Second World War.

Psychoanalysts, always the quarterbacks of Psychiatry, dominated the Department of Psychiatry at the University of Virginia, influencing its teaching and practice of Psychiatry.

Not every member of its department was an analyst. Some were eclectic; however, no theory of the mind was more respected than the psychoanalytic and psychodynamic theories.

Today, due to factors too complex to be adequately explained in this medium, psychoanalysis is somewhat less popular; however, all but the most inflexible psychiatrist will affirm that a fundamental understanding of psychoanalysis is unsurpassed as the most advantageous basis of understanding the mind.

Dr. Vamik Volkan, a training analyst, later to become internationally acclaimed in Psychoanalysis, formerly a student of Dr. Abse, was the Director of Psychiatric Residency Training. He was a difficult task-master, but fair in his dealings with residents, and a gifted teacher.

Dr. Richard Garnett, the Psychiatry Department's most senior clinician, was my outpatient supervisor. He was the faculty member with whom I met weekly to discuss the nature and complexities of each of the outpatients under my care during my second and third year of training of the three-year psychiatric residency.

Dr. Garnett was the psychiatrist to whom medical school faculty members were most often referred. His calm, accepting, understanding personality made him an excellent therapist and professor.

Dr. Garnett may well have been the most refined and brilliant, but the most humble member of the faculty. He was distantly related to the Norfolk Academy and Camp Greenbrier Garnetts mentioned earlier.

My fellow psychiatric residents, all bright and uniquely talented, came with varied backgrounds and skills. One had practiced family medicine for years after serving in the Army. Another had been a University of Virginia Student Health physician for a number of years. Another, internationally educated, had been a Neurosurgery Resident in Philadelphia.

Only two other fellow residents, like me, had come into the psychiatric residency directly from an internship.

During our first year, each of us was chosen to care for specifically assigned inpatients hospitalized on the well-known "Davis II and Davis III Wards." These patients were the most seriously ill.

We also followed an every-other-night call schedule, covering the emergency room and emergent issues among the inpatients.

During the second year, we spent months on the Consultation-Liaison Service, answering consultation requests sent by attending physicians and house staff on any patient in the University Hospital needing psychiatric intervention. It was a challenging and fascinating educational experience.

We also rotated through Neurology, learning to distinguish between symptoms caused by physical lesions in the central and peripheral nervous system and those symptoms that were largely psychiatric.

The third and final year consisted of opportunities to treat patients in nearby Western State Hospital where chronically severely ill mental patients were hospitalized. We could also elect expanded outpatient treatment, and additional time in Neurology, Consultation-liaison Service, Child Psychiatry, and research.

Two exceptionally fine educational opportunities arose during my psychiatric residency.

Without much fanfare, in fact without my understanding how it occurred, I received an extra monthly stipend throughout my residency from the University Hospital as a Research Assistant in Medical Educational Research.

To the best of my knowledge, I was the first occupant of the position. Clearly, it must have been from and with the good will of Dr. Harry Muller, Chairman, Department of Surgery, the scholar by whom I was directed to the Dean of Duke University School of Medicine.

It was understood, as I understand it now, that as time permitted during my psychiatric residency, I could seize any opportunity to study the pedagogy of medical education at the University. The reader will forgive me, I pray, for using the endearing term, "the University," the most important name by which the citizens in the Commonwealth of Virginia name the University of Virginia. More can be said about the University.

Two publications came from medical education research, "House Staff as Teachers," and "Pedagogy for House Staff," both appearing in the Journal of Medical Education.

Dr. Virgil S. Ward, my mentor and dissertation advisor in my PhD studies in the Curry School at the University, kindly helped me conduct a series of lectures for surgery house staff designed to improve teaching.

The second exceptional opportunity, also largely unanticipated, was the fulfillment of my wish to develop a college and graduate level course in mental health at the University and to teach it during my psychiatric residency.

The Beginning of My Mental Health Course

The proposal to teach Mental Health fell on receptive ears in the Curry School administrative offices, but the conservative administration in the Medical School needed to be convinced that the course would not interfere at all with my responsibilities as a psychiatry resident. Thus I taught Mental Health in the Medical School on Wednesday nights from 7 to 9:40 pm.

I want to spend some time describing the experience of teaching Mental Health, because I immensely enjoyed it. Much of what I learned from teaching Mental Health for four decades, I apply in my treatment of Active Duty Soldiers.

Fourteen students enrolled in my first Mental Health class. It was later to become identified as one of the University's "large classes."

Mental Health met for its first three years in the Tumor Clinic, a small amphitheater style class room in the basement of the Old Medical School at the University.

It was an ideal arrangement for me at the time. I could walk from the Tumor Clinic to the Emergency Room in two minutes if I was needed; fortunately, that rarely if ever happened while I was teaching Mental Health.

I was reading in depth during the day much of the same material I was teaching to my Mental Health students at night. I often presented cases for the class to discuss. The clinical teaching model, sometimes called the "case study" model in business schools, was well received by the Mental Health students.

"When she gave her thirteen-year-old heart to me, then as now three years her senior, it was forever."

A good editor, as a matter of course, will see this manuscript, as these pages will reveal, is Dottie's story, one of unswerving love, dedication, energy, strength, and integrity.

When she gave her thirteen-year-old heart to me, then as now three years her senior, it was forever.

The combination of Dottie's love and my mother's prayers strengthened both of us for the wonderful journey we have been traveling together as man and wife for sixty years.

Dottie graduated from Granby High School, Norfolk, Virginia, with honors, was elected the Most Talented in her large graduating class, and then really lived her life for me and our children, consciously choosing to place us ahead of herself and her ambitions.

Unfortunately, much of Dottie's contribution went unrecognized. For example, she "took in children" when we lived on Old Copely Hill, making it possible for other student wives to seek employment. She cared for those children with the same firm tenderness our children received. It was exhausting work for a mother already stretched to her limits.

She prepared all our meals, kept the apartment clean, and did all the washing and ironing. She was a very good mother and a wife whose limitless love infused my life, as essential as oxygen and glucose.

If my words reflect doubt on my love for Dottie as the central theme of my life, then I have failed as a husband and as a reporter of the truth.

Dottie helped put the pieces of my life back in place. Medical school was at last completed. The internship fell into place. The psychiatric residency was accomplished.

A patient in the Norfolk General Hospital read the announcement of the opening of my practice. Forty years earlier, in the same hospital, this patient gave birth to a son whom she loved, for whom she prayed, and in whom she instilled hope. Now she was content.

"Dr. Robert S Brown is pleased to announce the opening of his office for the practice of psychiatry in Charlottesville" were the last words Johnnie Louise Beale Brown read before her perceptive eyes closed to the light of this world forever.

Peace of Mind

The most important peace, peace of mind, comes when the pieces of one's life are put into place.

Peace of mind is elusive and may be short lasting. Its greatest value may be its quality as a benchmark, a standard by which to measure an ongoing process with which one quells unrest.

Is peace of mind difficult to define? Is it like the familiar definition of pornography: 'I don't know how to define it, but I know what it is when I see it?'

Based on my studied observations, peace of mind is a consequence or indirect result of working hard to improve one's relationships, the willingness to sacrifice self-interest, and the joy of sharing the pursuit of one's dreams and hopes with someone whose love is limitless.

Theologians will testify there is no peace of mind without faith. With this position I cannot disagree.

Philosophers hold there is no peace of mind without knowledge. With this position I cannot disagree.

Soldiers assure us there is no peace of mind without the sacrifice of war to bring peace on earth. I have seen the result of this universal truth. With this position only the most irrational can disagree.

Soldiers suffer silently.

We owe our freedom to Soldiers. We owe them respect, support, and authentic appreciation.

We thank our Soldiers for assuring our independence and sovereignty without which we would have no privilege of seeking peace of mind or the pursuit of happiness.

The seventeen people mentioned in this chapter were essential influences without whom the pieces of my life and the peace of my mind could not have been achieved. Many more faces, names long ago faded by time, belong to the same or similar account.

Norman Burak, then a fellow first-year medical student barely known by me, now an accomplished Ophthalmologist and Emergency Medicine Specialist, nominated me in 1963 to be class president of the Medical School Class of 1967. We have remained fast friends these past 51 years.

Dr. George Minor, Hal Warner and the Jenkins Brothers helped me pay for my medical education.

Dean Ralph Cherry believed I could direct the McGuffey Reading Clinic. Dr. Harry Muller and Dean Analyn believed I could lead the first Duke University School of Medicine Office of Medical Education Research.

Dr. Burke Smith, Dr. Wilfred Abse, and Dr. Vamik Volkan were my influential teachers, along with Dr. Richard Garnett. Dr. Virgil S. Ward tirelessly supported each academic step I took.

Dottie loved me through crisis after crisis, through good times and all the other times. Bobby, David, Nancy and Clinton, God's irreplaceable gifts, were and remain our greatest source of joy.

This I know and this I will never forget: there is no peace of mind without the love and help of those whose lives touch ours and whose lives we reach out to love and help. It has been said that "happiness is directly proportionate to the quality of all of one's relationships." What I am describing here is beyond being happy. I'm talking about an inexplicable peace of mind that endures and transcends and defies mere understanding. It is a peace that energizes and animates. One does not go to a dictionary of psychology, as Ernest Becker remarked in <u>Denial of Death</u>, to find its meaning. One more likely learns about it in philosophy and theology upon which deep reflection is enlightening and gratifying.

18

WAR ON RELATIONSHIPS

"I am being taken off the promotion list"

Wednesday Morning Group, 0800-0930

SSG (STAFF SERGEANT) Wes Franklin, the first to speak, looked sad and tense.

This stocky Soldier spent a year in the hospital for a serious injury to his face during his first combat deployment to Iraq. Shrapnel pierced his chin, fractured his jaw, and damaged his vocal cords in its deadly burning trajectory down his throat.

"The group knows I don't like to complain," he said in muffled, nasal, moderately inarticulate post-injury speech, "but I need your help."

"What's up, big guy?" said Master Sergeant (MSG) Keith L. Johnson, the Soldier the group identifies as its father figure.

"I was wounded in combat. I needed medication that I've had to stay on. I gained almost 100 pounds from medication. Now they are flagging my record because I failed the tape test and weigh-in.

I am being taken off the promotion list because I'm overweight."

"Dr. Brown, you know that is not right"

The group became annoyed. I could hear cursing and vulgar speech.

"Dr. Brown," said MSG Johnson, "you know that is not right!"

MSG Johnson continued. "Soldiers are deployed when they are overweight. Being overweight does not keep them out of combat. Hell, I was deployed on Nitroglycerin."

Someone else shouted sarcastically, "The US Military is downsizing. They are looking for any reason to kick us out."

I could feel the tension in the group mounting.

"Some crazy things go on over there"

"The news doesn't talk about the war any more," someone said with disappointment.

MSG Ken Compton, Mortuary Affairs, a Soldier with 29 years of active duty, said, "Recently, I was told we are processing the remains of more CIA agents than Soldiers at Dover."

MSG Guy Goodson, a 38 year old recovering alcoholic with 3 combat deployments, a cheerful looking man of medium build, said, "Some crazy things go on over there."

The group paused to listen.

"I hand-delivered $50,000 in $5 dollar bills to an Afghan tribal leader. Do you know what kind of receipt I got?

The tribal leader made his mark on a paper napkin."

The other group members shook their heads in disbelief.

"What about SSG Franklin?"

"What about SSG Franklin?" I asked. "He appealed to the group for help."

MSG Goodson smiled. "Franklin is one of my Soldiers. I have him covered," he announced with self-confidence.

"You have me covered?" inquired SSG Franklin.

"Yes, I was going to tell you after the meeting. The Command Sergeant Major (CSM) is removing the flag. You are still on the promotion list."

SSG Franklin, as well as the group, was amazed how a career in danger of ending abruptly could be saved so simply.

MSG Goodson spoke again.

"The CSM took the time to review your case in detail. I asked him to review your ERB (Enlisted Record Brief).

It is pretty evident that you had undiagnosed and untreated PTSD for years. You went back on three combat deployments after you spent all that time at Walter Reed.

Man, you are a fucking hero."

SSG Franklin is a modest man from Alabama, the kind of person who chooses to ride on the back of the bus.

He stared at the floor in disbelief.

His lips moved. Softly, he said, "I ain't no hero."

We all felt a sense of relief. The session ended with a strong sense of relief. It was a good feeling.

Tuesday Afternoon Group, 1400-1530.

"How much of who you are now comes from where you were and what you did in combat?"

"My life is changed forever," said SFC (Sergeant First Class) Mark Highgard, a 27 year old, twice-married, attractive Soldier who is devoted to his 2-year-old daughter.

This physically fit young man has a thoughtful, reflective outlook. He was in a good mood today, one of a few good days for the chronically depressed Soldier with PTSD.

Addressing the group, he asked, "How much of who you are now comes from where you were and what you did in combat?"

Group members answered pensively.

"I can't do things ... not like I used to. I can't go anywhere in public and feel relaxed," said SSG Darby.

I was not pleased by what SSG Darby said. It is sad and discouraging, but I was pleased that he was the first member of the group to answer the question on the floor, an important change for this introverted, avoidant Soldier.

He continued. "I try not to get upset. Sometimes I get so mad it causes a headache. When I get like that, I can envision myself hurting somebody…but I've never done it."

SSG Darby is physically frail appearing.

Several weeks ago, I asked if he had lost weight. "About 15 or 20 pounds," he said, "but I don't know why. I seem to eat all right." I urged him to be checked out at the Active Duty Clinic.

"I spent a total of 12.5 years in the combat zone, just about half the time I have been in the Army," said MSG Ken Compton, a Soldier born in Puerto Rico.

Sex and Masturbation

"My interest in sex is gone," said SFC Mike Ford, a Soldier in the midst of a painful divorce. He spoke without feeling. His face looked blank. I detected no regret or any other emotion, unless it was protective numbness.

SFC Ford's statement, without apparent intention, gave the group its topic to focus on in detail today.

"I have had no sex for the past 5 months," said a group member, "but masturbation still works.

It worked in combat. Porn was everywhere over there. You could buy anything in Iraq except a car or a house!"

SFC Highgard, getting back to his original question, more than trying to change the subject, commented, "Thinking about combat now is much worse than while we were in combat."

It was too late today for lamenting combat. The topic du jour was sex!

"Sex starts with emotional connection," said SFC Mike Ford.

He continued. "I shut off my emotions so long ago that I fear starting them back up again."

"I even pull the female move," said another Soldier in the group.

"What's the 'female move?'" I asked.

"Sometimes, I fake an orgasm."

The group laughed knowingly.

"Sometimes I'm just not in the mood. I want to get it over with."

SFC Ford said, "Masturbation doesn't require emotion. It's an easy release."

He continued. "Sex is a chore. Don't lay on me. Leave me the fucking alone. I don't want to be touched."

SSG Bobby Davis arrived. He teaches Ordnance on the night-shift that ends at 0230. He appeared sleep-deprived. The group knows he can't fall asleep immediately after his shift ends. It is understood why he has trouble arriving on time.

SSG Davis reminds me of a large, soft Teddy Bear. He is gentle. I've never seen him lose his temper or even appear upset.

SSG Davis picked up the gist of the conversation quickly and added, "I find that I can buy more time with a kiss. If I give her a kiss once in a while, I can put off having sex. She's okay with that."

SSG Darby said, "Part of me is like the Incredible Hulk. I try to keep that part in. I'm always angry."

He continued. "Even when I'm laughing I'm still upset."

"I wanted to suck-start my 9 mil"

SGT Keely Jones spent the last six-months in a psychiatric medical facility for his severe depression and PTSD. Recently, Keely returned to our MTF (Medical Treatment Facility). His previous psychiatrist was no longer available. Keely became my patient.

It is often difficult for a Soldier "to start all over again with a new doc."

I could sense his emotional discomfort. Craning his neck in 180 degree arcs, Keely was making a threat assessment of my office. He wondered if it were a safe place? His blue eyes and bright white teeth were made prominent by his dark reddish hair. He had faced inexpressible horror in combat.

Keely, wearing his camouflage ACU (Army Combat Uniform) and tan combat boots, stood 6 feet tall; his average weight was well distributed over his medium frame.

"Before I was hospitalized last year," Keely said, strangely smiling, "I was going to suck-start my 9 mil."

My mind created an unwanted visual image that confused me. Nine millimeter pistols are worn by officers, not by enlisted NCOs (Noncommissioned Officers). Years ago on active duty, I was 9 mm- qualified on the firing range.

I repeated Keely's statement. "You were going to suck-start your 9 mil?"

Keely continued, responding to the perplexing expression my face communicated.

"Yes. You know, put it in my mouth and pull the trigger. I wanted to commit suicide. That was my plan."

"You must have been feeling devastated, Keely," I said.

"I was an MP in Afghanistan. We carried 9 mm pistols."

Keely was smiling again. Was this inappropriate affect, the kind seen in severe mental illness? Was this a counter-phobic defense, warding off unbearably unacceptable feelings?

"I saw a lot of bad stuff in Afghanistan.

It was the worst of my three combat deployments.

I was very anxious.

My filter was getting thinner and thinner. Someone would say something and I'd get into a physical altercation.

I got very paranoid.

My flashbacks were increasing.

The worst part…I lost 3 dudes. There was a daisy-chain…155 mm shells connected into IEDs.

A lot of bad things happened.

I can't get it out of my mind.

I avoid loud sounds, like kids screaming. I connected to kids screaming for their life in Iraq and Afghanistan.

I'm numb.

I cried at my mother's funeral. It was the first time I cried in a long time.

My mother just died. Alcoholism. She had cirrhosis of the liver.

My dad is also an alcoholic.

I was their only child. They adopted me.

They sent me back early from Afghanistan before my mother died."

If Keely had real feelings about his losses, he was not sharing them.

Keely continued. "I have a lot of trouble concentrating. I zone out.

I'm really conscious of my surroundings.

I always think people are following me. I don't know why.

I'm very irritable."

Keely returned to scanning my office again.

"Keely," I kindly inquired, "are you still having suicidal thoughts?"

"No, Dr. Brown. My suicidal thoughts are gone."

Relieved and pleased to learn that his thoughts and plans to harm himself were no longer present, I asked, Keely, "How did you get rid of your suicidal thoughts?"

He smiled again. This time it seemed more real. "I got rid of my suicidal thoughts when I got rid of my wife. She was crazier than I am.

She left me last year, thank God.

It is over."

"Keely," I said, "I am very pleased you have given up the idea of taking your own life. I believe you are competent to give and to withhold information about suicide."

Passing Keely my professional card on which I wrote my cell phone number, I said, "Keely, will you call me if your suicidal thoughts return? Will you call and talk to me about it?"

He took my card. He stared at it, even pored over it.

The smile was gone. He looked authentic for the first time. He spoke thoughtfully.

In a way that expects no answer, and slowly, Keely said, "I don't believe a doctor has ever given me his cell number. Thank you." Leaving my office slowly, he no longer felt threatened. Attachment began.

"MSG Ken Compton has been to Hell and back"

Death is no stranger to Ken, a Senior NCO (Non-commissioned Officer) one of whose MOSs (Military Occupational Specialty) is 92 Mike or Mortuary Affairs.

This delightful Puerto Rican American Soldier, nearing the end of 30 years of honorable military service, reminded me of Shakespeare's profoundly true statement, "When sorrows come, they come not single spies, but in battalions."

Ken's wife returned to their home in the mountains of Puerto Rico months ago to assist in a family crisis.

For the first time in their long marriage, he was separated from his wife without the fellowship of Soldiers he had known on seven combat deployments.

His young adult son, severely injured in a single car accident, was to be bed-ridden for a year.

His mother and father were both hospitalized for medical illnesses.

His father died unexpectedly.

His house in the U.S. has been on the market for months and "was not moving."

Ken sat before me. Here is a professional Soldier, I thought, the kind of Soldier we all respect.

"I find myself crying for no reason," Ken said.

"I cry anywhere, even when talking to my students."

"It got so bad the other day, I left class."

He reached for the Kleenex.

I silently waited for Ken to continue.

"After I left my class, I heard one of the other instructors say, 'MSG Compton has been to Hell and back.'"

Another long pause.

"I got my pink slip this week. My contract is cancelled. It's not so bad. All the contracts in our department were cancelled, and I'm leaving any way."

"Ken," I said, "you have a right to cry! You have a need to cry! I think it is wonderful you can cry!'

Looking puzzled, Ken needed me to say more about crying.

"How fortunate are the combat Soldiers who can cry," I said.

"Too many Soldiers permit themselves to have only one emotion to express. Do you know what that one emotion is, Ken?"

"Anger," he said. "In my case, I have a lot of tears and lots of anger as well."

"Be thankful you can cry, my friend. It will do its intended job. It will also reduce your anger."

This Soldier is intellectually sharp. He appeared to be pondering whether to accept my pronouncements or to debate me.

I changed the subject.

"How is your lovely wife, Ken?" The tactic worked.

"I saw her last week when I went home for my father's funeral. It was the first time in 6 months. We talk 2 or 3 times on the phone every day."

He continued. "She has done a wonderful job caring for our injured son. She has done a wonderful job repairing our home. She is a wonderful person. She knows I love her. She is pleased to be back in our home at last."

His thick white, bushy moustache emphasized his smile as he talked about his wife. Their marriage has flourished. They successfully managed their frequent separations. Their parenting, like their marriage, is anchored in their faith and in their faithfulness to each other.

"You know, Dr. Brown, 2 of my 3 children are in the Army," he stated proudly.

I congratulated Ken on his marriage and on his children.

"My children have never embarrassed me."

After a long pause, with a look of uncertainty on his face, Ken's disposition changed. He looked more serious.

Ken reached into his pocket, unfolded a letter-size sheet of white paper and passed it to me. He made no comment.

I read the letter out loud.

"To Whom It May Concern, this is to document the actions of Ken Compton on 29 Apr 2013. Ken is a co-worker and we spend a lot of time in the office working at our desks.

The afternoon of 29 Apr 13, I was returning to the office and observed Ken sitting at his desk in what appeared to be a trance. He was sitting upright in his chair; his face was flushed and his eyes were open and tearing.

When I asked what was wrong he did not respond. I asked several more times before another co-worker came up and started speaking Spanish to him. Still there was no response; we even knocked on his desk; still no response.

Finally, after several minutes of him not responding, he just snapped out of it with a confused look on his face.

We asked him if he remembered us talking to him; he said no. He still appeared disoriented, so we kept an eye on him until he left work.

The office supervisor stopped by his house after work to ensure he was okay.

He came to work the next morning and still could not recall the events from the day prior.

This was the first time I had witnessed Ken in this condition.

If you have any further questions feel free to contact me."

(Signed by the Soldier's Supervisor who also provided his e-mail address and phone number, offering to assist further if needed).

"Ken," I said, "what do you make of this?"

"I guess it's true. I do not remember it. They would not lie about something like that.

I have no memory of it, none at all."

A similar episode occurred a year earlier. Ken was driving from one military post to another, one hour away. He put his car on cruise-control and drove safely.

Ken did not did not take his car off cruise-control as he approached the entrance to the other military post.

An alert driver, coming from the opposite direction, blinked his lights.

Ken instantly reacted, slowed his car, and averted potential problems. He had no memory for events of the preceding hour in his car. This was more than "highway hypnosis," a common form of distraction while driving long distances.

He was referred to a neurologist, placed on driving restrictions, and thoroughly evaluated.

The neurologist diagnosed "Transient Global Amnesia." Eventually, his driving restrictions were removed. Fortunately, he had no recurrences while operating his car.

"Ken," I said, "this reminds me of the driving episode last year. What do you think?"

"Yeah, I guess it does. I don't know what to make of it. It's the first time I have zoned out in the past year."

Ken looked discouraged.

"Ken, will you go back to your Primary Care Provider in our hospital, show him this document, and get his recommendations?"

"Yes, I will go there as soon as I leave your office today."

"I'll give you a consultation request form to take to him.

Ken, do remember what you were working on in your office last week before this incident occurred?"

"As I said, I don't recall the incident itself, but that afternoon I was writing a report."

I asked Ken to tell me about the report he was writing. I also wanted to know his feelings about the report.

"There are lapses in our training of Mortuary Affairs.

We have an immediate need to start training commanders to prepare for the removal of the remains of Soldiers killed in action.

The problem is the attitude of the commanders. They don't want to think about it; they are afraid that if they think about it, then it will cause the death of one of their Soldiers.

I know it sounds crazy. That is the way the commanders think. Of course, they want to bring all their Soldiers back home, alive and well."

"Is this something you feel strongly about?" I asked.

"Yes, I feel very, very strongly about it."

"Ken, I believe you have a type of PTSD called 'Dissociative Subtype.'

It is important that you and your wife understand the limitations this severe form of PTSD places on you."

Ken reminded me that we had already arranged for his care to be transferred to the VA near his home in Puerto Rico.

"Share this note from your co-workers with your wife, Ken, as soon as you reach your home."

"I know what this is, Dr. Brown. I sat next to a guy in our group a month ago who had the same thing. We kept calling his name and he did not respond.

He just sat there, staring into space until he woke up."

"Yes," I said, "you are correct. I remember it well.

He was all right after that. The group was very kind to him," I said

"I know it's serious. It will be another way that my wife and I can be closer," Ken said smiling.

I asked Ken how he would explain "Dissociative Subtype" of PTSD to his wife.

"She already knows about PTSD. She came here with me last year for one of my sessions with you.

You explained PTSD to her. You gave us 3 or 4 DVDs on PTSD."

"Ken, 'dissociation' is a $50 word. What does it mean to you?"

Ken looked around my office. He was getting one last good look at my office walls plastered with military operations maps of Iraq and Afghanistan.

He was less concerned about his subtype of PTSD than about leaving one of his safe places.

We were going to be saying goodbye.

He had not forgotten my question.

Ken stood up and took my hand.

"You always quote somebody that says the mind controls the brain.

I guess my mind lets me space out…do things I don't remember. So far, my brain has not let me do anything really bad."

There were glistening tears welling up in Ken's brown eyes.

He said thanks with a bear hug. We were sad together. We were parting for good. Ken left slowly.

Tuesday Morning Group, 1000-1130

"A word can ruin it"

MSG Norris, an articulate, intelligent Soldier, is soon to retire after 22 years in the Army. He is a large man, well over 6 feet tall, with a shiny bald head, medium blue eyes and a very caring smile.

He addressed the question on the floor, "What is the effect of war on relationships?'

"It is difficult to have a good relationship with anybody. A word can ruin it.

I'm always looking for something that sets me off. That triggers me. I see it as conflict. Any conflict is war. It takes a while for me to realize I'm in it.

My girlfriend and her sister are staying with me. They go out every night. They called to say they could not find their way back so they were going to stay in a hotel. Later that night, I called the hotel. They were not there. They were lying to me."

His facial expression depicted anger.

"I can blow this out of proportion.

They can say something that has no congruence. Red flags wave in the air."

SGT Tom Quincy, whom we call Q, responded.

"I don't care how you see me, you have to respect me.

My 16 year old son said he doesn't respect me because I don't work…I don't have a job like his mother.

I told him to get the fuck out of my house."

Q is permanently disabled, a victim of an Iraqi IED that nearly took his life. To his credit, Q is a full-time college student who spends time coaching Little League soccer and basketball. The group lauds him for being a good father.

CSM (Command Sergeant Major) Paul York, reared on a Tea Plantation in Africa, a Hindu, spoke up, moved by Q's encounter with his son. He is a small, tan-skinned Indian whose dedication to the Army and his family is matchless.

"How come they don't know what we've been through?

My kindness is taken as weakness."

SFC Tommy Kennedy, a forward sniper whose PTSD has been nearly unrelenting for 2 decades, described worsening problems with an unfriendly neighbor, a "bitchy older woman who calls the sheriff too damn often.

If you want to know what war does to relationships, have us bring our wives in here. They will tell you what it does."

MSG Norris stated, "We think about everything in terms of survival.

A lot of guys volunteer to go back to combat because they feel more comfortable there.

Most of us have ED (erectile dysfunction). It takes a lot of understanding on the part of a woman to understand and accept that…

There are a lot of unfaithful wives.

Many Army wives, not just the young ones, are getting plastic surgery…you know…tummy tucks. They are becoming fit, getting their teeth straightened.

My wife is 40 years old. She just got a tattoo!"

Q said, "I change my relationships like crazy. I don't stay with anybody."

"What is the ideal relationship for a Soldier with PTSD?

I asked the group to ponder what they would consider the "ideal relationship."

Inherent in this challenge is their conception of the woman, (since all Soldiers in this group are men), best suited to be the wife of a Soldier struggling with combat-induced PTSD.

The following list is a composite of the "ideal wife." Every Soldier shared his opinion.

1. The good wife of a Soldier with PTSD must be "strong."
2. She must be "educated" on what we expect her to be.
3. This ideal woman must "care" about what we are going through.
4. She must "know" when to leave us alone.
5. She must "accept" that we are the ones with the problem.
6. She must "understand," when we are harsh, that it is unintended
7. This very special woman must be "faithful."

SFC Tommy Kennedy, a man of strong, unyielding convictions, said, "My first two wives cheated on me."

He then asked the group, "What is a healthy relationship?"

Following a long silence, SFC Kennedy answered his own question. "The ideal relationship is the one we built in the combat zone.

We compare all relationships with the bonds we have in combat. How can I bring my wife in the fox hole with me?"

This may be the crux of the matter. Eerie images invoked by this casual but critical question rushed into the minds of Soldiers perplexed by unfamiliar vivid mental pictures.

The unanswered question hung in the air as rhetorical.

MSG Norris said thoughtfully, "We create impossible standards for others.

I have to keep my circle small.

I make my circle much smaller. I don't let people in."

The group acknowledged the same constraints.

SFC Kennedy said, "If there is a positive side to PTSD, it is clarity. I don't want to lose it.

I see the world for what it is. I see people for who they are.

PTSD is like a light switch that is switched on. You don't want it switched off.

Since I got PTSD, two things are nonnegotiable, dependability and honesty.

Never lie to me. Kick me in the balls, but do not lie to me."

"My kids saw me like this. My 13 year old daughter started crying"

MSG (Master Sergeant) Hector DeVala apologized for "bothering" me with "so many problems."

Too upset to hear my reassurance, the Soldier humbly, often tearfully, repeated his request for forgiveness. Was this a penitent wrongdoer addressing his Priest? What happened, I wondered.

Hector is and looks like a Hispanic Soldier. He has short black hair, piercing dark eyes, clear olive skin, all are dark, but not as dark as his mood. In his combat boots he stands 67 inches tall and weighs about 135 pounds. On better days he appears physically fit.

He wears a Combat Action Badge over the left pocket of his camouflage uniform, an Airborne Combat Patch on his right sleeve, and a Ranger Badge at the top of his left shoulder. These insignias testify he is a proven combat Soldier, immediately commanding the respect of all those who know their meaning.

Today, Hector is like a shadow of himself. I have never seen him cry so continually, look sadder, and tremble with feelings of helplessness.

I strained to hear his hushed, tense voice.

"I took my wife and kids to the Steak House. It was a celebration of my wife's recovery from surgery.

Something didn't smell right.

I felt like something was going to happen that's not supposed to happen.

I get anxious around people.

I didn't feel right.

I didn't trust the people behind me.

I had my back to the door, something I never like because it makes me anxious. One of the kids switched places with me, not knowing why.

I was getting so anxious I was drenched in sweat within 10 minutes of being seated.

The food came out.

The kids saw this."

LT Toms

Hector continued talking. "When my wife cut into her medium rare steak, blood came out.

Instantly, I started throwing up.

I had to get out of there.

My kids saw me like this. My 13-year-old daughter started crying. My kids ask why I'm this way.

LT Toms appeared at once in my mind, just as real as if he were there in person.

I could see him, like he was really there. His face was as clear as day. I could tell you his last 4 (Social Security digits). I did his paper work in Iraq.

I could see him bleeding."

I picked a box of Kleenex, slowly passed it to Hector, and waited between long tearful pauses for him to speak.

"This happened the day after I saw you two weeks ago. I can't get it out of my head.

LT Toms was screaming, 'Don't touch my feet…don't touch my feet…don't touch my feet.'

He was bleeding profusely.

I'm not a medic. I'm a fueler.

It was the second day of the war in Iraq. My convoy was carrying 4,000,000 gallons of fuel for the Tank Brigade invading Baghdad.

My convoy, trailing the Tank Brigade, carried the only physician.

The Tank Brigade met unexpected resistance. The Iraqi tanks had a superior position on top of a hill. They fired down on our tanks.

The causalities were med evaced by helicopter back to our position. My team helped the doctor triage the wounded.

"It was the longest day of my life"

"It took four men to lift LT Toms' litter from the helicopter.

The doctor told me to apply tourniquets to the LT's legs.

The doc had a look on his face. To me, the look on the doctor's face meant bad news, very bad news.

The LT was in shock, too.

A lot went on that day.

It was the longest day of my life.

I had taken a course in Basic Life Support and a six-month course in San Antonio in Combat Trauma.

Manikins and real life are not the same.

I was not prepared for what I embarked on.

We are always in the rear. We were moving into Baghdad. It was rough. There were tanks on each side firing at us. Our fuel tankers had bullet holes. Fuel was leaking out.

It was the longest 18 hours of my life."

"I tried to apply tourniquets"

"We were taking care of Iraqi casualties, too.

There were so many bad days there.

Everything that happened those 9 months was terrible.

LT Toms was wearing a tanker suit. A big shoe tag was attached to the front of his uniform: "LT TOMS, 531st Armor," and his last four.

Field dressings had been placed on his lower legs.

Blood was dripping…really pouring… from his legs into an empty MRE (Meals Ready to Eat) box with a black plastic trash can-liner inside the box.

I tried to apply tourniquets.

The LT was still screaming, 'Don't touch my feet!'"

Hector stopped. It was difficult for him to continue telling LT Toms' story.

After a long pause, as if violating confidentiality, Hector whispered, "LT Toms had no feet.

I could see bone. Heat had melted the skin off."

"Thank you for your service"

"The LT had blond hair and blue eyes. He grew up on a farm in Nebraska. He looked like a kid just out of college.

"What is your favorite sport?" I asked him.

'Polo,' he grunted painfully.

"Hang in there. We're going to take care of you," I responded, trying to sound confident.

I couldn't stop the bleeding.

His eyes were wide open, but he was not responsive.

I closed his eyes with my hands.

It was all I could do for him."

Hector, staring at the floor, suddenly stopped talking.

The silence was soothing like a pleasant cool breeze on a hot day.

Neither of us spoke.

Finally, I said, "Hector, what happened next?"

"I said a prayer.

Thank you for your service.

He was just a kid.

He didn't have a chance to live life.

His eyes were wide open, Dr. Brown.

He didn't have a pulse.

He died from loss of blood.

Forgive me, Dr. Brown. I'm sorry to bring all my troubles to you."

Looking deeply into his eyes, eyes that at last looked back into mine, I said, "Hector, you honor me with your burdens.

There is no place in the world I would rather be this very moment than right here with you. I am on sacred ground when I hear what you did to help your fellow Soldier.

Thank you, Hector, for trying to save LT Toms' life."

"I was there to try to save his life...even if it was only 5 minutes of life.

I couldn't tell him he had no feet."

Another long pause.

Hector's tears were like sworn statements of witnesses in a capital murder trial.

"Nobody knows about the good things we did over there"

Still puzzled by Hector's repeated petitions for forgiveness, I asked if he felt guilty.

"I did the best I could. That's what helps me.

What was the purpose, Dr. Brown?

Was it a punishment?

What did I do wrong?

I want to be successful for my family.

I tried to save LT Toms' life.

Why was a bunch of fuelers in a situation like that?

Why did I break down in front of my family?

I can't tell my family about LT Toms." His body was heaving with tears of remorse.

Hector, like many fellow Soldiers, was struck by the strange irony of his own mental imagery.

"I remember everything, every detail of the terrible things... but I hardly ever think of the good things.

Nobody knows about the good things we did over there. From helicopters, we dropped thousands of tons of food, thousands of Teddy Bears, and thousands of soccer balls.

We even dropped food in hot zones (unsafe combat areas where dangerous retaliation lurked)."

A parched, irrational guilt longed for water. I was the water boy and coach.

"Hector, my friend, you did nothing wrong," I said.

"Sometimes the most we can do for another person is limited to witnessing their suffering.

You were more than a witness for LT Toms. You gave him words of encouragement.

You did not abandon him.

It is punishing to witness the death of a young Soldier, but your earnest unsuccessful attempts to save the LT's life were selfless and noble. You did all you could do, more than you were trained to do. You did not abandon LT Toms. You have no rational reason to feel guilt. You deserve no painful retribution.

LT Toms was already in shock when he was assigned to your care."

Truth is often helpful. Distortions in cognition are always unhelpful. At best, Hector was confused by his own feelings.

Nonjudgmentally, I said, "Hector, the management of a patient in shock with catastrophic multiple traumatic amputations outside a university trauma center is almost always unsuccessful.

You tried to save the LT's life. I agree completely with your statement, you did your best.

No one could have done more for LT Toms than you did. You did as well as a trauma surgeon."

Hector was listening.

"It felt like a break down at the Steak House, but I believe it was a break through.

You have carried these painful vivid memories of LT Toms since 2003.

You never shared these memories with me until today.

Without the Steak House experience, another year may have passed without the relief that will come from working on ways to find peace with the LT."

"What can I tell the kids, Dr. Brown?"

"They are so proud of you, Hector. The relationship between a Soldier and his children is treasured."

"I can't tell them the gory details, Dr. Brown."

"The gory details belong to you. None are too gory to reveal to me. You must hoard none of the gory detail of war, Hector."

"My 20-year-old son can hardly wait to join up. He wants to be a Soldier like me."

"Is there a greater compliment, Hector?"

"I don't want him to go through what I have seen, Dr. Brown."

"When your children see you suffer, what can you say?" I asked.

"I can tell them it is because I am a Soldier who fought in war for my country."

"I can think of no better answer, Hector. Can you say anything about your treatment?"

"I've tried to hide that part of it, Dr. Brown."

"Many Soldiers refer to psychotherapy as training or taking classes. Your treatment is called Cognitive Therapy. In many ways, it is very much like taking classes in how to improve thinking."

"That's a good way of putting it. I could say I am taking classes to help."

"What could you say about your prognosis? Do you plan to improve?"

"Yes, I can tell them I am hopeful."

"What can you tell your children about who caused your problems?"

"I don't understand, Dr. Brown."

"Did your children cause your problems?"

"Of course not, Sir. They had nothing to do with it!"

"What could you say about that, Hector?"

"I can tell my children I love them very much and that my problems came from combat. They had nothing to do with causing it."

"Hector, you have been a wonderful 1SG. You put your Soldiers first, ahead of all else. You have done the important work of a 1SG for 20 years. Now it is time to begin the healing process. Do you agree?"

"Yes, Sir."

"If LT Toms' mother and father saw what you did for their son, they would be so thankful. "Hang in there. We are going to take care of you" was so caring, so encouraging. Every word you said and every act you performed demonstrated you loved the wounded Soldier you tried to help.

Hector, you gently closed their son's eyes, prayed for him, and thanked him for serving.

Hector, can you imagine what it would have been like for the LT to die without you?"

Someday Hector's children will know the truth of his situation. What a great day of celebration that will be!

19

WHO COULD ASK FOR ANYTHING MORE

It was a day that changed my life

PATHOLOGY, THE STUDY of the effects of disease on the human body, is a major second year course in medical school. Our Pathology course was divided into Gross Pathology and Neuropathology.

One of the more interesting pedagogical practices in the teaching of Gross Pathology was the requirement to observe, up close, the complete performance of an autopsy of a recently deceased person.

No less fascinating, Neuropathology examined the effects of disease on the human brain.

"Brain Cutting" describes the day brains collected at post-mortem examinations delicately reveal their anatomical secrets in the knowing hands of well-trained Pathology Residents, supervised by their even more well-trained Pathology Professors.

I will return to "Brain Cutting" later in this chapter. It is relevant to a Cognitive Science course I taught at the University at the invitation of several Echols Scholars and University Scholars, the University's best undergraduates.

Almost 5 decades ago, as a second year medical student, I was privileged to enter the Morgue of the University Hospital. Some of what I saw all those years ago remains vividly in my memory.

Looking back, it was a day that changed my life.

Three Autopsies: their relevance requires a more detailed explanation

In 1965, the Morgue was located in the basement of the Old Medical School Building. It could have been a movie set for a splendid Sherlock Holmes mystery, dull and dim.

Dark green shades kept in the indelicate. The thick, heavy shades also kept out the sun.

Bright hanging lights, the kind seen in surgical operating rooms, illuminated each of three autopsy tables.

The remainder of the Morgue, about the size of a two-car garage, was faintly lit.

The Pathologists, each assisted by black apron clad, experienced, and plain looking older middle aged men, proceeded in a hushed, systematic manner.

Old, noisy window fans, perched just above the three green shaded windows, created distracting sounds more than they removed unpleasant odors peculiar to post-mortem examinations.

The smell of formaldehyde competed with pungent odors of exposed intestinal content. The latter won hands down.

I experienced a strange combination of fear, fascination, excitement, and dread. Here were scenes of the human form previously unbeheld and unimagined by me.

As mentioned earlier, three unrelated men, ranging from 24 to 35 years of age, all accidental victims of tragic traffic collisions, were undergoing extensive post-mortem examinations.

Their lives were ended prematurely by the blunt force of motor vehicles clashing at high speeds.

My 3 Pathology Lab partners and I stood close to one Morgue table.

The Pathologist showed us the striking evidence of a condition the 3 victims had in common.

"Had these young men lived long enough, they would have died from coronary heart disease.

Feel the outside of these blood vessels circumscribing their hearts."

Each of us in white lab coats and tight-fitting rubber gloves softly touched the unbeating human heart. The act of touching the dead seemed more priestly than medical.

Bright yellow fat glistened in the intense light. Its abundance around the heart was ominous.

Even thru the thickness of our rubber gloves, we felt the irregularities of plaques, made of calcium and cholesterol, beginning their slowly deadly occlusion of essential blood vessels that nourish the heart.

Years later, this toxic condition was referred to as the direct result of a "life-style disease."

Genetics play a role, but reversible factors have an enormous effect on heart disease.

Physical inactivity, poor diet, smoking, excesses of anything, combine to ramp up the risk of coronary artery disease, still the leading cause of death in America.

"This can't be just psychological"

After watching the autopsies, I became concerned about my own health.

I purchased the thin, paperback, <u>Royal Canadian Air Force Physical Fitness Manual.</u> The workout, mostly calisthenics, took no more than fifteen or twenty minutes, required no equipment, and I was able to do it every evening at home.

It was surprisingly grueling. I worked up a sweat in no time.

Shortly after starting the exercise commitment, I rediscovered a sense of wellbeing I had not known since I was an athlete.

Every athlete will understand this unique feeling. It was more than the "runner's high," thought then to be the result of endorphins, chemicals in the brain associated with pleasure.

I was a busy thirty-four-year-old, second year medical student, husband, father of Bobby, age 10, David age 7, Nancy age 6 and Clinton only 4 months old.

Exercise psychophysiology was not in my curriculum; however, I started reading the relevant literature as time permitted.

I learned later that an article in the New England Journal of Medicine reported a seven fold increase in endorphins when exercise-naive women spent weeks riding stationary bicycles.

Another article, however, proved that the sense of wellbeing resulting from aerobic exercise was not produced solely by endorphins. Runners finishing a race still reported a strong sense of wellbeing even after they were injected with a chemical that blocks endorphins.

I was convinced that the feeling was too real, too authentic, too similar, in fact identical to the feeling I last experienced thirteen years earlier when I was physically fit.

"This can't be just psychological," I reasoned with myself. But how can I prove it?

If physical exercise causes significant mental health changes, how can I confirm it? What can a lowly medical student do? I had no research grants. I had no time to spare.

A very cold night in January

"Volunteers needed as subjects in a study of exercise and depression," read the announcement I placed in the Daily Progress, the Charlottesville daily newspaper, in the winter of 1965, a very cold one, as I recall.

Fifty people from 15 to 70 years of age answered the advertisement. We met in the Old Medical School Auditorium. The volunteers, a motley crew, many with stark white hair, were seated, scattered apart in the large room.

"Please move down front," I requested. Slowly the group gathered in the right front side of the auditorium.

"Thank you for coming out on a night like this. We are studying the effects of exercise."

A hand shot up. "What exactly do you mean by exercise, Sir?" inquired a middle aged, round faced, overweight woman.

"Exercise is any physical activity you perform voluntarily and intentionally for its own sake. For example, we are asking you to keep an exercise journal, one that I will give you, in which you record any kind of physical activity you choose to do for a minimum of thirty minutes a day, three days a week, for ten weeks.

The exercise can be walking, nature's best exercise, jogging, dancing, calisthenics, just about any exercise you can think of.

Ideally, you will work up a sweat when you exercise for thirty minutes.

For me, I know that I am exercising appropriately when I sweat on my brow.

Some people do not sweat easily under any circumstances. I believe this is more often true of women than men. Hopefully, you already know whether you are a non-sweater."

Depression

"The ad mentioned depression," a somber, white haired, thin man, irritability in his voice, queried, "but you have said nothing about depression."

"Thank you, Sir, for thoughtfully bringing that to my attention.

Those who decide to participate in our study will read and sign an informed consent stating that the risks and benefits of exercise are explained, that they have been cleared to exercise by their physician, that they will indemnify the University, and that they will take a depression test at the beginning and at the end of the study."

"Who will get the results of the depression test?" the same man asked, perhaps even more irritated.

"We will protect the confidentiality of everyone who participates in the study. The only person who will know the depression score will be the subject him or herself. After the data are collected, names will be deleted from the results.

Let me explain it for the benefit of everyone. I am going to give you the CES-D depression test, a self-report of the symptoms of depression. It was developed by the Center for the Epidemiological Studies of Depression. It is brief, taking less than five minutes to complete.

I would like you to take the test tonight.

I will send you home with an exercise journal, ask you to write in the journal the answers to the questions that appear there about your exercise program.

My name, address, and phone number is printed on the front of each exercise journal. Call me when you have questions about the project.

When you return in ten weeks, you will re-take the CES-D. Your results will be given to you."

Everyone who came to the Old Medical School Auditorium that night took the depression test and went home with an exercise journal. Most of them returned ten weeks later, re-took the depression test, and turned in their exercise journals.

I had no control group, volunteers who did not exercise for ten weeks.

Forty of the original 50 volunteers returned with their completed exercise journals. All those who returned reported they had exercised at least thirty minutes at least three days weekly for ten weeks.

All those who exercised reported they were less depressed, a finding confirmed by significantly improved depression test scores.

It was a tiny step for science, but I was encouraged by the results.

"Jogging for the Mind"

For the next four decades, I investigated the effects of exercise on the mind as Agatha Christie pursues criminal suspects. I also discovered a variety of ways to persuade people to discover the benefits of exercise.

Thirteen years after my first research, and after many years of collecting data, <u>Physician and Sports Medicine Journal</u> published my research entitled, "The Prescription of Exercise for Depression."

In July 1978, <u>Time Magazine</u> mentioned my work in an article called "Jogging for the Mind."

Psychoanalysts would sense a causal relationship between my exodus from the Football House on Rugby Road in 1950 and my sustained, if not compensatory, interest in exercise's effects on the mind.

Isn't it strange how our regrets and shame may help improve our lives?

I knew in my heart there is little one can do to improve the functions of the mind that is more reasonable and more effective than regular aerobic exercise.

Exercise releases BDNF (Brain Derived Neurotropic Factor)

BDNF causes neurogenesis and synaptogenesis.

In common sense terms, BDNF causes the development of new brain cells and new or optimized connections (called synapses) between brain cells.

Antidepressant medication has a similar effect on the brain, but exercise is much more robust.

The credit for this discovery goes to Dr. Fred Gage of the Salk Institute.

Dr. Gage made the discovery of BDNF in laboratory rats exercising on a "treadmill" in their cage, using non-exercising rats as his control group.

No, you do not have to get on a treadmill in a cage to increase BDNF in your brain. You do not have to run the Boston Marathon, unless you need the T-shirt, to get a good level of BDNF.

BDNF is there for the taking.

BDNF is there for those who just want to take a nice walk.

"Is gardening alright for exercise?"

Several years ago I was a guest on a radio talk show. The subject was exercise.

A woman called in from a mid-western state. The sound and nature of her voice suggested she was a senior citizen. She was inclined to be serious.

"Is gardening alright," she pleaded, "for exercise?"

Almost bringing tears to my eyes, I replied, "Gardening might well be the best exercise of all.

Gardening may also be the strongest evidence of God…to put a tiny seed into the earth, attend to its needs, and behold its vast productivity.

Gardening teaches trust, because what you plant is what you reap.

Your daily attention to the needs of your plants demands exercise that may well make you sweat.

Gardening may strengthen your character by regularly taking care of something that needs your attention."

A long pause followed. With tears in her voice the caller, barely above a whisper, said "Thank you."

How Does Exercise Affect the Mind?

Most scientists will tell you that exercise is a good thing. Most scientists will agree that no one knows exactly how exercise exerts its positive influence on the mind.

I agree with this position.

However, it is a splendid time to offer competing hypotheses.

My hypothesis is that exercise is hot stuff.

Thirty minutes of moderate exercise, such as brisk walking, raises the core body temperature to 104 degrees Fahrenheit. The core body temperature is measured at the tympanic membrane or eardrum.

As the core body temperature rises, the circulation to the brain increases with it. As the circulation increases in the brain, the metabolism in the brain increases with it.

Imaging studies of the brain are capable of identifying metabolic rates. It is well established that depression is often associated with poor or lower than normal metabolic rates in specific areas of the brain.

If you have not been exercising five days weekly for thirty minutes daily, do not stick a thermometer in your ear and run down the street.

Having your best interests in mind, it is likely your neighbors will request an emergency psychiatric examination.

Carefully put away the thermometer, trying not to spill the mercury.

When your core body temperature reaches the optimal degree, you will begin to perspire. Some perspiration is insensible, hardly noticeable.

Don't expect profuse sweating, the sauna effect, unless you are in a sauna.

Sitting or baking in a sauna is not desirable because it does not release adenosine, a chemical uniquely associated with exercise that dilates blood vessels and thus enhances desirable circulation.

Chemicals derived from adenosine are used emergently to dilate blood vessels in patients whose coronary arteries are occluded or plugged up, causing a heart attack or a stroke.

If you have not been exercising five days weekly for thirty minutes daily, pay a visit to your family doctor.

Ask, "Doctor, how much exercise do you get?"

If he or she says, "Oh, I run around all day taking care of my patients," then rudely interrupt and state, "No, I mean the time you dedicate just to exercise to clear your mind, to work up a sweat."

Apologize for being rudely direct. Then ask your physician for approval for you to exercise.

You are likely to be advised to start low and go slow. Follow that advice to the very letter of the law.

Memorize the law: start low and go slow!

I hope you noticed that I have refrained from using "mind" and "brain" interchangeably. I like what William James, a Harvard physician and philosopher of the 19th Century, said about the mind.

"The function of the mind is to control the activities of the brain."

Sadly, too often, as in the case of combat-induced Posttraumatic Stress Disorder, the activities of the brain overwhelm the mind.

Information processing is impaired when the mind becomes helplessly the victim of an over-active brain.

The subjective experience of the mind bewildered, dumbfounded, and bowled over by the activities of the brain is precisely the cause of the symptoms we come to identify as mental disorders.

The central purpose of the healing process, in my professional opinion, no matter which treatment model is followed, is strengthening the mind.

At the risk of being simplistic, it can be said that psychotherapy or "talking therapy" is directly attentive to the mind, while psychopharmacotherapy directly impacts the brain.

It is fascinating, however, that imaging studies of the brain demonstrate that both forms of treatment effectively change the brain.

Cognitive Behavioral Therapy (CBT) developed by Aaron T. Beck, University of Pennsylvania, the most widely accepted form of psychotherapy, emphasizes the cognitive aspect of the mind.

It is an appealing form of psychotherapy, free of adverse side effects, and it is equal to if not superior to antidepressant medication for Major Depression.

The Prescription of Exercise for Depression, a Case History

Physical exercise may well be included in behaviors represented by the "B" in CBT (Cognitive Behavioral Therapy). The combination of CBT and aerobic exercise, for example, may well be a potent combination treatment for depression. The following case history illustrates its effectiveness.

Despair hung over the family that sat before me as the early morning fog clings to the Blue Ridge Mountains.

"I don't know where to begin," said the mother of her college student son, wringing a small white handkerchief between her tiny hands. "He is president of his fraternity, enrolled in one of the best Ivy League colleges, and his grades have been excellent... until now."

His father, dressed in a dark blue business suit, stocky, and confident, his voice raised, said, "Let me explain it.

He has always been on the honor roll, dean's list, whatever you want to call it. He is studying electrical engineering, and even his summer job pays more than most people earn in a year.

He called home two nights ago and said he is no longer interested in college, or jobs, or anything, for that matter. His mother and I are baffled. We want to know what is wrong with our son... he is only twenty-one years old and he should have no worries in the world."

"I have everything in the world that I could want," the attractive, young-looking son quietly said. "I have no reason to be feeling this way; that's really what's making it worse for me...the fact that I cannot understand why nothing has any meaning for me.

I find that I enjoy nothing. I want to sleep the entire time. I haven't been to class for weeks...I just don't know what's wrong with me."

His eyes did not meet mine. He spoke as if in a soliloquy. His head dropped into his hands.

His parents were silently shouting, "Do something for our son."

To their credit, his parents had taken him to their family doctor the day before, and no medical explanation could be found.

Calling him by his name, I asked if he recognized the following quotation, "I have of late, wherefore I know not lost all my mirth; forgone all custom of exercise."

"It sounds familiar, Sir. Could it be Shakespeare?"

"Yes. It is from Hamlet, Act II, scene II. It is one of the best definitions of depression," I said.

"Frankly, I am relieved, Sir, to learn that I am depressed. I thought there was something wrong with me as a person."

He needed treatment, but he also needed it delivered as a crash course in order to get him back to college.

He was one of the most cooperative patients I ever treated. Twice weekly we spent one hour in CBT (Cognitive Behavioral Therapy) in my office, and twice daily he exercised.

Like many depressed patients, he felt worse in the morning, so I had him go from his bed to his bike, a stationary Schwinn bicycle. There was a dose-response curve: the beneficial effects of the physical exercise in the beginning lasted only several hours.

He climbed back on the Schwinn for another 30 minutes in the afternoon. An antidepressant was prescribed also for this, his first episode of depression.

The combination treatment of CBT, exercise prescription, and medication was successful. The following semester, the young patient returned to college, flourished, and stayed in touch with me for a while over the years.

Will physical exercise of moderate exertion on a daily basis for at least 30 minutes, at least five days weekly, cure all depression?

No, but it makes a contribution that is under-appreciated. It decreases irritability, improves sleep, increases cheerfulness, and its place in the field of psychiatry is no less important than its proven value in cardiology.

I have never treated a physically fit depressed person

Recently, I attended a University of Virginia Medical Alumni Association meeting as the Class of 1967 Representative. I'm the guy who is told about the best things going on at the Medical School so I can include it in my annual fund-raising letter to my classmates.

I raced from work, drove 2 hours, arrived late, took a seat on the back row next to a pleasant woman, and tried to stay awake.

Dottie joined me for the reception that followed the meeting.

Standing around a tall table, libations in hand, the pleasant woman next to whom I tried to remain awake during the meeting joined us.

"Did you teach a class at the University 30 years ago?" she asked. "I believe I took your class."

"I'm always pleased when a former student greets me," I replied. "What do you remember from my Mental Health course, may I ask?"

"You stressed the importance of physical exercise," she replied without hesitation.

"I believe you said that in your practice of psychiatry, for many years, you had never treated a physically fit depressed person."

I turned to my wife. I said, "Dottie, get this nice woman's name and address. If she did not get an A in Mental Health 30 years ago, I want it changed!"

Dottie said, "I'll drink to that." We all raised our glasses, aware that a little red wine may be healthy.

If physical exercise is so great, you may well ask, why are not more people exercising to improve their sense of wellbeing? They are; more people are exercising now for health and well-being than in the recent past.

We are told that Samuel Johnson, the 18th Century intellectual genius, walked the streets of London for his depression.

Charles Dickens is said to have walked all night long on some occasions for his depression.

William Wordsworth poetically memorialized the golden daffodils while out walking for his depression. He was often accompanied by his sister, a good exercise partner. It inspires us to find someone with whom to share the benefits of exercise.

Picture 500 university students each semester eagerly attending to a patient interview

"Mental Health Adjustment" was offered by the Curry School at the University as both an undergraduate and graduate course.

I taught Mental Health for 39 years under several different professorial titles, ranging from "Instructor" to "Professor of Education."

The course belonged to the Curry School, but it was the College of Arts and Sciences students whose attendance nearly burst the enrollment at the seams.

I included Mental Health in Chapter Thirteen, The University, but the "Exercise Option," and patient interviews, two of its most appealing scholarly endeavors, are reserved for this section of Sacred Ground.

Picture 500 university students each semester eagerly attending to a patient interview.

The large auditorium was hushed. "Will you tell the class what led you to my office for psychiatric treatment?" I asked.

The patients had given their informed consent to be interviewed in front of my class. They came without duress, but with some natural hesitancy and anxiety or stage fright.

The telling of their stories, with minimal or no prompting, took about an hour.

The round of applause from the grateful class at the conclusion of the interview did more for my patients than a promotion at work.

The thoughtful questions raised by the Mental Health class were even more thoughtfully answered by my patients.

Many of the students were planning careers in psychology, medicine, or health related fields. Across the board, the students were intellectually and emotionally intrigued by the patient interviews.

With very few exceptions, my patients wanted to return for follow-up interviews, perceiving it as helpfully interesting.

Some student questions opened up new insights for me to later explore with my patients.

"The Exercise Option"

Academic freedom was never more appreciated. Academic freedom was never more enjoyed. It was delightful to teach Mental Health.

I was permitted to teach what I believed.

What I believed is what I learned from my experience with failure and disappointment.

What I believed is what I learned from my patients.

What I believed is what I learned from teaching and coaching at the Norfolk Academy.

What I believed is what I learned from graduate school, medical school, and post-graduate training.

I believed that students learned what made sense to them.

I believed that I could only teach what made sense to me.

Students approach learning as economists approach the market. It has a lot to do with dividends.

I knew that regular aerobic exercise is profoundly beneficial for the body and the mind.

I offered academic credit for exercise! Yes, and I repeat it here: I offered academic credit for exercise.

Eye brows of deans of the College of Arts and Sciences rose higher than the stock market. Unlike the stock market, these eye brows stayed up.

Criticism spread like an Hepatitis epidemic.

Two people supported me. The Dean of the Curry School prevailed against the tide of criticism. Thomas Jefferson was said to have sat up from his tomb at Monticello. He loudly applauded the sheer single-mindedness of it, and sang the "Good Old Song."

"It sounded too good to be true"

My Mental Health students quaked with anxiety when I announced that the "Exercise Option" was on the table.

"One-third of your final grade," I said the first Wednesday night of class, "may come from the "Exercise Option," one-third from the mid-term exam, and one-third from the final exam."

It sounded too good to be true. In fact, it was unbelievable at first.

The "Exercise Option" was described in the Mental Health Syllabus for all to read, but I had to repeatedly explain it.

The University is renowned for its Honor System.

The "Exercise Option" I said, "will fall under the Honor System. It will be pledged work.

I warn you in the beginning, the "Exercise Option" will consume 30 minutes of your time three days weekly for 10 weeks.

You will also be required to come to the First Day at the Track and Last Day at the Track."

A hand went up. A student asked, "Sir, what is the 'First Day at the Track?'"

"You will meet your TA (Teaching Assistant) at the University Track. We will record your vital statistics, time your 2-mile walk or run, and answer your questions about the "Exercise Option."

You will keep an Exercise Journal published for this class, record your mood before and after your exercise, list the type of exercise you select, and the name of your exercise partner, should you choose one.

Each week, your TA will read and sign your Exercise Journal."

Appropriate consent forms and releases were executed.

It was too good. It was true

The Mental Health "Exercise Option" went well, swimmingly well.

I never determined whether the Mental Health enrollment reached standing-room only proportions because of its accomplished instructor or because A's for exercise were for the taking.

If the reader has any preconceived ideas on this question, they are not being solicited at this time.

Fortunately, there were no injuries.

Remarkably, only one somewhat questionable adverse outcome arose from the exercise option in its four decades.

When Dottie became my Office Manager, I told her I had no "personal mail." Among her duties was "mail call."

A confidant once told me the University administration had mail call each morning. In the days before electronic communication, important issues were conveyed by the US Postal Service.

My mail call, admittedly, was likely a bit smaller than that attended to by the host of University vice-presidents and assistant vice-presidents. It was no less important to me.

Dottie separated the mail and placed it on my desk each day by noon.

Ordinarily, I read my mail leisurely, usually in the early afternoon after returning from exercising at U-Hall.

"I would read this letter before you leave, if I were you," said Dottie, looking grim and serious.

Dottie placed the letter in my hand.

"Dear Dr. Brown:

I am writing to you from the Charlottesville-Albemarle Joint Security Complex (jail).

I was jogging for Mental Health on the median strip of the 250 Bypass.

A Police Officer slowed down his car and started to speak to me. I could not hear him for the traffic, usually busy that time of day.

'Get off the median strip,' he shouted.

I like the median strip because the grass is soft there. It is a good place to jog.

Suddenly, I heard a loud crash.

A car struck the Police Officer's car from the rear.

Why should I be blamed for his unsafe driving practice?

I can think of no good reason why I should be in jail.

I enjoy your class very much, Sir. I hope to see you next Wednesday."

All good things…

One morning, an e-mail from the dean of the Curry School caught my eye.

It was a "dear john" letter.

The words are in the blurry part of my memory now, but the sudden pang of disappointment lingers.

It had something to do with the incorrect presumption that I knew the budget was no longer available to support my Mental Health course.

It included words of appreciation and a promise that, in the future, a fitting way would be found to recognize my years of service.

It appears now, a decade later, that the fitting way is still under consideration.

According to the dean, he appreciated the high road I took in my written reply to his missive.

A 39-year habit is hard to break.

I spent Wednesday nights teaching Mental Health at the University more than half my life.

Over those years, cumulatively, I taught 30,000 students.

Thirty thousand fine young students instilled hope in me.

Some of my Mental Health students are even civil to me nowadays.

Screechingly, this good thing called Mental Health came to an abrupt and unwanted end.

Two Dave's and a Steve

Max Tufts, a World War II US Marine Corps pilot, was one of the finest men I ever knew. Max was a descendant of the family who founded a university bearing that name. Max was a stocky, blond headed man with caring blue eyes.

He loved his family, his farm in Warrenton, Virginia, and Sandy Side, his estate on Cape Cod.

Max was a generous, sensitive, and loyal friend.

For years, Max wanted me to meet "Doc Murdock," a close Warrenton friend.

Dr. Murdock Head, a man about whom many books should be written, built his dream, "Airlie," an unsurpassed conference center in Warrenton, Virginia.

I always thought about my Mental Health students when I met interesting people. "This is somebody the class needs to meet," I said to myself.

Murdock Head, an invited guest speaker to my students, was a remarkable speaker. The class loved him. The class was enthused by the story of his life.

Murdock Head was enthused by the students. His financial contribution to the Curry School was one of its largest up to that time.

Murdock Head's friend, Dr. David Snyder, an Orthopedist, was a surgeon in the Vietnam War.

Dr. Snyder's friend, Steve Rozel, a World War II Army pilot, built his own helicopter at 75 years of age.

When Dave and Steve were Mental Health visiting speakers, they stayed on as members of my teaching team.

The last Dave, Dr. David Peterson, a licensed professional counselor, created one of the earliest and most successful "day hospitals" in Virginia. Dave also held a degree in theology.

The two Dave's, Steve, and I worked as a team during the last years in the life of Mental Health.

The loss of these treasured friends was no less sad than the loss of the students.

Brain, Mind, and Behavior

Debbie Pink, now completing her residency in Psychiatry in Canada, had been a Mental Health student, and then a Mental Health TA, one of 26 TA's, when the course was being pronounced terminally ill.

Debbie was one of the best of the best students, an Echols Scholar and a University Scholar.

"Why don't you take the most interesting parts of Mental Health," she asked, "and teach it as a seminar for a small group of the University's most successful students?"

I liked the idea.

"I will take responsibility for setting up the course. You can teach it on the Lawn," Debbie said.

Here we must return to Thomas Jefferson's tomb for a brief explanation of the University's founder's deepest thoughts and fondest wishes for his University.

Mr. Jefferson was so intimately involved in the construction of the University that he specified the precise mixture of sand to concrete in the mortar holding together the bricks he selected for the Rotunda.

From Monticello, he closely observed the construction of the University through a telescope.

The University Lawn, I believe, was Jefferson's idealized replacement for the happy childhood home he never knew. His father died when Jefferson was only 14 years old, an age close to that of the entering class in 1819.

Jefferson designed beautiful rows of student rooms separated strategically by faculty houses. He wanted a "father and son" relationship between the faculty and students. Education for women slowly reached the University in the mid-twentieth Century.

I never dreamed I would teach a class on the Lawn.

I named the course Brain, Mind, and Behavior.

Each student selected a book from a list of scholarly texts ranging from philosophy to religion. The course requirements were simple: read their text, write a critical review of the text, distribute their review to their class mates, and present and defend their review.

The course was listed in the Department of Psychology as Cognitive Science.

Students wishing to join me at "Brain Cutting" at the School of Medicine found it fascinating. For example, we discussed the

Amygdala as the brain's center for the "fight or flight" response to stress.

"Show us the Amygdala," I asked. The Pathologist obliged, pointing with the tip of his long, wide, sharp blade to the right temporal lobe and then to its match in the left temporal lobe.

The pre-medical students, of course, had the most interest in "Brain Cutting."

For our weekly seminar, we sat around a rectangular shaped table on the first floor of Pavilion VIII on the Lawn. Faculty lived on the second floor, I believe.

The discussions were enlightening. Books on philosophy of mind intrigued us. The joy of learning was humbling.

The students became people to me, people I got to know, people I got to like.

Dottie invited us to the house for dinner and discussion.

David Magoon

David Magoon, a tall, friendly scholar with sandy hair, grey eyes, and a warm smile, approached me after Brain, Mind and Behavior class one evening.

Almost apologetically, David said, "I have to write a senior thesis. Will you be my thesis advisor?"

"What an honor," I replied.

"My mother has Parkinsonism," David said. "I want to write about Parkinsonism."

This began a meaningful, lasting friendship. David wrote and defended a first-rate thesis.

He stayed in touch with us. From Spain after graduation, he wrote nifty e-mails. When he came back to Charlottesville, we had breakfast at the Boars Head Inn.

We met his wonderful family. Both parents are Harvard Medical School graduates.

It was on to Harvard Medical School for David.

He completed the first two years of medical school, won the hearts of his class mates, and was already identified as superbly able in medicine.

Dr. Martha Magoon, David's mother, phoned us one night. Dr. Elbert Magoon, David's father, was also on the phone. It was very bad news, the worst I've heard in years.

David was dead. He had accidentally fallen from a roof in Boston. No foul play or alcohol was involved.

The shock, loss, grief were painful.

David's memorial service was held in the Dome Room of the University's Rotunda.

His ashes were spread by his family under a tree in front of Room 47 University Lawn, the room he occupied as a University Scholar.

On holidays, Dottie and I place flowers under the tree to honor David.

David J. Magoon's photograph is on my desk as I type.

We stay in touch with David's parents.

How rich my life has been made by the people I have come to know first as students!

Unexpectedly, remuneration for teaching Brain, Mind, and Behavior came to me from the Seven Society, the most respected, but unidentifiable, secret organization on the Grounds of the University.

Dr. M.C. Wilhelm

In my capacity as Clinical Professor of Psychiatry at Virginia, a privilege and pleasure for many years, I worked with Dr. M.C. Wilhelm, renowned breast cancer surgeon, as consultant to his Breast Cancer Clinic. Pat Trussel, his renowned Nurse, added considerably to the privilege of working with their patients.

Every Tuesday morning, I left my private practice to join Dr. Wilhelm and Pat Trussel at the University Hospital. One by one, I met with patients who, understandably, were confronting the emotional consequences of their diagnosis and treatment options. A caring atmosphere engulfed these women whose faith in Dr. Wilhelm was well placed, but their depression was besetting. As a treatment team member, I tried to exercise them back to a sense of wellbeing while making myself available, as needed, for ongoing individual therapy. It was a journey of hope.

For many years, supervising psychiatric residents, two hours weekly, usually on Friday afternoons, in our living room with Dottie serving tea and fellowship, was one of the most intellectually challenging events of my week. These bright, young, ambitious professionals with "lean and hungry looks" have minds of steel and prefer debate to glib talk. Some became lasting friends. All were excellent.

Completing the Narrative Arc

From observing three autopsies to research on depression, to offering academic credit in Mental Health for physical exercise, to teaching, at their request, the University's brightest students on the Lawn, a course called Brain, Mind, and Behavior, to learning at the feet of unsurpassed students like David Magoon and Psychiatric Residents too numerous to remember by name, to loving a wife who loves me as I love her…who could ask for anything more?

20

No End in Sight

"I don't see how I can go on like this"

THE ROUND SAD Asian American face of the 26 year old single Soldier sitting uncomfortably in front of me in my office could not have been more disheartened.

Large black eyes, from which tears flowed endlessly, told me more about his sadness than his own few carefully chosen words.

SGT Joseph Harobi, nick-named, "Bataan," stood no taller than 5 feet 7 inches. His thick black hair was "crew-cut," short. Militarily, he would be judged somewhat "overweight," but not disqualifying.

Bataan is a combat medic. He wishes not to recall his combat traumas. He distracts himself by staying busy, avoiding reminders of combat, and preferring emotional numbness to all other human emotions.

He is intelligent, articulate, and penultimately sensitive when the iron doors hiding his feelings are even slightly parted.

A month ago, Bataan was hospitalized for severe depression. He had suicidal thoughts and he had a detailed plan to end his life.

He was released from the psychiatric hospital yesterday. His anxiety was worse. His depression had not lifted. He still had suicidal thoughts. He no longer had a plan to take his life.

"Every time I try to relax, my mind cannot erase my thoughts. I feel overwhelmed.

I don't see how I can go on like this."

Reassuringly, I asked, "What is the 'this' you just referred to?"

To my great shock and approval, Bataan said, "Do you want to hear my story?"

I had been treating Bataan for three months. He mostly talked about pain caused by stress fractures in his shins. Until today, he had no interest in talking about the inexpressible pain caused by his combat trauma.

"He never had any money on pay day"

"Jack was my best friend.

He was 17 and I was 18. We met at Fort Gordon, our first duty station. We were both combat medics.

We became good friends. I don't know why. We were very different people. We came from very different backgrounds.

Our friendship started with teasing. I always teased him about his lack of money.

He never had any money, even on pay days.

What do I do when I'm broke? I call my mother and dad.

'What are doing for your birthday, Jack?'

He was doing nothing because he had no money.

'It's your birthday, man. I have money. It'll be my treat,' I said.

We went out for dinner. We had a very nice time. I picked up the tab. Then we went bowling. We had a lot of fun. I picked up the tab."

That evening Bataan learned why Jack had no money, even on paydays.

Each payday, Jack sent his entire pay check to his disabled parents who had 4 other children at home.

"At the end of the evening, Jack said, 'Bataan, I haven't celebrated my birthday in 15 years. Thank you.'

That's when our friendship really started.

From then on, each time we met we hugged and said, 'I love you, brother.'"

Bataan was on a mission in my office

Bataan cried in brief intervals. Each pause ended with vigorous blowing of his nose.

He filled an entire small trash can next to his chair with a whole box of Kleenex drenched with his tears.

Each nose blowing episode was like the end of a stanza of a mournful funeral dirge precisely played by a military band marching in cadence.

Bataan was on a mission in my office. He perceived his mission, telling me his combat trauma story, as emotionally dangerous but as "mission essential."

"This is not easy," he said. "I'm afraid I'll completely lose control of myself.

In the hospital, they kept telling me I had to tell my story.

This is the third time I've tried to tell it."

Bravo and Alpha Companies were in the same sector in Iraq, close enough for Jack and Bataan to often meet and talk. When possible, they talked at length, once for 2 and half hours.

Jack and Bataan, both in the same regiment, were deployed to Afghanistan, 2008-2009.

"Jack was the youngest combat medic to win a CAB (Combat Action Badge)"

Bataan's legs, by no means previously still, now really started rapidly moving up and down.

From his appearance, it could have been a prisoner interrogation scene under blinding bright light. Mercilessly, the captive is demanded to disclose his secrets, but Bataan was the interrogator as well as the prisoner.

Using the Soldier's nick-name, I offered reassurance, suggesting he need not continue his report if he felt a later time would be less stressful.

"No," he stated abruptly in a raised voice, "I came to tell my story today."

Bataan continued. "Jack was the youngest combat medic to win a CAB (Combat Action Badge). You only get that award if you have actually been engaged in the shooting war.

Jack was the medic for Bravo Company.

I was the medic for Alpha Company.

Bravo Company went out on a night mission.

I went to bed.

I was awakened in the middle of the night by a knock on my door. It was my Platoon SGT.

My Platoon SGT said, 'I don't know how to tell you, Bataan, but Bravo Company was hit pretty bad. There were 3 deaths. There were scores of injuries. Jack is dead.'

I didn't believe him.

It must be a sick joke.

'Don't fuck with me right now, SGT.'

But this was no joke.

I fell to my knees. My hands covered my face.

I started throwing things around, yelling 'I hate this place.'

My God, he was so young!

I was furious!

I still wanted to believe it was a joke. I kept expecting him to knock on my door.

I kept expecting Jack to say, "Hey, let's go eat."

"Doc, start bagging up body parts"

"My Platoon SGT needed me as a medic to rush to the scene of the attack.

I had to triage everybody to see who could be saved.

One Soldier had disfiguring burns.

We had to set up a perimeter to make sure no more attacks would take place."

Bataan described the scene. It was too sickening and ghastly to ever be forgotten.

"Doc, start bagging up body parts."

It was an order from my Platoon SGT.

I felt like a robot mechanically picking up anything resembling parts of a human being."

A long, silent pause filled my office. We could have been in a funeral home.

Bataan was staring into space.

"Fifty yards away, I spotted a Soldier.

There was a name tape on the flak vest (protective body armor) over an ACU (Army Combat Uniform).

I raced over to it.

It was Jack's name tape.

It was Jack's body. Thankfully and mercifully, he died instantly for his country."

"We only have six trucks"

"I remember in training telling Jack I was afraid that I would fail as a medic.

Jack said, "What you wouldn't think of! You will do fine. If I can do it, you can do it, Brother."

I put Jack's body into a body bag (Human Receptacle Pouch).

With help I put the bag into the truck.

I cried.

"Put those bags in the HUMWV (High Mobility Multipurpose Wheeled Vehicle, a four-wheel drive military automobile, commonly known as the HUMVV)," the Platoon SGT shouted.

'We only have 6 trucks. We will need the trucks to take the men back to our FOB (Forward Operating Base).'

I disobeyed the order.

I got in the truck. I held Jack's remains all the way back to the FOB.

Before Jack's death, I knew by far he was going to be one of the best in the Army.

Why him?

Why did Jack have to die?

Why do so many dirt bags get to live?

Jack got the MSM (Meritorious Service Award) for that night.

I cried hysterically at his memorial service when they did roll call. I cried the entire night.

I cried for the rest of the deployment.

When I got home, I hoped they'd send me back to combat quickly.

He was such a good person to die.

Every time I feel happy, I feel guilty."

Jack's Mother

"Jack's mother called. Would I come up for the first anniversary of Jack's death and speak?

I respectfully declined.

I was drinking lots of alcohol. It was the only thing that stopped the nightmares.

Two years after Jack's death, I visited him (his grave).

I saw Jack's mother afterwards. We hugged for 5 minutes without a word."

Another long pause.

Bataan continued. "I spoke on the phone to Jack's mother yesterday. I said I love you. She said I love you."

"Jack's heart was so pure"

"Bataan," I said, "this is the third time you have told your combat trauma story. It was not easy. It took courage to tell it today. I am honored by you to hear it.

What meaning does the story have for you?"

Bataan looked puzzled.

"When you told your story the first two times, were you asked what the experience means to you?"

"No, sir. I've never thought about its meaning."

"It's the meaning we give to our experiences, Bataan, that determines their influence on us," I said softly.

The expression on Bataan's face suggested deep pondering.

"What does it mean to you today to have known and lost Jack?"

Bataan paused thoughtfully and said, "I wish he had not died. I wish he would call."

"You celebrated his birthday, his first celebration of his birthday in 15 years," I said.

"Is there anything you can do now related to celebrating his birthday?" I asked.

Silence.

"I always call his mom.

I send gifts to his siblings on their birthday.

I was a bratty kid. I was given everything as a kid.

Jack's heart was so pure.

I could tell him I fucking hated the whole world. By the end of the conversation, he would have convinced me I had no hate in my mind.

I miss him so much."

Bataan's legs were not bouncing up and down now. He was grieving.

"What can you celebrate now, Bataan?"

"You celebrated Jack's birthday, Bataan, What can you celebrate now?"

"They have dedicated an Aid Station to Jack."

"What can you celebrate, Bataan?"

"I never thought about it."

Another long pause.

"I can celebrate his life.
But I miss him so much."
I calmly said, "Jack is here in so many ways."
He looked up.

"You picked up his remains on sacred ground"

'Jack is here in you," I said.
"Jack is here in his mother.
Jack is here in his father and 4 siblings."
Bataan appeared to be listening for the first time.
"Jack was killed taking care of wounded Soldiers," I said.
"You picked up his remains on sacred ground.
All of us need to celebrate Jack's life.
Our nation needs to know the Jack you knew.
Our nation needs to celebrate Jack's life.
Jack showed you how to live.
'If I can do it, you can do it, Brother.'
That priceless encouragement came from Jack's heart."

Do not let his death hold you captive

"You were sent to Jack like a messenger.
You brought good cheer to Jack.
Bataan, you brought celebration where poverty had resided with his family.
Poverty and disability held Jack and his family captive from his third birthday.
Do not let Jack's death for his country keep you from celebrating his life.
Do not let Jack's death hold you captive.
You have the spirit of generosity, Bataan.
I will never forget Jack," I said.
"I know him because you knew him.

Jack's family will never forget you."

Sitting quietly, our stares of recognition comforted each other.

"Regrettably," I said, "there is no more Kleenex left for either of us."

Bataan smiled.

Intensive Outpatient Treatment Program

Together, we drew up an individualized treatment plan.

On Mondays, Bataan attends our Traumatic Grief Group.

On Tuesdays, Bataan attends our Post-Deployment Combat Stress Group.

On Wednesday mornings, Bataan attends our Post-Deployment Combat Stress Group.

On Wednesday afternoons, Bataan attends our Spiritual Domain Group.

On Thursdays, Bataan attends our Dream Interpretation Group.

On Fridays, I treat Bataan individually, using Cognitive Behavioral Therapy.

A treatment contract was executed bearing the signatures of Bataan's command, Bataan, and myself.

We do not expect a smooth, steady, unbroken line of improvement. We are informed that recovery will follow a jagged, up and down slope.

Good and bad days are ahead. He will not face them alone. Our session ended with hope.

"Another episode..."

"I had another episode today. I guess that's what you call it," said Raul Gomez.

Raul is Hispanic, a SGT, six feet 3 inches tall, 225 pounds. He was seated in his usual position near the window in the semi-circle of the group in the group therapy room.

His legs were anxiously moving rapidly up and down. He was slumped backward in his chair. His eyes were sharp, penetrating. His pupils were enlarged.

His fellow group members, sensing the nearly crippling anxiety in his voice, looked in his direction, but said nothing.

"What happened?" I inquired.

"I was seated in my cubicle at work, looking at my computer. This E-7 (Sergeant First Class) walked up behind me and slapped me on my shoulder.

Nobody walks up behind me and touches me; I thought they all knew that at work.

I blanked out and don't know what I said or what I did.

Six, seven, eight months ago it would have been worse.

You remember, Dr. Brown, when you first met me…I had just knocked out an E-7 who walked up behind me. You put me in the hospital."

I nodded in agreement.

"He got into your space," a fellow group member reassuringly said.

"The First Sergeant said I threatened to stab him, but I don't remember that part.

I have some memory of throwing my in-box across my cubicle; the papers went everywhere.

I was ready with my fists.

I flew into a rage…a blind rage. People had to pull me off him.

My 1SG (First Sergeant) told me to leave…to get outside and cool off.

I got in my car and drove around Post.

I replayed in my mind different endings…all the ways I could have ended the episode…like going to jail, to the SRMC (local psych hospital), going AWOL.

I took my meds and did a lot of deep, deep breathing.

At one point, when I first went outside, I thought about waiting for him to come outside the office…I thought of running over him in my car.

I'd call my wife and then parallel park my car and run him down.

I thought of punching him and I thought of beating him with a computer…but I didn't do any of those things. In that way I am better.

At 1330 I went back to work.

The 1SG called me in his office and brought in everybody who was affected by the episode.

I was still angry. I stared at the floor and kept up the deep breathing. Everybody said they were sorry.

At 1345 I told the 1SG I had to go to group. He said well…go. I was coming here to group, no matter what he said."

"Did the 1SG explain to your co-workers that your reaction was related to your combat experience?" I asked.

"The Army just deals with what they see. They don't care why you act that way."

"They look down on you when you go for treatment," a group member said. The group agreed.

Following the public display of emotion, including the expression of anger described by Raul, inevitably there is a period of shame, guilt, and sadness.

"When you were alone, did you cry?" asked a group member.

"I used to be a non-crier, but now I know it is so good for you to cry…to let the pressure out. It is like pressure that will burst a pipe if it builds up and has no release.

It is worse when you are alone, just you and your mind. I was a big violator of that…I stayed away from people and I made myself worse because so many thoughts went through my head."

SGT Raul Gomez is better. He knows the importance of the difference between thoughts and actions. Admittedly, he has a long way to go, but he is on the right track.

How horrifying must have been the combat trauma that causes his intolerance of being touched from behind!

How terrible must be the anxiety he is learning to contain!

How vulnerable he must feel!

How fortunate we are to witness his step by step recovery!

Is this the Traumatic Grief Group, Sir?

SGT Pamela Jenkins, a 27-year-old Soldier, just under 5-feet tall, small frame, dark-brown eyes, olive complexion, wore a quiet, vacant expression on her face. In her right hand she held several damp, crumpled, white facial tissues.

She wore the Army Combat Uniform, named "ACU's" by Soldiers.

She had been crying. Her eyes were red.

Five Soldiers, all men who have been deployed and lost a close friend in combat or a relative back home, were seated in Group Room A. Their chairs were arranged in a semi-circle. LTC O'Quinn, my co-therapist, sat in front near the windows on the far wall, almost part of the semi-circle. I sat up front.

"Is this the Traumatic Grief Group, Sir?"

Welcoming the new patient to the group, I invited SGT Jenkins to take a seat.

For the sake of our new member, each Soldier gave his first name.

"This is a low-pressure group," addressing SGT Jenkins. I spoke quietly. "We have only two rules. Can anyone here tell SGT Jenkins what our group therapy rules are?"

Almost unanimously, the group said, "The rule of confidentiality...what is said in group stays in group."

I waited, but no one announced the second rule.

"The second rule, SGT Jenkins, is just as important as the first one: you don't have to talk if you don't want to. Soldiers tell me they often learn more from listening to what other group members say. Ideally, it's the combination of talking and listening that helps Soldiers deal with the loss that precedes grief."

Another Soldier arrived. He was 15 minutes late. I said nothing, but, looking at him, I extended my left arm so I could easily see my watch, and dramatically shook my head disapprovingly.

"I really love my husband"

After "going around," a group therapy method of having its members briefly describe recent significant circumstances they encountered since the last meeting a week ago, I turned to SGT Jenkins.

"Can you tell us, SGT Jenkins, why you joined our group?"

I was pleased but surprised that SGT Jenkins did not hesitate to tell her story to her new fellow group members.

"I really love my husband. We were married...." The SGT stopped suddenly, mopping tears from her eyes and cheeks.

"We were married 7 years. He had been deployed once before we were married and 5 times since our marriage. I was deployed 3 times with him. We were both 88 Mikes...truck drivers.

After each deployment, he liked to party. I do, too...but there is a limit. Even though we still loved each other very much I came to believe our differences could not be reconciled. I divorced him.

We continued to see each other. We still made love. I became pregnant with our son.

On his sixth deployment, we talked or skyped every day. He was really excited about having a son.

We were deployed out of Fort Hood. We lived off-post. I had trouble with our landlord, so I moved out. I found a better deal just across the street.

My old landlord called me on my cell. I was angry with her and resented her call.

My old landlord said, 'There are some people here looking for you."

I said tell them to go away, and I hung up on her.

She called right back. She said, 'These people are military.'

I said, 'If they are military then they already know where I live.' I was going to hang up on her again, but quickly she said, 'There is a chaplain with them.'

My heart sank. Suddenly, I was out of breath. I felt I couldn't breathe. I knew what the chaplain was going to say. My world was shattered. I called my mother. She lives in Seattle."

"I went to Dover"

"My husband's truck was hit by an IED.
 I went to Dover and took his remains to California to bury. I'm crying now, but I was just going through the motions then. I felt numb.
 Three months after his death, our son was born.
 I had to be hospitalized for depression after his birth."
 "Did you feel guilty for divorcing your husband?" asked one of SGT Jenkins' fellow group members. It was a question on everyone's mind.
 "No, I have never felt guilty over the divorce. I gave him 3 chances. I was convinced he was not going to change.
 I have not felt guilt, but I have felt regret that we did not have more time together."

"Last week was the first anniversary of my husband's death"

The group, attentive to every word SGT Jenkins said, felt empathy for her, a fellow Soldier going through what they fear and dread. Vividly, they see a chaplain knocking at their own front door.
 They can see the military vehicle parked in front of their own home. They can see the smartly dressed casualty assistance officers and chaplain bringing bad news to their own spouse.
 SGT Jenkins, now crying between every word, said in very sad terms, "Last week was the first anniversary of my husband's death."
 Her fellow Soldiers, her new group members, men of sadness, familiar with grief, were grieving with her. No one was startled by the shrill, clashing sound that interrupted the painful silence when one of her fellow group members slammed his cell phone into a metal trash can.

In the pitch of anger, he shouted, "We give our fucking lives over there, and who gives a fuck when we come back?"

He had buried one of his Soldiers who committed suicide. His mother died the day he returned home from combat. Two years ago, his infant son died in his arms.

He was filing his grievance, filing it with anger-near-rage. Pathetically, he was loudly filing his grievance in a trash can.

SGT Jenkins, seated three feet from the trash can, continued her narrative.

"I went to my husband's grave in California as a memorial to him last week, and then I flew to Fort Hood where his unit held a special service in his honor.

They engraved his name on a wall at the main gate."

"I wanted to find out everything I could know"

"At Fort Hood, I talked to members of my husband's unit.

Maybe it's part of my problem, but I wanted to find out everything I could know. How did he die? What happened? What went wrong? Did he die instantly? Did he say anything before he died? Did he die alone? Was someone with him when he died?

Another Soldier, I found out, someone in his unit was with him when he died. They told him I wanted to see him, and to speak with him. He agreed.

After the memorial service at Fort Hood, they pointed him out to me. He was about 10 feet away. As I walked up to him, I could see tears in his eyes.

He hugged me for 15 minutes. We did not say a word. It is very hard to explain. We felt each other's sadness. I could feel my husband's presence.

He told me that when the IED exploded it threw my husband 200 feet from his vehicle."

"I ran to him," he said. "He was still alive...still breathing...but he was injured internally.

I held his hand. He could not speak.

'Don't leave, Joe…don't go, Joe…please don't leave us, Joe.' I kept pleading with him, even after he slowly closed his eyes and his breathing stopped. I stayed with him until he was MedEvaced in a helicopter."

The group respectfully did not speak.

The SGT's crying stopped. I sensed her relief. I also sensed her strength.

"SGT Jenkins," I said, "I'm sure I speak for your fellow group members and for myself when I thank you for sharing your grief with us today. It was not easy, but it was important.

I sense your strength is returning. I sense your strength throughout your entire terrible ordeal. You are to be congratulated for your bravery and courage.

Lovingly, you took your husband's remains from Dover, Delaware, to his grave in California, a very sad journey. You bore his son 3 months after your husband's death in combat. You went back to his grave for the first anniversary of his death. You went to Fort Hood for his unit's memorial service and you met with the last Soldier to see your husband alive.

I can't tell you how many Soldiers struggle with the painful memories of a battle buddy who dies in their arms or while holding his or her hand. None of them get over it. None of them get used to it. None of them ever forget it.

You have completed the trip from Dover to the hugging arms and warmth of the Soldier who witnessed the last moments of your husband's life.

For this group, and for yourself, you bring to us your precious grief. Thank you, SGT Jenkins."

"Dr. Brown, your son Michael is on the phone for you"

Two days before Father's Day, my office phone rang.

The kind and efficient Ms. Diggs of our clerical staff said, "Dr. Brown, are you with a patient?"

Ms. Diggs knows that I never refuse to speak to a Soldier.

"Yes, I'm with a patient, but what do you need?" I asked.

"Dr. Brown, your son Michael is on the phone."

I have 3 wonderful sons, Bobby, David, and Clinton.

Without hesitation, I said, "Put him on," having no idea I had a son named Michael.

"Dr. Brown, this is Michael Shumata. How are you?"

"Michael, my friend, how in the world are you?" I asked with joy in my voice.

"I'm fine, Dr. Brown. I'm in the waiting room at the airport. I'm flying to Afghanistan."

My heart skipped a beat. How I wanted to say so many things to this wonderful Soldier, my son!

"Michael," I said, "I am with a patient. Let me give you my cell number. How long before your flight?"

"I think I have 3 or 4 hours.

I have a new phone and lost your cell number," Michael said. "I wanted to wish you a Happy Father's Day."

I thanked Michael and gave him my cell phone number, and asked him to call me back in an hour. I hung up. I tried to refocus my attention on the Soldier in front of me, but it was not possible.

I had no way to reach Michael by phone. I did not have his number.

My mind starting filling up with so many memories of Michael.

Michael Shumata

I well remember Michael. He was terribly, if not permanently, disturbed by the trauma of combat in 3 deployments to Iraq.

He was there in the beginning of the war. "We shot anything that moved when we first went in to Iraq. Baghdad was our destination. Saddam Hussein was our target.

The ROE (Rules of Engagement) changed quickly. Soon we had to be shot at twice before we could shoot back, it seemed," he said during our first session.

Michael, a stocky, fit, fast, and well-coordinated 27 year old African athlete, was a humble, kind soul. He came to America on a college tennis scholarship, graduated, and enlisted in the Army.

All his family remained in Africa, in a small country run by a ruthless dictator.

Michael spoke with a thick British accent, but his sincerely friendly smile was universal.

He married an African American woman with 2 children. It was not working out for Michael.

An IED at an American Army Post

It was a dark, cold, inclement night in February. Michael, redeployed less than 6 months from his third combat deployment, was driving to his apartment, not far from our Medical Treatment Facility.

His mind was troubled by domestic discord, wondering if he had done the right thing to leave his wife and her children, and to live alone "to think things out."

"Am I just too suspicious," he thought, "or do I have good reasons for my mistrust?"

There had been angry exchanges between the couple. The "shouting matches," occurring with each meeting, were escalating.

His eyes were on the road, but his mind was on his marriage.

"Dr. Brown," he said with a deep voice in a thick British accent, anxiety leaping from his eyes, "all of a sudden there was a large IED in the middle of the road last night. Just outside the gate here.

I immediately turned my truck away from the IED, trying to dodge it."

His truck spun out of control, turned over 3 times, and landed upright.

"A Policeman was directly behind me.

I was not injured. I was scared to death."

The Policeman, a recently discharged Soldier, knew intuitively what had just happened in front of him. Michael was reassured, not arrested, by the understanding Policeman.

"I'm going to write this up," said the Policeman, "as a back spasm. Have a good day."

Walter Reed Army Medical Center (WRAMC)

I did not know Michael well at that time. The IED incident occurred less than a mile from our Army post. The IED was a visual hallucination. The experience is called a "flashback" when it happens to Soldiers with PTSD.

"Michael," I said kindly, "I believe we need to hospitalize you."

Michael said nothing.

"If you were my son, I would hospitalize you. I want the best for you. Do you understand, Michael?"

"Yes, Dr. Brown, but I don't like it. I don't want it on my military record," he said.

I explained that Behavioral Health records, not a part of a Soldier's military record, are maintained separately and confidentially. Future employers, I explained, cannot by Federal law ask a former Soldier if he or she received psychiatric treatment except for violent behavior.

Two weeks later, Michael returned from WRAMC (Walter Reed Army Medical Center) much less anxious. He looked relaxed and fit, joined the Wednesday Morning Post-Deployment Combat Stress Group, and spent the next 4 years improving.

Exaggerated Startle Response

Like many Soldiers, Michael suffered from prolonged autonomic arousal after his return from combat.

Michael tended to be irritable. He had difficulty falling and staying asleep. He had difficulty concentrating. He was hypervigilant. I saw no Soldier whose startle response was more exaggerated than Michael's.

Michael's African home country was not known for its slim, athletic world-class distance runners. When Michael was suddenly stressed, however, I believe world running records would be handily broken.

Out of breath, one day Michael rushed into my office.

"We were loading profile-type targets into the back of a truck for the firing range. I wasn't paying much attention to the job.

All of a sudden, one of the profiles assumed an upright position in the truck. It looked exactly like a Hodgi.

I ran here as fast as I could, Dr. Brown. It's the only thing I knew to do."

He had run two miles in less than 10 minutes, seeking safety in my office.

Another occasion was even more remarkable.

A Post Run with a General Officer

Like all active duty Army Posts, our Post has cannon for ceremonial occasions. Cannon is also fired at the end of each day. Its boom can be disturbingly loud, even at great distances.

Michael, running in formation with his unit, found the pace comfortable, not in the least demanding.

Michael was not informed, however, that the cannon is fired during a General Officer run each time a mile marker is passed.

Imagine the shock to Michael's nervous system, already more tightly strung than a Gibson guitar, when the first mile marker was crossed.

Instantaneously, Michael was mentally transported to a potentially deadly scene in Iraq by the unexpected, loud cannon fire.

Witnesses said Michael ran faster than a speeding bullet.

Leaving the formation, he darted into the nearest building to "take cover."

The group laughed heartily, hearing about his record-breaking speed days later in the safe and secure group therapy room A.

From Green to Gold

It is said you can't keep a good Soldier down. Michael is a good Soldier.

He made the difficult decision to end his marriage. Fortunately, his marriage ended on friendly terms.

He worked long and hard on his challenging combat-induced PTSD.

Michael picked up his tennis racket for the first time in years. It was like transfusing an anemic patient with all the missing components of his blood.

What satisfaction it brought to observe this man getting back on his feet!

Michael was selected for OCS (Officer Candidate School).

He graduated from Fort Benning as a 2nd Lieutenant and was sent to Hawaii as a finance officer.

Michael stayed in touch over the last 2 years.

He did not hesitate when ordered this week to Afghanistan.

There is no end in sight.

Michael remains in my heart.

I hope to hear from him in Afghanistan.

Michael is like so many wonderful people in our Army.

21

Suffering: A Handbook on Understanding PTSD

If there is a single theme connecting all the stories shared by our brave Soldiers in this manuscript, it is suffering.

In particular, the witnessing of suffering of others may cause unrelenting emotional pain and overwhelming, pervasive feelings of helplessness. Should the witnessed suffering be that of a battle buddy, then the intensity of the trauma is even more severe because it invokes the intolerable loss of an attachment that may influence survival.

Furthermore, the suffering of combat-induced PTSD has several distinct characteristics that set it apart from suffering in general.

First, it may be life-long. No research, to date, has a settled answer to the question most often asked by our Soldiers fighting terrorism in Iraq and Afghanistan, "Will I be like this the rest of my life?" I am convinced it is not life-long when the attachment between the therapist and the patient is mutually trusting, the distortions of thinking are minimized, the truth of the situation is discovered and the truth is accepted.

The severity and the frequency of the trauma also distinguish combat-induced PTSD that may well be unique to 21st Century War. No war spares sacrifice and suffering. However, our 21st Century War is too often associated with atrocity that is savagely cruel, outrageously brutal, intentionally wicked and unending.

Explosions cause approximately 90% of all injuries in Iraq and Afghanistan. The IED (Improvised Explosive Device) is the signature weapon of this war. Methods of delivering the IED are limited only by the evil imagination of our enemies. The explosives may be strapped to a child, a woman appearing as if pregnant, an animal, an automobile, or buried in the ground or placed in harmlessly appearing boxes.

The enemy is identified by no uniform, no military base, no battle field position and no code of ethics.

Mortar attacks may plague our troops, ranging from seldom or infrequent to continual. In many instances, combat trauma occurs with such frequency that unimaginable emotional resources must be summoned up to preserve sanity.

It is difficult to prepare our Soldiers to fight terrorists. It is equally difficult to psychologically heal our Soldiers when they redeploy from the dangerous 21st Century War.

A group of Army Chaplains, for example, were prepared for combat cruelty by watching a film of an actual beheading. The realism of the mutilation, more than one observer could psychologically process, haunted him throughout his deployment. In combination with his combat experience, the film caused PTSD that required intensive and prolonged treatment before it remitted.

A common irony among many Soldiers in the midst of combating terrorism is the thought, "I'm here to help these people who are trying to kill me." This perception inevitably influences the meaning Soldiers give to their combat traumas. Combine this perception with the perception that "America has forgotten 21st

Century War and will never know what I suffered," and the gloom is further saddened.

The Brain's Response to Trauma

There is a psychological "daisy-chain" effect to the suffering from our 21st Century War in the Middle East. The inevitable memories of witnessing terror acquire a magnetic attraction for even the most subtle element associated with the original event or trauma. Initially, the common element is outside the awareness of the individual, further complicating the recovery of the Soldier.

For example, any element associated with the original terrorist-induced trauma can, in an instant, confuse the brain, convincing the Soldier that the original horror is happening again. Because the original trauma was "high stakes" or life-threatening, the brain errs on the side of safety.

The speed with which the transaction occurs in the brain is measured in Nano-seconds.

The brain sees that its job, above all else, is to keep the Soldier alive. Suffering encountered in false alarms, commonly called "flashbacks," is a very small price to pay, as the brain sees it, compared to being unprepared for the next life-threatening attack.

What are some of the "common elements" of a terrorist-induced trauma? There are many common elements, but they are not infinite. It could be an olfactory stimulus, the time of day, specific weather conditions, auditory or visual stimuli, each acquiring the power to cause or trigger a "flashback."

In therapy, Soldiers are taught to identify their "triggers," or an element in common with the actual trauma that now has the power to confuse the brain, making it falsely believe the trauma is happening again.

Soldiers who become adept at identifying their "triggers" develop a rational understanding of what previously appeared to be chaos. Improvement in PTSD speeds up when the triggers are identified.

Senseless Loss

Our Soldiers come home from 21st Century War feeling vulnerable.

In combat, two things kept them feeling strong and protected: their weapon and their battle buddy. If given a choice, a battle buddy is of far greater value than any weapon.

It may be argued that no human relationships are more intense than those formed between Soldiers in combat. Without hesitation, battle buddies leave no fallen Soldier behind. A battle buddy will lay down his life for his friend.

"Attachment" is the term that best describes the relationship between battle buddies. The loss of a battle buddy is the loss of a significant attachment figure.

Psychologically, the loss of a parent, spouse, or child may not be more traumatic. The grief it engenders is emotionally draining and may seem endless, bringing with it confused feelings of guilt, remorse, even shame. Too often the guilt is unidentified and the grieving process is delayed or becomes a source of pathology.

In a peculiar way, the loss of identity or the loss of self-confidence is strongly associated with the loss of attachment.

No one returns from combating terrorists without being changed in some fundamental, identifiable way. The ill-defined loss of the pre-traumatic self, for many Soldiers, causes grief that is puzzling. It leads to a protracted sense of loss that is disturbing, but remains largely in one's unawareness.

The Magnitude of the Problem

It is likely that 2.5 to 3 million American military personnel have been deployed to Iraq and Afghanistan since 2001. Whatever the actual number, it has been large. Most of those deployed are Soldiers.

Approximately one-third or 1 million of our deployed military will develop PTSD (Posttraumatic Stress Disorder) from combat.

The 2014 estimate is increased to one-third to 40%, a staggering number.

PTSD, a serious mental disorder, can be severe. It is characterized by episodes of re-experiencing the worst symptoms associated with the original trauma, efforts to avoid thoughts or other reminders of the trauma, and autonomic nervous system arousal.

More recent changes in the <u>American Psychiatric Association Diagnostic and Statistical Manual, Fifth Edition</u> include updated symptoms, such as reckless or self-destructive behavior and persistent negative cognitions and mood alterations. The changes, however, are little more than nuanced alterations of the descriptions of suffering of those afflicted with PTSD.

Of the 1 million military suffering from PTSD, only one half or less seek or accept therapy.

Some assumed that one half of those likely to get PTSD would recover without treatment, thereby leaving 15-20% requiring treatment for PTSD. Support for this assumption is lacking. More likely, the 412,500 or one half of those refusing treatment, suffer with PTSD on their own rather than risk seeking treatment.

Reasons for declining psychiatric treatment are complex and will not be addressed here. However, the reader is reminded that SFC Ronnie Marks, Chapter One, was alienated by his family when he disclosed at a family picnic that he was being treated for PTSD.

The Army cannot be faulted for Soldiers declining treatment for PTSD. To the contrary, the Army has made huge investments in manpower and facilities to treat PTSD and TBI (Traumatic Brain Injury), conditions for which there is an 80% over-lap of symptoms.

The Purpose of this Chapter

The purpose of this chapter is to clarify and synthesize the Soldiers' stories in order to help identify and understand the psychological costs of the current 21st Century War to save American lives.

I will be the first to point out several weaknesses of this manuscript.

First, even though the doctor/patient encounters were large in number, estimated to be up to 12,500, the Soldiers telling their trauma narratives come from one active duty Army post, and as such they may not be representative of Soldiers in general who have been deployed to Iraq and Afghanistan.

I believe the Soldiers I treated, however, are fairly representative of active duty Soldiers across the Army because they often served at multiple Army posts before I saw them for diagnosis and treatment.

Another potential weakness of the work is that it does not address the issues of seriously physically injured Soldiers.

It is exceptional when a seriously injured Soldier is assigned to the active duty Army post where I am employed. My work has largely been with Soldiers who were spared significant or disfiguring injuries.

For the most part, my patients were physically healthy but plagued with PTSD and mild concussion or TBI (Traumatic Brain Injury).

On the other hand, spared of physical injury, looking healthy but having PTSD or TBI is one of the features that worsen the problem: Soldiers with a serious mental disorder such as PTSD or TBI tell me they are often misjudged and misunderstood because they appear otherwise physically normal.

Death, the ultimate price one might pay for one's country in combating terrorism, is neglected in this work, the reader might protest.

For the families of those who have lost a loved one in 21st Century War, I have the greatest respect and admiration. It is a topic beyond the scope of this work, worthy of sentiments transcending the psychological costs of combat.

However, I have tried to deal respectfully with the lasting pain and sorrow of the death of a battle buddy, one of the most significant attachment figures for a Soldier in combat.

In summary, this work is solely about the psychological consequences our Soldiers endure, in their own words, combating terror.

I assumed the role of transmitting their stories of suffering to our nation that we might be more intimately informed of the emotional cost of 21st Century War. As a result of learning from these Soldiers themselves, we may come to honor, love, and respect our military even when the war is no longer reported as important news.

SUMMARY OF THE PSYCHOLOGICAL COST OF 21ST CENTURY 21st WAR

The following list of psychological problems, some of which may become permanent forms of compensable disabilities, is not meant to be exhaustive or complete but rather representative of the problems presented by Soldiers whose stories are told in this manuscript.

1. **Significantly Damaged Sleep/Wake Cycle**
2. **Significantly Damaged Personhood as Observed by Others**
3. **Significantly Altered Memory**
4. **Significant Impairment in the Capacity for Intimacy**
5. **Significant Injury to the Spiritual Domain**
6. **Significant Damage to the Soldier's Sense of Self**
7. **Significant Adverse Changes in Temperament**
8. **Significantly Damaged or Lost Sense of Basic Trust**
9. **Significantly Damaged Capacity to Relate to Others**
10. **Persistent Emotional Turmoil**

Each psychological problem listed above will be discussed primarily in the words Soldiers used in describing them to me. It is the emotional suffering, day and night, often for years, that is the focus of this section. Its intention is to inform the public of the psychological cost of our 21st Century War. The author's hope is that the nation will come to understand, comfort, admire, and respect our Soldiers upon learning, first hand, what these Soldiers endured.

1. **Significantly Damaged Sleep/Wake Cycle**

In the final analysis, falling asleep at night in one's own bed is an act of trust. Trust itself is closely aligned with self-confidence. Soldiers with combat induced PTSD, their self-confidence shattered and their sense of trust nearly destroyed, dread the coming of night. Always conscious of the danger, Soldiers check doors and windows throughout the night.

Robbed of sleep for three months, the CPT in Chapter One could not rid his mind of a "picture," a horrifying scene of two Soldiers dragging between them their wounded buddy whose brain matter escaped from his head. The two Soldiers pleaded with the CPT, mistaking him for a medical officer, to "Save our Brother."

The CPT confessed that he "froze for a moment" beholding the actual wound and irrationally blamed himself for failing to save the mortally injured Soldier. Guilt flowed from the error in his thinking leading to intractable insomnia.

When the CPT realized his purpose was to comfort the wounded Soldier's two friends, in acute grief over the loss of their friend, not to save the life of the mortally wounded Soldier, his sleep returned.

The CPT required little or no therapy. Seen in the gym months later, the fully recovered CPT attributed his improvement to 3 facts: "I got my thinking straight, I got my sleep back and I got back into exercise, Sir."

The CPT's case, sadly, is not typical. Most Soldiers with PTSD have no happy ending of their insomnia. They struggle with a significantly damaged sleep-wake cycle for years. Refreshing sleep eludes them.

Nightmares, frequently reenactments of combat trauma, are too often terrifying for Soldiers with PTSD. Our numbers are small, but Soldiers who openly discuss the details of their dreams and nightmares in our weekly Dream Interpretation Group appear to recover some improvement in their sleep.

Some Soldiers, such as Gunnery SGT Seth Johnson, find that caring for and sleeping with a pet dog decreases the frequency of nightmares.

PTSD causes a state of nearly constant physiological and psychological arousal, a condition that is not commonly associated with normal sleep.

Too often, Soldiers with PTSD learn that ingesting ethanol reduces or stops nightmares, and thus alcohol abuse and dependence replaces nightmares.

Normally, voluntary muscles are temporarily paralyzed during REM (Rapid Eye Movement) or the stage of sleep most commonly associated with dreaming. Some Soldiers with combat-induced PTSD develop REM Behavioral Disorder, a condition in which the large or voluntary muscles are not paralyzed while dreaming.

Both the Soldier and his bed-partner are surprised and frightened by the Soldier physically acting out the dream in REM Behavioral Disorder. Soldiers with this sleep disorder may physically strike the bed-partner, but have no memory of it upon awakening. MSG Keith L. Johnson invited me to interview his bed partner whose nocturnally inflicted bruises puzzled and disturbed him.

Further complicating sleep is the surprisingly high percentage of cases of Sleep Apnea in Soldiers redeployed from Iraq and Afghanistan. Acceptable explanations for this phenomenon have not yet been provided.

According to recent research, chronic loss of refreshing sleep may result in irreparable harm to the brain and may be a contributing factor to cognitive impairment.

Picture a sleep deprived Soldier, stressed out at work, troubled at home because he cannot relate to his wife, uncomfortable in public, intolerant of crowds in stores and at shopping centers, anxious driving in traffic, prone to realistic nightmares, and you may begin to sense what having combat induced PTSD is like.

2. **Significantly Damaged Personhood as Observed by Others**
Soldiers redeploying from Iraq and Afghanistan with combat-induced PTSD are seen and told, by others important to them, that they are no longer the same person they knew and loved before deployment. By inference, these Soldiers, sensing rejection, feel permanently impaired or damaged as people.

Personhood, as used in this section, primarily refers to the perception others have of Soldiers changed by 21st Century War. Examples of the adverse effects of being told by others their personhood has changed may be found throughout the text, but are emphasized in Chapter Four.

"I feel like a stranger in my own home," typifies the feeling of alienation. One Soldier said, "Even my own mother said she did not know me now."

These Soldiers long to be accepted. Instead of acceptance, however, remarks about being a changed person are perceived as painful denunciation.

All the experiences contributing to these Soldiers' personhood, from childhood to combat, have been reordered by trauma. Now a stranger to him or herself, to family and friends, what is left?

What is it in combat, one might well ask, that brings about the marked changes in people we call Soldiers that volunteer for military service and are deployed to combat terrorists?

It is the central question this work attempts to answer.

If I knew precisely the cause of such life altering suffering, then I might hasten the healing process, but I confess that I do not know.

But this is what I have learned from our Soldiers. They have not been born, given a name, loved by a family, educated and enlisted in the Army to be indifferent to death.

They have been taught to love their fellow men and women. They have been taught to value life. They have been taught to protect women and children.

They have been taught to be sensitive to those in pain.

They have been taught to endure hardship in order to help others.

As Soldiers, they have been taught to lay down their life for a friend, an act described biblically as the greatest form of love.

Is it so difficult to understand then that witnessing killing for its own sake by those indifferent to the value of life causes a living Hell for our Soldiers?

Is it difficult to understand why our Soldiers can have no peace of mind when their minds have been filled with indelible images of actual memories of inhumane killing more horrible than they could have imagined?

Frankly, I am amazed that only 15 to 20% of our Soldiers who return from 21st Century War request treatment for dreaded PTSD! The new estimate of 40% returning with PTSD may be more accurate.

Our decent men and women have witnessed the indecent acts of terror. Some of their worst memories include the terrible acts of senseless brutality of Iraqis on Iraqis and Afghans on Afghans.

Our military, thank God, makes no attempt to turn our Soldiers into insensitive witnesses, unaffected by brutality, murder, and destruction.

Yes, the War on Terror comes at high emotional costs.

Would we have accepted it on any other terms? I think not.

3. **Significantly Altered Memory**
"Why do I have trouble remembering things I need to remember, but I can't forget things I don't want to remember?" This question is frequently raised by Soldiers with combat-induced PTSD.

Cognitive changes associated with PTSD include difficulty with attention, concentration, and memory. Often it is tough to separate the symptoms of PTSD from mild TBI (Traumatic Brain Injury or Concussion). In TBI, cognitive changes are even more dramatic than in PTSD.

It has been shown that the average person can keep 7, plus or minus 2, variables on the screen of awareness at one time. The standard phone number, 7 digits, and one's Social Security number, 9 digits, for example, demonstrate easily recalled information.

Soldiers with combat-induced PTSD recall trauma memories every day and they relive the combat trauma on the anniversary of the trauma. These memories are costly, taking up much of the available space of awareness. The result is impaired concentration, inattention and impaired memory.

Combat trauma memories are powerful. As one Soldier said, the memory of the trauma is just as painful as or worse than the reality of the trauma.

The attention of Soldiers with PTSD is extremely sensitive to their life threatening trauma memories and even to subtle reminders of the trauma memories. Little else captures their attention in the same way. As a result, they appear and they are too often preoccupied and inattentive.

The "thousand mile stare" is the term that best captures the PTSD Soldier's inattentiveness.

It is common for Soldiers with PTSD to lose car keys, forget appointments, and even forget identification cards required for admission to a military post.

An intelligent Soldier with combat induced PTSD said, "I forget how to spell simple words when I'm typing."

All Soldiers with PTSD tell me, "My mind is always occupied…I can't clear my mind. That's why I stay busy. PTSD is a terrible thing. You don't know when it will kick in."

Imagine the disappointment of a spouse whose husband forgets wedding anniversaries, children's birthdays, or other important dates.

Another important consideration of combat-induced PTSD is the question of accuracy of the trauma memory itself. Too often, self-incriminating memories distort the factual recall of important trauma memories.

Psychological relief from the suffering associated with the recall of trauma memories requires addressing the truth of the trauma. Distortions must be minimized. Often, this requires repetitive retelling of the trauma. In this way, memory of the trauma events is more accurately recalled.

"I'm still losing things," said SFC Albert North, a divorced 38 year-old Soldier with PTSD and mTBI (Mild Traumatic Brain Injury or history of a concussion).

"I've lost my fucking brain. I can't keep anything...lost my memory. Every day I struggle with something. I'm so focused on looking for danger I lose things. I lost my car keys and found them 2 months later in the grass in my backyard. They even had rust on them. I have no idea how they got there."

Memory is vital to a normal, healthy life. Trauma memories occupy the mind of Soldiers with combat-induced PTSD. A mind filled with thoughts of danger from 21st Century War is focused primarily on safety issues. There is little respite from scanning their environment for perceived threats they believe they must avoid.

4. **Significant Impairment in the Capacity for Intimacy**
Up to eighty percent of Soldiers with combat-induced PTSD report erectile dysfunction. Sometimes, erectile-enhancing medication is helpful; however, more commonly it is of limited value because Soldiers with PTSD have low libido or low interest in sex and are intolerant of physical closeness.

"Emotionless sex" was the term used by one Soldier described in Chapter Eight. He struggled for 3 years before he was able to have "passionate sex" with his wife. "It only happened after I became desensitized to combat, when combat became secondary...not primary, in my mind; then my family became primary."

The Soldier said he started to improve when he realized "the doctors are taking care of me...I started to accomplish things. It built my confidence. My emotions returned. I was able to love..."

Patient education and couples counseling are the most effective ways to resolve this impairment. Unfortunately, misunderstanding goes unaddressed and many couples suffer needlessly. Too often, relationships end.

Combat deployment is difficult for Soldiers and family alike. "Absence can make the heart grow fonder," but it can also be disruptive. Wives face demands few can understand who have not had close contact with the military.

Some Army wives achieve a level of independence that the redeployed Soldier finds staggering and discomforting at home-coming. The old proverb, "No one can step in the same river twice," tells us that change is inevitable. The home and the family the Soldier left 12-15 months earlier will not be the same upon his or her return.

The Army provides education and social support for the wives and children, but nothing can replace the deployed spouse.

There is a period of adjustment when the military spouse deploys and an even greater, more stressful period of adjustment when the spouse is redeployed. Established routines are necessarily altered when the Soldier returns.

Many Soldiers tell me they "emotionally shut down for weeks" before they are deployed, preparing themselves for the painful separation. Many Soldiers have even greater difficulty opening back up emotionally upon return home (redeployment).

Soldiers with combat-induced PTSD have little energy for relationships, even less for intimacy. Managing anxiety and depression is necessarily exhausting. Much time and energy is spent trying to hide their emotional problems from spouse and children, fearing they will be seen as "weak."

A significant number of Soldiers come in for PTSD treatment only after being threatened by their spouse: "if you don't go for help, then I am leaving this marriage." Under these circumstances, I encourage the spouse to come in as well to tell me what the Soldier is like as a spouse and parent.

Intimacy is also threatened by sexual self-stimulation Soldiers resorted to while deployed. Pornography was readily available at low cost. It provided temporary relief of sexual tension. It required no attention to a partner. Easily habitual, self-stimulation may become preferable to actual spousal intercourse, only adding to marital discontent. This issue requires more elucidation, more study.

One Post-Deployment psychotherapy group openly discussed the advantages and disadvantages of masturbation. The Soldiers said, referring to sexually stimulating materials, "you can buy anything in Iraq except a house or a car."

Some Soldiers with combat-induced PTSD, isolated and angry, regrettably choose self-stimulation over intimacy after returning home. In depth interviews of these Soldiers reveal they have lost confidence in their ability to please their partner and are ashamed to admit their impotence.

Unless directly approached by the health care provider, this topic, a common source of marital discord, may go undetected and untreated.

Most cases of intimacy issues of the type experienced by our Soldiers with PTSD are resolved successfully as long as they have an interesting and interested partner.

On the other hand, there are important, yet to be understood, puzzling aspects of the damage done by combat to the capacity for intimacy.

Without regard to age, even young, otherwise healthy Soldiers are returning from 21st Century War only to be given the diagnosis of "hypogonadism."

Hypogonadism results from low testosterone, the male sex hormone.

Secondary or acquired hypogonadism is a complex endocrine disorder. Stress may affect the hypothalamus which affects the pituitary gland's release of hormones that influence the biosynthesis of testosterone.

It is also known that long-term use of narcotic pain medication will lower the testosterone level in males of all ages.

The usual treatment of hypogonadism is testosterone replacement therapy. Many Soldiers whose stories are reproduced in this text, however, tell me they are disappointed in the treatment available for their low testosterone. Testosterone replacement may have harmful physical side effects.

It is hoped that more attention in the near future will be devoted to identifying the specific causal relationship between combat-induced PTSD and hypogonadism. The development of effective treatment for combat-induced hypogonadism is needed without further delay.

5. **Significant Injury to the Spiritual Domain**
The effect of 21st Century War has been highly costly to the spiritual health of our Soldiers.

First Sergeant Barry Walker, Chapter Ten, put it this way: "Once you go over there, you are changed. The circumstances of combat challenged my beliefs. Seeing inhumanity in Iraq scarred my soul. The inhumanity of Iraqi people killing each other was more than I could take."

1SG Walker continued: "I lost my faith. My sense of truth was not the truth. I felt like Adam and Eve after eating the apple. I saw the ugliness."

Fortunately, at the funeral of an admired old man from his childhood, 1SG Walker encountered a childhood friend, now a minister, who inspired him to find a "new faith."

Americans are not reared to kill. Even killing in combat can result in major, lasting attacks on one's conscience. "Is it a sin to kill in combat?" "What I did was wrong. There is no forgiveness."

Killing children in combat is intensely and uniquely disturbing. One Soldier said, "I will never get over shooting a child in combat, even if he was trying to kill me with an AK-47."

"It's surreal. You go from killing in combat to flying home in a matter of hours. World War II was bad, but the Soldiers came home on ships. It took weeks, not hours, from combat to home."

"It is the thought of what we did in combat that upsets us, Dr. Brown. Our children may not love us if they knew."

I repeat, it is the meaning we give to our experiences that determine their effects upon us. Many of the meanings we assign to our experiences come from our spiritual values.

Our spiritual values come from our parents and grandparents, from our education, and from those we admire. A young woman recently told me that her father was never in her life because he was in prison. She hastened to say, "My track coaches became my father-figures."

Only a few Soldiers enjoyed a good relationship with their fathers. In many cases, grandparents became important parental substitutes for many men who became Soldiers.

Returning from combat in Iraq or Afghanistan is described by some Soldiers as "being born again." The Soldiers who have found a meaningful way to have their spiritual needs addressed upon redeployment appear to cope more effectively.

Chaplains have an important function in assisting Soldiers in their spiritual domain, do their work well, and are appreciated by the Soldiers they help. Collaboration with Chaplains in the treatment of Soldiers with PTSD at our medical facility has been of great value.

Our former Post Chaplain, now retired, co-leads our weekly Spiritual Domain Group. He is readily available for consultation on matters of the spiritual domain.

6. Significant Damage to the Soldier's Sense of Self

It is a truism that "war changes people." Based upon in-depth evaluations of large numbers of Soldiers redeployed from Iraq and Afghanistan, reported in this manuscript, 21st Century War may change people as much if not more than previous wars.

"You lose something over there," a Soldier said in Chapter Twelve. It is a common theme among returning Soldiers. "Where do I fit in...I have this feeling of horrendous responsibility (for the deaths of his hand-picked personal security team)...I don't fit in any more."

It is evident in their own words that Soldiers with combat-induced PTSD are perplexed about their sense of self. In their own words, Soldiers describe their longing for an acceptable identity.

"Who am I now after combat?"

"I am absolutely displeased with myself."

"I am too occupied with perceived dangers around me."

"I even take my gun to church. It ain't real safe anywhere."

"Roll Call is so sad because part of you is gone."

"Power is what I lost…I am different."

"Our integrity is questioned."

"People look at us different because of things we might have done or seen done during deployment."

One Soldier said, "I'm defined by my trauma."

A combat medic said, "It is not normal to see what we saw." As stated earlier, it is estimated that as many as 70% of combat medics will develop PTSD. "Nobody expected what we saw."

"A lot of times, I feel like the man who stuck his face in the cardboard cutout. You know, like the ones you have your photograph taken in. It could be a cowboy or whatever.

I don't want anybody to see my emotions. I don't want them to see the real me."

A senior NCO said, "You get to a point where you are no longer afraid to die.

At one point, I believed the only way to show respect for the men who died is to die myself."

In uncanny ways, significant guilt, much of which is irrational, keeps this good man from remaining fully alive. Now, for reasons largely outside his awareness, he leads an isolated, unrewarding existence, falsely thinking he does not deserve to live.

Hardly knowing how to address the changes wrought in him by 21st Century War, one Soldier said, "You lose something over there. I lost something. Maybe I am looking for what I lost over there."

"I don't fit in any more."

SGM (Sergeant Major) Hall said, "The other day I went back to the pond where I fished as a child.

A lady came out and asked me what I thought I was doing.

I told her who I was.

I told her that I fished there as a child.

'You can fish here today but don't come back.

The only reason I'm letting you fish here today is because I know your father,' she said.

I went to another fishing hole in my home county.

The same thing happened.

I don't fit in any more."

7. Temperament is Significantly Adversely Changed

Temperament is ordinarily defined as a "person's nature, especially as it permanently affects their behavior." Synonyms for temperament include nature, character, personality, makeup, constitution, mind and spirit.

One is familiar, for example, with the term "artistic temperament," referring to people in the arts who are emotionally reactive, gifted, hedonistic and experience extremeness of sociability and reticence.

Based upon the stories told by Soldiers with PTSD induced by fighting terrorists, there may well be a "PTSD Temperament."

SSG Cecil Upton, Chapter Fourteen, War on Temperament, is typical of the "PTSD Temperament." Cecil told the Tuesday Morning Group, "It bothers me that I'm not in control of my feelings.

"I can't sleep.

Things make me cry.

I don't know why.

Before combat, things would be make me sad, but I wouldn't cry about it.

I'm either mad quicker or sad quicker.

I'm more sensitive to animals since Iraq."

Cecil's heart went out to a mother bird that had used his attic to build a nest for her 3 unhatched eggs. His wife saw the situation entirely differently, ordering her son to block the mother bird's access to the attic and destroy the nest.

Cecil said, "I watched the mother bird try over and over to get back into the vent.

I got angry with my wife...but I did not tell her.

I thought she let those birds starve to death.

I thought what if I didn't feed you?

This happened yesterday. I could not sleep at all last night.

I cried alone."

Insightfully, a fellow group member observed that it was not the helpless state of the mother bird that upset Cecil. "Cecil felt she (Cecil's wife) should have known how sensitive he was to the situation."

Cecil is more sensitive to death, even the death of three unborn baby birds.

Cecil's story provides an opportunity to more closely examine what appears to be an irony regarding temperament.

He is typical of the majority of Soldiers with combat-induced PTSD in his increased sensitivity. Like many of his peers, however, he strongly feels the need to hide his sensitivity. In Cecil's own words, "I cried alone."

But here is the irony: when Cecil, like his fellow Soldiers with PTSD, is not in his sensitivity mode, he is "numb."

It is the emotional numbness of Soldiers with PTSD that tends to frustrate and annoy those around them. Spouses often complain, for example, "My husband has no feelings!"

Scholars who have studied PTSD identify "numbness" as a form of emotional avoidance. I believe it is more than avoidance. More specifically, it is an improvised emotional defense, failure to stop feeling.

One of the challenges in treating combat-induced PTSD is to teach the Soldier to modulate his or her feelings, to avoid the extremes of feelings and behavior.

Aristotle defined virtue as the habit of choosing the mean between the extremes of feeling and of behavior. Virtue is not innate, he said; it must be learned.

SSG Allen Turner, also introduced in Chapter Fourteen, represents the extreme degree of anger that also, sadly, comprises part of the "PTSD Temperament."

Ordinarily, Allen is a quiet man, introverted, and withdrawn, but when his highest moral principles are offended, his anger can be dangerous. Fortunately, only in the most exceptional circumstances has he ever acted out of anger.

An aggressive driver intentionally stopped his car in front of Allen's car, preventing the normal flow of traffic. Fortunately, Allen's wife quickly left the passenger seat of her husband's car. She raced to the offending driver with an urgent message.

"Sir, my husband just returned from Afghanistan. Please don't upset him. He may be dangerous." Her quick thinking prevented a likely ugly situation.

Another common part of the "PTSD Temperament" is typified by this statement, "I'm not happy with the person I am."

Marked sensitivity of the combat-induced PTSD Soldier is unexceptional. "My depression lingers all the time. It gets worse when the news gets worse. Any news about death makes me feel more depressed."

A Soldier whose best friend died in his arms in combat said, "I lost my whole weekend because I was depressed. It comes with anger. I got mad because the sun came up. I wanted it dark.

I'm talking about severe depression. It's been worse recently.

I could easily lie in bed all day. I don't want to take a shower.

I withdraw and wallow in my own misery."

Yes, combat-induced PTSD may have long-lasting devastating effects on temperament. One of the main goals in the treatment of this challenging condition is to materially assist the Soldier to acquire the skills to find comfort in living without extreme emotions.

8. **Lost or Significantly Damaged Sense of Basic Trust**

The ramifications of lost or significantly damaged sense of basic trust are almost limitless. It affects every aspect of one's life from the most trivial decisions to one's most intimate relationships.

Lost or significantly damaged sense of basic trust may be the most costly price our Soldiers pay in 21st Century War.

Once lost or badly damaged, basic trust is difficult to restore.

I see my job as a physician to Soldiers with combat-induced PTSD as someone who must, perhaps above all else, be perceived as a qualified listener who is first and foremost a trustworthy person.

Rule one for me, the therapist: be a qualified, competent and caring listener, perceived by Soldiers as a safe attachment figure because I consistently show that I respect and care for Soldiers.

Rule two, no surprises in what I say and do.

Rule three, I can be predicted. For example, I wear a blue blazer, shirt and tie every day. My tone of voice and demeanor is equally easily predictable. I don't give up on people or projects to assist Soldiers under my care.

CPT William Abram, Chapter Sixteen, said, "I have a different view of the world now. The world is a terrible place. There are a lot of bad people. I don't recall my former self."

CPT Bell, Chapter Sixteen, said, "Basic trust is nearly destroyed when women and children are turned into killers, but I was crushed by my wife's betrayal while I was deployed. It removed the last amount of trust I had left."

CPT Bell continued: "I always looked for the good in people. My mom and dad said that about me.

That is now changed.

I see people negatively. I look for their ulterior motive.

I sense danger in people. Danger is not the right word for it.

People are no longer trustworthy.

I was a very helpful guy. Now I steer away from people.

My character has changed.

I'm not as open."

SFC (Sergeant First Class) Bruce Carson, also Chapter Sixteen, said, "I have trust problems with people and with the world. I leave 3 lights on at night. My bedroom door is locked. I have little trust in myself. I lost my self-confidence."

SGM DeVala said, "I don't trust anybody."

SGM DeVala continued: "I sound paranoid.

I don't know what a person is going to do.

I drive very slowly, always cautious.

In the supermarket, I look for danger.

People get too close to me in the stores. I don't shop on paydays...too many people.

When people get close to me in public, my skin breaks out."

Terrorism succeeds when it destroys the sense of basic trust. It may be its most deadly weapon. Restoring basic trust therefore becomes our most important treatment objective. No matter how long it takes, I believe it is the essential first step in recovery from combat-induced PTSD.

9. **Significantly Damaged Capacity to Relate to Others**

Some forms of suffering permanently alter one's sense of one's self.

Research in child development describes attachment styles that are easily apparent early in childhood. These attachment styles or typical ways of relating to others and to the world are permanent, unless life-altering changes are experienced.

John Bowlby's research on maternal deprivation following WW II and Mary Ainsworth's refinement of Bowlby's work led to the identification of three attachment styles or forms of developing intense bonds or relationships: secure, anxious, or avoidant.

The application of attachment theory to Soldiers with combat-induced PTSD suggests that, regardless of their prior attachment styles, Soldiers with PTSD become anxious and or avoidant in their typical style of relating.

An important exception to this finding is the secure attachment that is maintained with fellow Soldiers with whom strong bonds were established during combat. Fundamentally, attachment is driven by survival needs.

Some say that one's happiness is directly proportional to the quality of all of one's relationships. If this is true, our Soldiers with combat-induced PTSD are the unhappiest people in the world because most of their relationships suffer.

The following Soldier statements, taken from Chapter Eighteen, tell why their relationships are unrewarding.

"I can't go anywhere in public and feel relaxed."

"My interest in sex is gone. I don't want to be touched."

"I either feel anger or protective numbness."

"I shut off all my emotions long ago."

"It is difficult to have a good relationship with anybody. A word can ruin it."

"I think about everything in terms of survival."

"Most of us have ED (erectile dysfunction). It takes a lot of understanding on the part of a woman to understand and accept that."

"We create impossible standards for others."

"I don't let anybody in."

"Never lie to me. Kick me in the balls, but do not lie to me."

"I get anxiety around people."

Human beings are made for relationships. It is the exceptional person who thrives in isolation. I have found a sequential pattern in restoring meaningful, healthy human relationships in the lives of our Soldiers with combat-induced PTSD.

The first significant relationship for these Soldiers is with their battle buddy. It was forged in combat. Too often, unfortunately, these relationships are not fostered upon redeployment. Too often they are separated by military orders, sent to different posts.

In so far as possible, I try to fashion myself as a person to whom the Soldier with PTSD may be willing to become attached. Recently, a Soldier told me, for example, that a map of Iraq on my office wall was like "seeing a map of my home town. It told me that you somehow knew me."

Once the Soldier with PTSD becomes meaningfully attached to me, he or she is willing to risk becoming attached to other Soldiers in Post-Deployment group therapy.

In group therapy the Soldier with PTSD discovers the universality of PTSD. "Climb aboard," one Soldier greeted a new group member, "we are all in the same boat."

By freely discussing their issues, these Soldiers in group therapy strengthen their attachment to me, the group leader, and to each other.

In the final step in this importance sequence, several times a year, spouses are invited to vegetarian chili luncheons prepared by "Mrs. Santa Claus," AKA "Momma Brown," following group therapy.

For many of the Soldiers who are able to complete the process, good relationship skills are acquired.

The bonds become permanent. They are fulfilling. One Soldier, driving home to Michigan for Thanksgiving, for example, totaled his car on "black ice." He called his family, and he then called me. Fortunately, he was not injured. I shared the information with his group, all personally interested in him.

10. Persistent Emotional Turmoil

One of the most discouraging emotional costs of the 21st Century War is the persistent reoccurrence of emotional turmoil and symptoms. A "good day," one of getting by without embarrassing anxiety, shame or depression, may be followed by a week of inexplicable instability.

Making sense of one's symptoms is the first objective of therapy. Every symptom has a rational explanation. Once that is understood, and the causes identified, the chaos fades away like invisible ink.

Recently, I presented a brief for the non-psychiatric professional staff of our clinic. An observant Internist was the first to reply to my question, how do you identify Soldiers who might have PTSD?

"They can't sit still," the Internist astutely observed.

Marked anxiety is discharged, often outside of awareness, by, among other symptoms, rapid leg movement: one or both legs move up and down speedily.

Most Soldiers with combat-induced PTSD also have at least one other psychiatric diagnosis along with the PTSD, referred to as a comorbidity. For example, it is not uncommon for Soldiers with PTSD to also have Major Depression.

Some Soldiers with PTSD are comorbid with Substance Abuse such as Alcohol Abuse or Alcohol Dependence.

In the case of depression, the medications approved for PTSD are also used for the treatment of depression. Many of these medications may cause erectile dysfunction in men. But no medication cures PTSD.

Substance abuse disorders require specialized treatment provided by ASAP (Army Substance Abuse Program), in which case the Soldier's commander plays a supportive role.

Panic Disorder is also a common comorbid disorder with PTSD. Cognitively, Panic Disorder is a catastrophic misinterpretation of the body's normal response to stress. It is best treated with Cognitive Therapy.

Soldiers with combat-induced PTSD from combating terrorists in Iraq and Afghanistan experience significant changes in their deeply held beliefs. The most troubling change is the persistent belief, "I am in constant mortal danger."

Our feelings and our behavior are influenced by what we believe and by the meaning we give to our experiences.

The deeply held belief, "I am in mortal danger," causes the Soldier afflicted with PTSD to be on guard, checking doors and window throughout the night, and remaining on high alert all day for possible attacks.

They expect the unexpected.

They also believe, "those I love are in constant mortal danger," and therefore "I must protect those I love."

"I must not rely on old, unfounded beliefs of logic and self-confidence; they will not help in my defense against terrorism."

"I must not turn off my alarm system."

"Only those who experienced combat in Iraq or Afghanistan understand me and can help protect me."

Deeply held beliefs are resistant to change.

Marked anxiety, deep depression, disturbed sleep, or destructive substance abuse commonly accompany these dysfunctional beliefs.

One may well imagine just how badly one must feel who sincerely believes he or she is constantly in danger of experiencing a horrible form of death or mutilation. It must be like waiting to face a firing squad, an electrocution, or the gas chamber.

Living in constant dread of death leaves little time for joy, intimacy, memory, sleep, or any of life's delicacies.

These suffering men and women need to be understood and comforted by our nation, the people they were defending when stricken with PTSD.

For the most part, I have found, during 12,500 doctor-patient encounters with these incomparable Soldiers, that healthy attachments can be restored when they become convinced that a trustworthy person values, admires, and respects them.

The healing occurs by degrees.

It cannot be shortened.

Each Soldier is unique.

When the traumatized Soldier is ready, each trauma narrative must be told, leaving out no detail, no matter how small

We are the honored listeners who are privileged to hear the combat trauma narratives. We must be prepared to contain, within ourselves, the strong emotions stirred up while hearing the unspeakable and while witnessing the suffering of the narrator.

When the narrating Soldier sees that the honored listener is not indifferent to his or her suffering, is moved by the suffering described, but able to contain it, healthy attachment begins.

Skip Ryan, a Harvard graduate and a gifted Presbyterian minister, spent a summer ministering to minority children in the inner parts of New York City. At the end of his term he asked, "How many of you children are Christians?" Surprised by the raised hand of a Hispanic boy, Skip asked, "When did you become a Christian?"

"When you learned my name," the 10 year old boy replied.

It is the equivalent of "when you learned my name" that the sorely needed first steps toward healing attachment begin for the Soldier with combat-induced PTSD.

Those of us who listen must be able to help Soldiers find meaning in their trauma stories that helps explain and, when possible, helps justify their suffering. Nowhere is honesty and authenticity more relevant than in helping Soldiers discover the truth of their combat trauma. It is most likely to occur when our nation learns the high emotional cost of 21st Century War to save American lives.

22

THE BURDEN OF UNCERTAINTY

The Physician becomes a Patient: "Bob, we need to discuss your echocardiogram."

I HAVE BEEN BLESSED with a long life and good health. I've tried to stay fit and conscious of the importance of a healthy life-style.

I have been blessed with a loving wife to whom I'm very happily married. Together, we have been blessed with 4 fine children, 4 fine grandchildren, and a fine great-granddaughter.

I have also been blessed by a rewarding career permitting me the fulfillment of my life-long dreams to be a Soldier and to be a physician.

I enlisted in the US Army Reserve on 25 OCT 1954. I came in at the rank of E-2 (Private) instead of E-1, because I had 2 years of Military Science at the University in its Army ROTC program.

Ultimately, I retired at the rank of 06 (Colonel) with 24 years of military experience, served on active duty during the first Gulf War, and was Acting Commander of the 531st Rapid Deployment Combat Stress Control Company, USAR. When I retired I was Chief of Professional Services, 2290th USAR 1000 Bed Hospital, Walter Reed Army Medical Center, Washington, DC.

I "maxed" the Army PT test at 61 years of age, running 2-miles in 15.29, and doing the push-ups and sit-ups well.

This text has already told the story of my love of medicine and my career as a psychiatrist and professor.

In short, I thought of myself as the "poster boy for fitness among those with greying hair."

A routine echocardiogram, my first ever, however, revealed a significant narrowing of my aortic valve. Dr. Robert S. Gibson, my cardiologist, and I were equally shocked. Except for an unchanging minor heart murmur and controlled hypertension, I had no symptoms suggesting significant medical problems.

Dr. Gibson sent me an e-mail. "Bob, we need to discuss your echocardiogram. Call me at home tonight."

The news was shocking. "You will have to have a catheterization of your heart, of course, and then we could do a stress test. A special blood test indicated that your heart is working harder than normal," Dr. Gibson said. "I suspect sooner or later, you will have to have the aortic valve replaced."

"What do you think we should do?" I asked.

"Bob, it's up to you.

"Dr. Gibson, I want to get it behind me."

"If I were in your shoes, Bob, that's exactly what I'd do. I will introduce you to John Kern, a fine surgeon who heads up our heart-transplant team. He is very good at replacing valves in the heart."

Meeting Dr. John A. Kern

If first impressions are important, Dr. John Kern, Professor of Surgery, University of Virginia, would have scored less than favorable in appearance.

His uncombed straight, dark hair covered his forehead in an unruly fashion. His unshaven face surprised me the Monday morning of our first meeting. A man of medium stature, estimated to be 48 years old, stared at me seriously through his dark horn rim eyeglasses as he firmly shook my hand.

It occurs to me now for the first time that he could have been up all night in the operating room. In fact, he was neatly dressed and groomed in all our subsequent encounters. There was something more commendable about Dr. Kern that I was to learn unexpectedly, and I will mention it later.

Trying to be funny, I said that psychological tests found little differences between psychiatrists and surgeons. Unsmiling, Dr. Kern said, "I've heard the same thing." He was unimpressed.

Dr. Gibson introduced us and left. I felt awkward, not knowing what to say.

"Do you have any questions, Dr. Brown?" Dr. Kern asked.

"Your nurse said I will not be returning to work for 4 weeks after surgery, Dr. Kern. I make my living sitting down. Does it really take 4 weeks to recover from heart-valve surgery?"

"We generally say 4 weeks but looking at you, I'd say you could probably go back to work after surgery in 3 weeks."

Dr. Kern's able assistants scheduled my cardiac catheterization, and set the date for my open heart surgery, 23 AUG 2013 at 0500, University of Virginia Hospital.

Leaving my Soldier Patients

"Don't die on me," one Soldier said when I announced to his Post-Deployment Psychotherapy Group that open heart surgery would keep me away from work for at least 3 weeks. The Soldier could not have been more serious. I was disturbed by his comment. It was a perspective I had not seriously considered.

Three weeks sounded like a long time! However, other providers agreed to accept responsibility for the care of my patients until I returned.

Any change for Soldiers with combat-induced PTSD can be stressful. Facing open heart surgery can also be stressful. In a certain sense, it was a "perfect storm." Both patients and doctor were under stress.

I found myself staying busy. I left work on 22 AUG 2013, the day before my open heart surgery, drove to Charlottesville, and took the Basic Life Support (BLS) skills examination, having already passed the on-line American Heart Association's factual knowledge portion of the examination. It was my good fortune to pass the BLS skills exam. It is a requirement for my job as a staff psychiatrist.

Fifty face-to-face patient encounters per week since 2005 meant I would miss 150 patient encounters in my anticipated 3 weeks of recovery from open heart surgery.

Instead of 3 weeks, however, for reasons explained below, I did not return to work with Soldiers for almost 3 months, missing approximately 600 patient encounters.

Despite strong words of discouragement, one colleague drove from our military treatment facility to visit me in the immediate post-operative period. What is more, two Soldiers came to see me while I was still in the coronary ICU.

I turned off my cell phone. I was too weak to help anyone. Soldiers stayed in touch with me on the Internet.

Several weeks into my recovery, a Soldier, facing an important deadline, needed a letter from me that I somehow found the strength to write.

A Rented Hospital Bed

Dottie and my son Clinton drove me home from the hospital on 29 AUG 2013. It was 6 days after successful open heart surgery for the replacement of a barely functioning valve with a new, miraculous "biosynthetic" aortic valve.

Merely attempting to seat myself in the car was a major endeavor. I had no energy, no appetite, and no idea how I could manage myself at home. In a word, I felt vulnerable.

"Home Health Care has already called," Dottie said. "They are sending over a rented bed for you, like the one you had at the hospital."

Sweat poured from the forehead of the middle-aged man who delivered the hospital bed. Regrettably, the hospital bed, older than the kind, industrious man who delivered it and set it up in our house, bore no similarities to the hospital bed I had in the hospital. We complained. The kind man, still sweating, came for its return the following day.

Lying flat in a bed of any kind increased my sense of vulnerability. Dottie had a recliner delivered. Its remote control provided a number of comfortable positions from which to choose.

It took several restless nights to confirm the truth. I could not sleep. At best, I got two or three hours of sleep at night.

The problem was neither the bed nor the new recliner. The problem was the patient.

Several hours of unrefreshing sleep in a borrowed bed was followed by respite-seeking in the recliner, comfortably covered with a bed sheet and a soft pillow. Then it was back to the bed an hour or two later. Weeks slowly passed before I woke up with daybreak, not at 0300.

I did not prefer to be alone.

I felt unusually secure in the presence of my youngest son, Clinton. I sensed his physical strength. I did not want him to return to his own residence at night. For a while, I needed him to sleep in a nearby room, Dottie in our bed, and me in the recliner or a bed we borrowed from my oldest son, Bobby.

Our bed was too high up from the floor, too tall, for me to access without a struggle. Even when I was assisted into our bed, I felt very insecure. I could remain there no longer than a few minutes.

It was a strongly felt need to be attached to those I love, those I perceived would protect me. Oddly, I had no idea what it was from which I needed protection, but that did not lessen the need.

I had no pain, no physical discomfort.

The evenings got me down. I dreaded the night. The bedtime ritual included taking medications, reassurance that a bell I could ring for assistance was within easy reach, a night-light, strategically placed, was functioning, and a light in the bathroom was left burning.

Something was wrong between me and my imagination. In the words of many Soldiers I treated for PTSD, I acutely sensed danger in the most unusual places and "I could see the second and third order of the consequences of the danger."

"I lost my sense of mirth"

My favorite television shows no longer appealed to me. If I read the newspaper, I turned immediately to the obituaries. The sports page carried the losing record of the University football team.

I tried listening to the audio version of <u>Great Expectations</u>. In the recent past, it seemed to shorten my car trips back to our military treatment facility on Sunday afternoons as I enjoyed a pleasant narrator reading one of the many Dickens stories I relished. The joy was gone. Several attempts to rekindle my interest failed.

I had no appetite for food or for just about anything else. In 5 weeks, I lost 20 pounds. I was not dieting.

Viewing my body in the bathroom mirror was distasteful. I did not want to go out in public. I was ashamed of the way I looked. My clothes no longer fit. It was embarrassing.

I wondered what was wrong with me. Years ago, I witnessed the same kind of rapid wasting in a previously strapping man, the spouse of one of my patients. He had developed Diabetes.

The uncertainty of my physical and emotional state was a burden. "Do I have Diabetes?" I asked Dr. Gibson, my trusted cardiologist, now functioning as my primary care physician as well.

"Let's get a fasting blood sugar, Bob, and a Hemoglobin A1C," Dr. Gibson suggested. "The hemoglobin A1C will tell us your average blood sugar over the past 2-3 months. The fasting blood sugar will tell us what your level is today."

According to the blood test results, thankfully, I do not have Diabetes.

For years, Dottie and I enjoyed going out for dinner. I dreaded the thought of it now.

A physician assistant (PA) on Dr. Kern's team, addressing my weight loss, said, "Forget about a heart healthy diet now. Eat whatever tastes good to you. I don't care what it is, if it tastes good to you, go for it!"

The first thing that came into my mind was a cold turkey sandwich from Foods of All Nations in Charlottesville. At one time in my life it was my favorite food, second only to Kit Kats, first encountered in the White Hart Royal Hotel, Chipping Norton, Cotswolds, England. It was splendid with tea.

Some years ago, Kit Kats were so tasty that I had to find a way to wean myself off the delicacy. A friend suggested I go "cold turkey." Dottie and I laughed loudly. I was already hooked on "cold turkey" sandwiches from Foods of All Nations, a bigger problem than Kit Kats.

In my post-surgical state, even Kit Kats lost their appeal.

"Nothing tasted good."

"Dottie," I complained, "this orange juice tastes too sweet."

"It's Simply Orange, the brand we have used for years," she replied.

"I don't care. It tastes entirely too sweet to me. Please dilute it with water, or I can't drink it."

Nothing tasted good. More specifically, nothing tasted right. Nothing tasted the way I expected it to taste.

I've always been conscious of my weight. After surgery, I dropped from 182 to 162. Ironically, 162 is an ideal weight for me. It places my BMI (Body Mass Index) in the normal range, but it was too much weight to lose in too short a period of time, as I said, in 5 weeks. What was worse, I was losing weight because I was losing my appetite. This is not a healthy way to lose weight.

Nearly 4 months post-surgery I learned something new about open heart surgery and weight loss. Strangely, it significantly reduced my burden of doubt.

"Hello, Dr. Brown. How are you today?"

Kerry, the friendly and competent director of the Cardiac Rehab Center near our military treatment facility, was taping leads to my chest. The leads carry information from my heart to his monitor where it can be observed while I exercise.

We have to weigh in before the rehab exercise begins.

"I remain baffled," I said, "how I lost 20 pounds in 5 weeks while I was recovering."

"That's easy to explain," said Kerry. "When I took my post-graduate training in cardio and pulmonary rehabilitation, the surgeon told us something I've never forgotten.

"Open heart surgery is very complex. They have to use so much anesthesia that the patient is almost dead. The excessive anesthesia causes many changes in the body. Some of the changes can last for months. One of the biggest changes of large amounts of anesthesia, he said, is that it kills taste buds. He said we tell the open heart surgery patients to eat whatever tastes good. If chocolate milk-shakes taste good, drink all the chocolate milk-shakes you want."

Knowing the effects of anesthesia on my taste buds helped me, admittedly rather late, to understand the loss of my appetite. It is a good example of how, at last, knowledge can lessen worry.

Uncertainty

My mind, no longer the steel trap under my usual tight grip, seemed to have a mind of its own. For example, it's been my long-time habit to review a pleasant experience once in bed at night as a way of falling asleep. It no longer worked.

Once I started to reminisce, my thoughts, no longer linear and logical, immediately developed into strange, usually unpleasant thoughts. These unwanted thoughts grabbed my attention.

It was not a matter of jumbled thoughts. It was a terrible experience, one I dreaded, one I did my utmost to avoid. Sometimes the panic it generated forced me out of bed.

Would these disturbing thoughts, ones that haunted me at bedtime, the ones for which I could not account, that drove me out of my bed at night, leak into my daytime thoughts?

For several weeks, I remained on high alert for this dreaded experience. Thankfully, it did not invade and contaminate my daytime thoughts.

Dottie said I was "super alert...nothing escaped your attention."

Her comments reminded me of "hypervigilance," a PTSD symptom, stemming from an aroused autonomic nervous system. Here the person is unduly and unnecessarily alert to all that is happening, deprived of the ability to relax.

"Bob, you are an entirely different person."

Another incident occurred during my gloomy stage of recovery from open heart surgery.

I had a routine follow-up examination with Dr. Gibson, my learned cardiologist. Dottie made it a point to come with me to my appointments, a new phenomenon that puzzled me somewhat, but I chose not to ask her why she wanted to be present.

I was burdened by the uncertainty of my health. I was gradually learning things about myself that concerned me. For example, I was "severely anemic" after surgery. My hematocrit, a laboratory measure of my red blood cells, had dropped 30 points to 24 percent. The normal hematocrit for my age and gender is 42 – 52 per cent.

I was discharged from the hospital on the 6th post-operative day with a hematocrit of 24. "Had your crit (hematocrit) been 22, you could not have been discharged. You would have been given another transfusion," the discharge nurse told me on 29 AUG 2013. It would have been my 4th transfusion.

Dr. Gibson instructed me to start taking iron pills twice daily to help treat my "severe anemia." Weeks passed and my hematocrit barely responded, adding to my gloom.

A wound infection developed. It required weekly visits to Dr. Kern who instructed Dottie on "wet to dry dressings twice a day."

"This wound must heal from inside out," he said. Faithfully, each morning Dottie packed 2 inch by 2 inch sterile gauze into the wound. Each evening, our son Bobby removed the gauze, cleaned the wound and repacked the gauze into the infected area of my sternal incision. Thankfully, it slowly healed.

Dr. Gibson, intelligent and articulate, chooses his words carefully. His stethoscope found its way first across my back, "breathe deeply" instructions were followed precisely, and then it moved to specific locations across my chest.

Appearing serious to me, Dr. Gibson said, "You are an entirely different person." I accepted his diagnosis, not asking for clarification. I had failed to hide my gloom, I concluded. Now even my cardiologist knows I'm depressed. It was a moment of defeat for me.

"Avoid Avoidance"

When the phone rang, Dottie would say, "Bob is sitting here right now. Would you like to speak to him?" I resented this intrusion of my space. I wanted to speak to no one and I wanted no visitors.

Small talk annoyed me. I saw no need for small talk.

Edith, my only surviving sibling, phoned. The phone was passed directly to me. I did not want to talk on the phone to Edith. She remains a lively, animated, adventurous soul who will be 90 in March.

"Bobby, how are you doing?" Edith, chipper as usual, asked.

I was not doing well, and I did not want to tell her how I was not doing well.

"If your pace maker is not working, Bobby, they can replace it," Edith said, attempting to be reassuring.

Yelling at Edith on the phone in anger, I replied "I don't have a pace maker, Edith! Do you not understand?"

Later, I apologized for hanging up on Edith.

Short-tempered, impatient and irritable: it dawned on me that I was developing an avoidant life style.

How strange, I thought, that I would withdraw into avoidance after preaching to Soldiers repeatedly, often in a raised voice, "Avoid avoidance!"

"I worry about things that can go wrong"

"You seem gloomy," Dottie said. "Your surgery went well, you have no major complications, and you are home from the hospital. What is bothering you, Bob?"

I did not have a good answer for her. The simple truth was that I did not know what was making me feel gloomy. Almost without thinking, I replied, "I worry about things that can go wrong."

Dottie did not press me for a better answer. She just continued to busy herself, addressing all my needs.

Casual statements about open heart surgery made by friends, family members and others replayed themselves in my memory.

Before I left work, I went to the hospital credentials office, making it known that I would be away for surgery but my Basic Life Support credentials would be completed later that afternoon.

The woman director of credentials, expressing concern and consideration, said, "I know you will do fine. My grandfather had open heart surgery. He had a heart-shaped pillow to hold up to his chest when he coughed. Actually, he had two heart-shaped pillows."

"Why did your grandfather have two heart-shaped pillows?" I inquired.

'He was given a second pillow because he had to go back to have the surgery done again."

Before I had the first performed, I found myself dreading a second open heart surgery.

Immediately after my 4.5 hour open heart surgery, I woke up in the Cardiac ICU. Good nurses were attentive. One of the nurses was told that another patient admission was headed to the hospital. When she was given his name, she commented to the other nurse, "He is coming back in for a third time since his open heart surgery because of recurrent wound infection."

I soon dreaded wound infections.

Dr. John A. Kern

The biblical Job said, "That which I feared has befallen me." A bloody discharge from my incision, a month post-surgery, had befallen me. I sent an e-mail to my heart surgeon, Dr. John A. Kern.

Maybe it was anxiety or perhaps some mild cognitive impairment commonly found at least temporarily among 60 per cent of open heart surgery patients; who can say? Nonetheless, I sent an e-mail to Dr. Kern on a Thursday morning. The subject of the e-mail was "Incisional Infection." However, I sent the e-mail with no message other than the title.

Immediately, I received the following reply from Dr. Kern:
From: "Kern, John A"
Subject: RE: Incisional Infection
Date: Thu, 26 Sep 2013 07:34:12 -0400
To: "Robert S. Brown"
Cc: "Alexander, Joan *HS"

Undecoded Letter
"Dr. Brown,
No message with this e-mail. Is everything okay?
Joan, can you check on him and let me know?
Dr. Brown, I am presently in the Dominican Republic on surgical mission trip."

Dr. Kern's prompt reply meant a lot to me. I did not intend to alarm him, but I can imagine the impact of an e-mail from a recent open heart surgery patient consisting of the subject line only. The fact that Dr. Kern was on a "surgical mission trip" raised my already high opinion of him to the highest echelon.

How selfless it is for a man of remarkable talent to travel to third-world countries to professionally serve the under-privileged!

Challenging Dr. Gibson

With time, cardiac rehabilitation, and a lot of support from my family, my strength gradually returned. In a word, I felt better.

Dr. Gibson's comment during an office visit in my gloomy period, "You are an entirely different person," tended to annoy me.

"Dottie, what do you make of the Dr. Gibson's statement that I'm entirely different?" I asked. First of all, I wanted to know if Dottie heard what I heard. I also wanted to know the meaning she gave it.

"I remember him saying it. I thought he was talking about the change in your personality after open heart surgery. Why do you ask?" she inquired.

"I didn't like it," I said.

At the next office visit I approached the subject directly with Dr. Gibson. I wanted to know what he observed in my personality that justified his observation

"Dr. Gibson, my good friend and my good cardiologist, do you recall telling me some time ago that I was 'an entirely different person?'" I asked.

Expressing little interest in my question, proceeding with his usual examination of my heart and lungs, he said, "Yes, I remember the observation."

"Will you tell me what you meant, Dr. Gibson?"

"You are an entirely different person. You have a new, highly effective aortic valve; all 4 echocardiograms after surgery show that your new valve is well positioned and doing a splendid job. It was only a matter of time. You elected to have the surgery sooner than later, but without it the chances of survival would at best be slim."

His explanation relieved my stress. For weeks, I mistakenly believed Dr. Gibson was referring to me as changed for the worse emotionally. I let a distortion burden me.

I can't tell you how many times combat Soldiers are described as "an entirely different person" by people who are important to them. I wonder if they, too, respond with perceptions that are burdensome, with painful, unnecessary misunderstanding and uncertainty.

Who Has PTSD Now?

In a number of ways, I found myself experiencing symptoms similar to those of the Soldiers under my care for the treatment of PTSD.

I was not equating open heart surgery with combat. It was much more subtle.

I had raced into the hospital for open heart surgery the day following my usual routine at work, and I had taken a Basic Life Support examination only hours before admission to surgery at 0500 the following morning.

Working as a staff psychiatrist treating brave Soldiers whose stories had pierced my heart for the past 8 years caused me to identify with the Soldiers to whom I had become attached.

The thought of my having acquired PTSD from working closely with Soldiers with combat-induced PTSD had occasionally entered my awareness earlier, but I quickly dismissed it.

Open heart surgery undoubtedly saved my life. It also temporarily robbed me of my psychological defenses. In my vulnerable state, the weakest weeks of my life, my busy-ness came to a screeching halt. My denial was no longer effective. I had to admit to myself that I am human. I am not indifferent to the suffering I witness.

I have PTSD.

Will my PTSD render me less effective as a psychiatrist treating Soldiers with combat-induced PTSD?

Will my PTSD render me more effective as a psychiatrist treating Soldiers with combat-induced PTSD?

I believe I have a new level of sensitivity to suffering.

I have a better understanding of the reluctance of Soldiers to seek psychological treatment.

I know how arduous it can be to find the best words that convey the meaning of thoughts, feelings and behaviors which are difficult to understand. I know the sense of security that comes from secure attachments to the few who are perceived as strong, protective and caring.

I know the feeling of safety that comes from limiting contacts of all types with as many people as possible.

I know the impatience evoked by small talk and the need to avoid it and people who engage in it.

I know the feeling of anger at perceived injustice.

I know how accurate information can reduce burdens.

I know how distortions in my thinking can cause unnecessary misery.

Most of all, I know what a privilege and honor it is to work with Soldiers who fight in 21st Century War to save American lives. Equally important, I now know it is necessary and urgent that our nation hear from our Soldiers themselves about the psychological burdens they volunteer to bear for our protection.

The End of Grief

On 12 NOV 2013, I happily returned to the work I love. Successful heart surgery was behind me. It was good to be with the Soldiers I had not seen since 22 AUG 2013. I very much missed being with them. It had been a much longer absence than I had anticipated.

Later, MSG Keith Johnson addressed the WED Morning Group.

"I stayed in bed, snug in my poncho liner, until 1430 on 21 DEC 2013, the 9th anniversary of the suicide bombing of the DFAC (Dining Facility) in Mosul, Iraq.

Something told me to go to the Walmart and buy a flagpole.

Flagpoles are not cheap. It cost me a buck 65."

"It only cost $1.65?" I asked.

The group, attentive to MSG Keith L. Johnson, laughed. Almost in unison, the group shouted "$165.00!"

MSG Johnson continued.

"I bought concrete mix and came back to my hooch (his term for the farm where he resides), to put up the flagpole.

I dug the hole, placed the pole carefully in the hole, and I installed motion lights to shine on it.

It was raining, so I didn't raise the flag until the next day.

It really makes me feel good to watch Old Glory up there waving in the wind. I look up at it many times…day or night…it doesn't matter. I just like to watch it."

A flagpole marked the end of an era for MSG Keith L. Johnson.

The purchase, installation, and the grieving ended in the rain.

It was the 9th anniversary of the suicide bombing of the Mess Hall in Mosul, Iraq.

At all military funerals in America, "Old Glory" is neatly folded and presented to the family.

MSG Johnson changes the subject when he is called a hero who remained in the Mess Hall through its destruction and great loss of American Soldiers, 21 DEC 2004. As detailed in Chapter Six, "I never saw so much blood" section, Keith Johnson, the African American from New Jersey, covered in blood and debris, saved lives.

For 9 long years, he has been covered in bloody memories that robbed him of his marriage, of emotional closeness to his children, and of his self-esteem.

The rain was his tears.

The flag is the funeral service for those he could not save in the Mess Hall.

It is the funeral service of his bloody memories.

The battle is won. The Star Spangled Banner waves victoriously over MSG Johnson's home and in his heart.

The group and I could tell by his voice, by his face and by his narration that this is the end of his grief.

We can only pray that all our Soldiers are blessed with such healing.

23

An After Word: How You can Help

A Natural Inclination

THERE IS A natural inclination for many Americans to support our Soldiers. I have seen civilians in airports walk up to our men and women in uniform to express their appreciation with a heartfelt hug or handshake, thanking them for serving our country in the military. It is touching to witness.

At the same time, in many cases, there is a feeling of awkwardness expressed on the face of both the man or woman in uniform and the civilian offering the greeting. It may be a sense of dread of feeling awkward that prevents many more Americans from being more hospitable to our Soldiers.

It is the feeling of awkwardness, ineffectiveness and ineptitude that I wish to discuss in this section.

Where does the feeling of awkwardness come from in the mind of the Soldier? How can it be overcome?

Where does the feeling of ineffectiveness or ineptitude come from in the mind of civilians? How important is it to master this feeling before our Soldiers can sense that our nation genuinely cares for them?

How important to our military is their certainty that our nation cares about them as people who risk their lives for our safety?

It is my thesis, based on hundreds of hours spent with our combat Soldiers, that there is no accomplishment more important to our national defense than determining meaningful ways of demonstrating our concern, support and understanding of our Soldiers and their families.

Why Combat Soldiers May Feel Awkward

No one returns from combat unchanged. Large numbers of Soldiers come home exhausted, haunted by memories that are unthinkable for most of us. Amazingly, and difficult to explain, however, is the fact that combat Soldiers often prefer deployment to the stress of life at home.

In the words of MSG Keith L. Johnson's underlying theme for <u>Sacred Ground</u>, "War is easy. Coming home is Hell." Recall that MSG Johnson was in the Mess Hall in Mosul on 21 DEC 2004 when a suicide bomber's explosion took the lives of many Soldiers. Some of the dead were his Soldiers.

Repeated inquiries of Soldiers expressing a preference for combat to the comforts of home enabled me to come to several important conclusions.

In combat, Soldiers are securely attached to each other, particularly to their battle buddies. Their survival depended upon their attachments.

In combat, each Soldier had a weapon. Many Soldiers continue to sleep with a weapon at home, but it does not make them feel safe.

It is not the weapon alone in combat, I conclude, that assured the Soldier's sense of security. It was the strength of their attachments that kept them alive.

At home, it is the absence of strong attachments with battle buddies that contributes solidly to the pervasive feeling of vulnerability. Soldiers often sense something important is missing, but they may not be able to articulate that it is the specific loss of these important attachments that grieves them.

The Soldier's spouse, also failing to understand the importance of strong attachments with combat battle buddies, are often puzzled by it and may even become jealous, baffled why their Soldier needs to frequently call or visit battle buddies. A further difficulty: Soldiers sense a strong need to protect their family, not to be protected by their loved ones. Soldier survival attachments are limited to Soldiers.

I consciously try to reestablish strong combat-like attachments between combat Soldiers in Post-Deployment Group Therapy. It is most successful when Soldiers first begin to perceive me as trustworthy, a qualified listener who cares about emotional and cognitive safety.

Soldiers may feel threatened when they are greeted by strangers. Combat taught them to expect the unexpected, to look for the unusual when things appear usual, and to always be on guard.

You can make your greeting warm and authentic when you approach the Soldier slowly, from a distance, nothing in your hands, a smile on your face and never from behind.

Even a dog can tell if you do not like it. Greet no Soldier if you have no true appreciation for their service.

Expect no real warmth in return. Many Soldiers feel confused and guilty. Often the guilt is excessive and irrational, further burdening the already sleep deprived, anxious and grieving Soldier.

Combat Soldiers without Attachments

SFC (Sergeant First Class) Stanley Wilson stands 6 feet 3 inches tall and weighs 240 pounds. He never smiles. The dark rings under his sleepless eyes are darker than his dark skin.

A man of few words, he stares down at the floor. Anyone can see and sense his immense suffering, but he is the last person to admit it.

This down trodden 38 year old unhappily married man, father of 4 children, has one of the toughest jobs in the military. He is a combat medic with 5 combat deployments to Afghanistan and Iraq.

Combat medics develop combat induced PTSD 3-5 times more frequently than other Soldiers. Only 3 out of 10 combat medics do not have PTSD.

This combat medic's chief complaint to his psychiatrist whom he is seeing as a mandate stemming from his potential for "provider (medic) impairment," is "My back." For SFC Wilson, it is okay to have a physical ailment. It is unacceptable to have emotional problems.

He does not speak spontaneously.

He may answer a direct question monosyllabically. More often he declares, looking now at the wall, "I'd rather not discuss that today."

I feel helpless. I want to help relieve his suffering, but nothing I've tried has helped. The first task, getting him to keep his appointments, was finally completed, but it took the better part of 2 months.

Six months ago, a case of beer every night was used by SFC Wilson to self-treat his unbearable nightmares. This led to a month's psychiatric hospitalization which stopped the drinking, but did little more.

Today, I read the above section, '**Why Combat Soldiers May Feel Awkward**,' to SFC Wilson. He listened intensively.

"SFC Wilson," I asked, "did you form any significant attachments when you were deployed?"

Without delay, without animation, SFC Wilson quickly replied. "My job was to save lives. My job was to make sure everyone came home. I couldn't show emotions. I did not want to get attached to anyone, because I might lose them."

It was more than SFC Wilson had said, at one time, than he had said in three previous sessions combined.

"I was the medic on a 15 member MITT Team."

"A Military Transition Team (MITT) is a 10-15 soldier team that lives with and trains Iraqi Security Forces (ISF), the Afghan National Army (ANA), and other allies in 21st Century war. The primary mission of transition teams is to advise the security forces of Iraq and Afghanistan in the areas of intelligence, communications, fire support, logistics, and infantry tactics. The aim is to make the ISF and ANA capable of conducting independent counterinsurgency operations, tactically, operationally, and logistically. When executing military operations with their Iraqi or Afghan partners, transition teams call for U.S. air support, indirect fire, and medical evacuation, whenever necessary." Center for Army Lessons Learned, US Army Combined Arms Center, Fort Leavenworth, KS.

SFC Wilson said, "The MITT Team was thrown together after I got over there. I knew no one. We worked with 3,000 Iraqi Soldiers.

We lost our MITT Team leader, MAJ Baxter. He was in the lead vehicle in our convoy. I was in the 3rd vehicle. They hit an IED. MAJ Baxter was almost cut in half."

Tiny tears, hardly visible, highlighted the dark circles under his eyes. In a barely audible voice, SFC Wilson said, "I should have saved him." His irrational guilt would not yield to logical reasoning.

A lot more challenging work with SFC Wilson must be accomplished.

I wonder if the 70% morbidity with PTSD would be significantly reduced if combat medics never served alone, but at least in pairs in order that life-saving and mind-saving attachments could be nurtured.

Sadly, SFC Wilson is the prototype of combat Soldiers without attachments.

A Soldier without meaningful attachments is nearly defenseless, the epitome of Soldiers who feel awkward, a feeling that persists long after the Soldier comes home from combat.

Why Warmly Greet Soldiers?

Even Soldiers with significant attachments may seem awkward and minimally responsive when greeted by strangers. It is not the way they want to be. It is not the way they would have warmly responded before their combat deployments.

Combat Soldiers live in a shrunken personal psychological space, one they can manage, much more reduced than the typically American 3-foot personal space.

The combat Soldier's shrunken personal space is difficult to penetrate, even more difficult to escape.

Isolated and avoidant, typical of so many returning combat Soldiers, is not what they want. It is self-imposed, mistaken as more psychologically safe.

Conveying genuine warmth through sincere greetings, even by strangers, over time and with consistency, may help Soldiers truly feel more at home.

On Being a Good Neighbor

How can being a good neighbor help combat Soldiers returning home from 21st Century War?

If there were a simple answer to this question it would be in two parts. 1. "Know the Soldier who resides in your neighborhood. 2. Know about PTSD and, if you can, learn about combat PTSD's common comorbidities, depression, panic attacks and alcohol abuse."

Luke, the "beloved physician," the Gentile author of the 3rd Gospel and the Book of Acts, recorded in 60 A.D. a brief encounter between Jesus and "a certain lawyer" who asked Jesus, "What shall I do to inherit eternal life?"

Jesus replies, "What is written in the law? What is your reading of it?"

"The lawyer answered and said, 'You shall love the Lord your God with all your heart, with all your soul, with all your strength, with all your mind,' and 'your neighbor as yourself.'"

Jesus said to him, "You have answered rightly; do this and you will live."

The lawyer then asked Jesus, "And who is my neighbor?"

Bible scholars suggest that the lawyer knew the scriptures, but did not know how to apply scriptures because they had not penetrated his heart.

The lawyer knew that Samaritans were hated by Jews since 722 BC when Assyria defeated the northern kingdom of Israel, sent the Jews into exile and brought in foreigners. Intermarriage between the Jews and Gentiles produced Jews in Samaria that were not full-blooded Jews.

Jesus answers the lawyer's question, telling him the parable of the "Good Samaritan."

In the parable, a man whose race was not identified traveled from Jerusalem to Jericho. He was robbed, beaten, stripped of his clothes and left half-dead. A priest saw the injured man, but did not stop to help. A Levite (those who served in the tabernacle) also saw the injured man, but offered no help.

"But a certain Samaritan who was on a journey, came upon him; and when he saw him, he felt compassion." The Samaritan attended to the injured man's needs, placed him on his own animal, took him to an inn, paid his bill and promised to pay more if necessary, upon his return.

Jesus addressed the lawyer with this question, "So which of these three do you think was a neighbor to him who fell among the thieves?"

The lawyer replied, "He who showed mercy toward him."

Then Jesus said to the lawyer, "Go and do likewise."

Who is Your Neighbor?

With few exceptions, in post-modern, deconstructed America, most of us are not good neighbors. Most of us don't even know our neighbors except in the most superficial ways.

Shamefully, I confess my own reticence to be good to my neighbors. I justified my behavior, lying to myself, that I was "too busy."

I share here an example of how I recently related to a neighbor. I am not proud of my response to my neighbor; I am recommending it as an example not to be followed.

A neighbor whose house is not a quarter mile from my home in Charlottesville tragically lost his young grandson. Three years ago, the child drowned in my neighbor's swimming pool.

I mentioned in Chapter Two that I spend, at most, approximately 48 hours each week at my home in Charlottesville.

I drove to my neighbor's house, intending to console him, someone who for many years was more than an acquaintance.

Several cars were parked in front of my neighbor's house. I felt awkward. I wondered what I would say, who would be there and what I would be interrupting.

Regrettably, I lost my nerve. I never left my car. I never went inside my neighbor's house. I just drove off.

Some weeks later, I went to my friend, apologized, told him what I had done and how sorry I was about the death of his grandson.

"Bob," my neighbor said, "that's alright. You are welcome to come to my home any time you like."

"He who showed mercy toward him" was the good neighbor.

Mercy is an interesting word. Today, it is most often used in criminal courts where the defense attorney pleads with the judge to show mercy on his client.

Interestingly, in the parable of the Good Samaritan, an attorney, searching for the answer to his question about inheriting "eternal life," is told to love God and love his neighbor.

The persistent attorney, however, is not satisfied. He is perplexed. The attorney then asks Jesus, "And who is my neighbor?"

The attorney answers his own question, after hearing the parable, that one's neighbor is the one that shows mercy.

Literally, the Good Samaritan, member of a hated minority, was a man of action, not a man of words alone. His actions met every need of the man who had been robbed, beaten, stripped of his clothes and left half-dead. It is said we don't remember the Good Samaritan for his good intentions but for his action.

Is showing mercy one way to welcome home our combat Soldiers? I believe the answer is yes and no.

Dictionary definitions of "mercy" are somewhat confusing. I list some of the definitions of mercy here:

"Pity." 1. Forbearance from inflicting harm, especially punishment, under provocation; compassionate treatment of an offender or adversary. 2. Disposition to exercise compassion or forgiveness; willingness to spare. 3. The power to be merciful; clemency; as, to throw oneself on the mercy of the conqueror. 4. A blessing as a manifestation of compassion. 5. Compassionate treatment of the unfortunate. It also includes kind or compassionate treatment of the suffering.

Soldiers, even those with the most severe forms of PTSD, do not want pity. They do not want sympathy. They do not deserve indifference.

The parable of the Good Samaritan begins with the command to love. It ends with a member of a detested minority, the least loved and the least respected in the attorney's community, loving his neighbor by showing mercy that included sacrifices of time, action and money.

Our returning combat Soldiers are responsive to people who care about them by knowing what they have paid for our freedom. Eventually, they will respond favorably to the merciful.

If there is a secret to becoming a good neighbor, it is revealed in the second part of Luke 10:33. "…and when he saw him, he felt compassion."

Does a Combat Soldier Live in Your Neighborhood?

The actual number of men and women who have been deployed to Iraq and/or Afghanistan is difficult to confirm. In round numbers, as previously noted, we are talking about a lot of people, easily between 2.5 and 3 million.

Most of us know a combat Soldier, or at least, we know someone who knows a combat Soldier.

Ask around your neighborhood until you find the name and address of a combat Soldier who has returned from Iraq or Afghanistan.

You may find a family who has lost a Soldier in 21st Century War. In either case, take food to the Soldier or to the grieving family. Make no small talk. Make your visit brief. You are there as a good neighbor. You are there as a good neighbor because you feel compassion for our Soldiers.

Ideally, have someone make the visit with you.

Introduce yourself as a neighbor.

Ask no questions.

Never ask, "Is there anything I can do for you?"

Thank the Soldier and the family and then leave.

It is unlikely that a one-time visit is sufficient.

Plan to return, always taking a gift (food is the best if you prepared it).

Always avoid small talk, ask no questions, show your gratitude, and stay no more than a few minutes.

Don't become a pest, but repeat your brief visits until you feel welcomed. That will take time.

Be patient.

What is Combat-induced Posttraumatic Stress Disorder (PTSD)?

You don't have to be a genius to know about PTSD. Having read this book, you already have a good idea what our Soldiers have endured.

First, learn to correctly pronounce PTSD. I am amazed at the large number of otherwise intelligent people who cannot even correctly pronounce "PTSD."

Let's get it straight right now. The "P" is for post or after the trauma. The "T" is for the trauma. In this case, the trauma is the horrible parts of combat in 21st Century War. The "S" is for the stress that the trauma produces. The "D" is for the disorder or medical and psychological condition that the stress causes.

Once you can correctly pronounce PTSD, then you need to have a high level of confidence in your understanding of the common symptoms it causes.

As mentioned earlier, the APA (American Psychiatric Association) published its most recent diagnostic criteria for PTSD in MAY 2013. The changes they made for PTSD from DSM (<u>Diagnostic and Statistical Manual of Mental Disorders, IV</u>) to DSM-5 include several new categories, details diagnosticians must ponder in correctly making the diagnosis of PTSD.

Fundamentally, every case of PTSD must have an identifiable trauma. In the case of combat-induced PTSD, the trauma is nearly always related to what happened in combat, acutely or chronically.

PTSD symptoms come from the trauma. Soldiers re-experience the trauma in a wide variety of ways including nightmares, flashbacks, dissociations and in any situation that reminds them of the original trauma. Often, there are multiple combat traumas that occupy the Soldier's mind.

Soldiers try to avoid situations reminding them of their trauma. They often become numb to avoid any feeling, fearing it may be overwhelming.

The body's fight or flight system of defense is over-active, disrupting sleep, mood, temper, memory and the capacity for intimacy.

PTSD can be severe. It can become chronic. It is almost always accompanied by depression, panic attacks and/or substance abuse, primarily alcohol abuse or dependence.

It is a common disorder. Seventy per cent of Combat Medics and Mortuary Affairs Specialists develop combat-induced PTSD. About a third, or more, of all combat Soldiers develop PTSD, but only half or less accept treatment.

Read this section repetitively until you believe you have acquired a basic understanding of combat-induced PTSD.

If you have a family member or friend who has served in the War of Terror who suffers from some of the symptoms of PTSD, go with him or her to a qualified behavioral health provider.

PTSD is like other disorders; the sooner effective treatment begins, the better the prognosis.

PTSD is nothing to be ashamed of.

We are a free nation. Need I remind you, dear reader, that "freedom is not free?"

We are grateful for the freedom our Soldiers assure. Thank God for our Soldiers.

We are proud of our Soldiers, an important emotion and strong cognition we need to convey to them.

What is Combat-induced Posttraumatic Stress Disorder Complicated by Depression?

PTSD may be largely understood as signs and symptoms of anxiety stemming from dysregulation of the autonomic nervous system.

Instead of a reasonable balance between the sympathetic and parasympathetic divisions of the autonomic nervous system, many PTSD symptoms are driven by over-activity of the sympathetic division.

The anatomical structure of the nervous system is comprised of two major parts: 1. the brain and spinal cord; and 2. the peripheral nervous system.

The autonomic nervous system is part of the peripheral nervous system.

The autonomic nervous system functions outside of one's awareness. For example, it regulates blood pressure, breathing and heart rate among its many other functions, while one is asleep or awake.

The sympathetic division of the autonomic nervous system prepares the body for "fight or flight," mediating its effects through the release of neurotransmitters such as adrenalin, for example.

The sympathetic division is vital during emergencies, dilating blood vessels in muscle, increasing heart rate and optimizing pulmonary function. Sadly, the redeployed combat Soldier's body and mind function as if in a nearly constant state of emergency. The sympathetic division is over-active.

The parasympathetic division uses acetyl choline, a chemical that helps transmit information from one nerve to another. It is one of a number of neurotransmitters in the body. The parasympathetic division functions importantly during ordinary, non-stressful times.

When therapy is successful, the sympathetic division of the autonomic nervous system winds down and the parasympathetic division ramps up. Eventually, the homeostatic balance is restored.

An over-active sympathetic nervous system responds favorably to prayer, meditation, mindfulness training, relaxation training with deep, slow breathing and to stable attachments or relationships that are perceived as protective attachments. As emphasized in this book, battle buddies in combat are understood by Soldiers in combat as more important to survival than their own weapons.

The cognitive model of depression, introduced by Dr. Aaron T. Beck, is associated with deeply held beliefs that lead to negative thoughts such as: "I am worthless, a failure. My past is bad. My future is dark, hopeless." It is these thoughts that contribute to a depressed mood.

These thoughts can be traced in therapy to one of two deeply held beliefs: "I am unlovable" or "I am incompetent."

Cognitive Behavior Therapy is equally as effective as antidepressant medication, and it is superior to antidepressant medication in preventing relapses of depression

Imagine the misery of a Soldier with both combat-induced PTSD and a Major Depression.

Both PTSD and Depression may be risk factors for suicide.

How to help a Soldier with both PTSD and Depression

Both anxious and depressed people avoid interactions with others. They tend to withdraw from people and become socially avoidant. It is important to be neither intrusive nor indifferent to the suffering of these isolated and avoidant Soldiers.

Encourage a depressed Soldier with PTSD to exercise by inviting them to go for a walk with you. Start low and go slow. Be satisfied with small beginnings, like a walk around the block. Increase the distance over time and try to make it a regular practice.

You know that exercise increases the release of BDNF (Brain Derived Neurotropic Factor) in the brain. You know that BDNF is associated with neurogenesis and optimization of synaptic connections, two potent antidepressant phenomena. No antidepressant medication, valuable and necessary as it may be, can achieve the same beneficial effects of exercise.

Say nothing to the Soldier that is not true, recalling that Soldiers detest incompetence as much as small talk. Saying nothing is better than being inconsistent with what you said earlier.

Depressed Soldiers may view the world as unfair. Refrain from debating.

A carefully chosen honest, positive remark can be helpful, but it may fall on deaf ears, be dismissed, deflected or discounted. Refrain from debating.

Encourage the Soldier to keep a positive daily log in which he or she writes down positive comments received and, most importantly, how he or she responded.

A positive daily log is used in CBT (Cognitive Behavioral Therapy). It can become powerful evidence to refute the Soldier's view of him or herself as worthless.

In the final analysis, it will not be a technique or a skill that helps Soldiers with combat-induced PTSD complicated by depression. What will help most will be compassion that precedes becoming a good neighbor.

What is Combat-induced Posttraumatic Stress Disorder Complicated by Panic Attacks?

Those who suffer from panic attacks will tell you that a panic attack is one of the most miserable feelings of which a human being is capable.

The first panic attack or "herald attack" is perceived as the worst feeling ever experienced. It is never forgotten. One cannot actually diagnose Panic Disorder if the patient cannot recall their "herald attack."

The experience of a panic attack may be devastating. Victims of a panic attack may be convinced they are going to die, lose their mind or something worse. It is not unusual, for example, to have the rescue squad extract the patient from their car and rush him or her to the ER where the diagnosis is not a heart attack, but a panic attack.

Cognitive Behavioral Therapy is effective with most patients with panic attacks. The cognitive model of a panic attack helps the patient understand what may otherwise seem baffling.

A panic attack, according to Dr. Beck, is a catastrophic misinterpretation of the body's normal response to stress.

Recall that Soldiers with combat-induced PTSD are keenly perceptive. Always alert to danger, they sense danger much sooner than others. It is almost like ESP (Extrasensory Perception). They not only have an earlier sense of danger, but they sense the "third or fourth order of consequences of danger."

It is understood that sensing danger, the Soldier's nervous system is alerted, preparing for "fight or flight." In other words, according to Dr. Beck, whose contributions I greatly respect, the Soldier catastrophically misunderstands his or her body's normal response to stress.

The panic attack, not understood, comes to be dreaded and feared, further contributing to avoidance, to isolation and suffering.

The good news about panic attacks is very encouraging. They will not kill you. They will not cause you to lose your mind. The more panic attacks you can have, the sooner you can learn they are harmless. They are the result of misunderstanding that your body is protecting you from partially perceived danger.

How to Help Soldiers with Combat-induced Posttraumatic Stress Disorder Complicated by Panic Attacks

Google "Academy of Cognitive Therapy." On their home page, find a photograph of Dr. Aaron T. Beck, founder of Cognitive Behavioral Therapy, and a way to identify a fully qualified cognitive therapist in your state.

You are a good neighbor. Should you learn that the Soldier residing near you suffers from panic attacks, offer to assist him or her in locating a suitable therapist.

What is Combat-induced Posttraumatic Stress Disorder Complicated by Alcohol Abuse or Dependence?

Soldiers soon learn that drinking alcohol helps them feel calm and more confident. It also helps them "sleep" and it eliminates nightmares.

This is a "yes, but" set of true statements. Yes, ingesting ethanol makes most people feel calm and may improve self-confidence. It eradicates nightmares. Yes, this is true, but alcohol destroys normal sleep architecture and will inevitably damage the liver and will have adverse effects on the brain and other vital organs.

A Soldier, distraught by discovering his wife was "sexting another man," drank beer until intoxicated. Regrettably, the Soldier reported, "I had a panic attack while I was drunk. It was the worst feeling in the world." He had to be hospitalized.

Unfortunately, many Soldiers mistakenly believe that beer is less harmful than other forms of alcohol. Ethanol is the form of alcohol in all alcoholic beverages. One 8 ounce can of beer contains the same amount of alcohol as a shot of whiskey or a glass of wine.

A former patient, mistakenly believing it was essentially harmless, drank beer throughout the day, never to the point of intoxication. He was self-employed. His wife was concerned about his drinking, but he saw no detriment in drinking beer pretty much all day because he never got drunk and he continued to work.

Imagine the shock when he was told that his liver was permanently and significantly damaged. His first liver transplant failed. It was life-saving when his second liver transplant was successful, soon to be 20 years ago.

Alcohol destroys normal sleep. Alcohol, an anesthetic, was used along with opium, before 1846 as the main way to reduce pain during surgery.

The discovery of anesthesia is a fascinating story, not to be told here in the detail it deserves. Ether was first synthesized in 1640, but its anesthetic properties were not recognized until 1846, although Dr. Crawford Long of Jefferson, Georgia, little known outside Georgia, had been using it as a surgical anesthetic since 1842.

Alcohol eliminates nightmares. Sadly, alcohol also eliminates normal sleep. I tell our Soldiers not to expect to have refreshing sleep until all alcohol and all caffeine is stopped.

Soldiers with PTSD complicated by alcohol abuse or dependence are less likely to improve. Based on my experience as a psychiatrist to the military, effective treatment of PTSD cannot begin until the alcohol issues are addressed honestly and resolved successfully.

The Army's Substance Abuse Program (ASAP) is a major asset. Skilled ASAP staff has a good success rate in assisting Soldiers in their recovery from alcohol and drug abuse. ASAP works collaboratively with Behavioral Health providers and with the Soldier's command.

The National Institute on Alcohol Abuse and Alcoholism has established a set of guidelines or recommendations in managing the use of alcohol. These recommendations are intended for adults not known to suffer from a mental disorder such as PTSD or depression. In my opinion, Soldiers with PTSD, panic attacks, depression or alcohol-related problems must avoid alcohol until their mental disorder(s) are successfully treated.

The National Institute on Alcohol Abuse and Alcoholism define safe levels of alcohol consumption for men as 4 or less standard drinks per day and 14 or less standard drinks per week. They recommend 3 or less standard drinks per day and 7 or less standard drinks per week for women. If you don't drink alcohol, then don't start. If you do drink alcohol, you may impair your health, because its risks far exceed its benefits.

How to Help a Soldier with Combat-induced PTSD Complicated by Alcohol Abuse or Dependence

Too many of us make alcohol an important part of our social life. It is not a good idea to serve alcohol to Soldiers returning from Iraq and Afghanistan, certainly not as you first welcome them into your neighborhood.

Choose not to be judgmental in discussing alcohol.

Should a Soldier or Soldier's family confide in you regarding alcohol-related problems, encourage contacting Alcoholics Anonymous and provide them with AA's phone number available in the telephone directory. The Army Substance Abuse Treatment Program (ASAP) strongly encourages Soldiers to attend AA meetings.

For two years, I unsuccessfully treated a Soldier with combat-induced PTSD. His mother became ill in another state. He went to her bedside and became embroiled in a family debate over breaking his promise not permitting her to be sent to a nursing home where, after two days, she passed away. Too angry to grieve, he resorted to alcohol.

Unknown to me, he had been imbibing large quantities of alcohol even before coming for treatment. Finding no answer for his grief or his PTSD in alcohol, he finally acknowledged suicidal thoughts with a plan to take his life. He was admitted to an inpatient treatment facility.

This week, he celebrated one year of sobriety. His response to treatment of his PTSD over the past year has been gratifying.

Summing up How You can be a Good Neighbor to Soldiers with PTSD

Effective treatment of combat-induced PTSD, even in the hands of experienced and skilled therapists, is difficult, taxing and perplexing. It can also be the most rewarding work of one's career.

Among many other reasons, treating combat-induced PTSD is tough because it is almost always combined with depression, panic attacks and/or alcohol abuse.

Being a good neighbor to Soldiers with PTSD does not mean becoming the Soldier's therapist. It means something far more important than therapy.

It means exactly what a "certain Samaritan" did two thousand years ago in the Middle East. He felt compassion for a person who had sustained life-threatening injuries, circumstances likely leading to PTSD.

Moved by compassion, the "certain Samaritan" demonstrated love for a person in need. It is not described in the book of Luke as a miracle, but I think it is best understood in no other way.

It is miraculous in that the good neighbor to the person in need was the most detested by the Jews.

It is miraculous in that compassion saved a person's life.

It is miraculous in that the compassion of a good neighbor remains one of the most powerful forces in the world.

Paradoxically, I cannot presume to tell you how to be a good neighbor. I am convinced, beyond any reasonable doubt, however, that being a good neighbor to our combat Soldiers can work miracles.

24

Bringing it Together

"It was akin to a discovery, an important discovery"

My memory of providing psychiatric treatment to Soldiers since 2005, the Soldiers whose stories are told in this book, is recalled less from the dates than from the buildings we occupied as a Medical Treatment Facility (MTF) on an active duty military Post.

The first building was a small brick stand-alone building, across the street from the hospital. We were there about 3 years.

The second building, a series of trailers conveniently connected to each other, housed the Department of Behavioral Health on a large parking lot adjacent to the hospital for the next 18 months.

The size of the accommodations expanded as the number of Soldiers needing treatment increased.

Finally, we moved into the hospital.

About the second year in the hospital building, while conducting a diagnostic psychiatric interview of a Soldier being seen by me for the first time, I finally understood the truth of the reality of the combat trauma being shared with me. In that moment, the Soldier and the doctor were together as if the trauma was happening right in front of their very eyes.

It was by no means the first time that a most difficult-to-describe set of feelings, images and perceptions had engulfed me while listening to a Soldier's story.

Spontaneously, never before having realized it ...never before having uttered it, I solemnly said to the Soldier, "I feel like I'm on sacred ground while talking to you."

I was touched, emotionally, cognitively and, yes, even spiritually.

It was akin to a discovery, an important discovery.

At last, I had a name for what I had felt and thought so many times earlier while hearing Soldiers tell their combat stories, their near-death experiences and their unwanted familiarity with the experience of death.

Speaking softly and slowly, I continued. "You put your life on the line for me. I want to put my career on the line for you."

The Soldier's tear-filled eyes stared into mine. They stared into my soul. The visual communication continued, uninterrupted by words. Words would have detracted from the meaning of the moment.

Soldier and doctor were both astonished. We both sensed the value and importance of a relationship or attachment that was being formed.

I reached for a small wooden box on my desk. It holds my professional cards on which one finds my professional identification and address and this phrase: "The finest gold is refined in the hottest furnaces."

I wrote my cell phone number on the back of my card. I passed the card to the Soldier. "This is my cell number," I said. "I want you to call me any time you wish to speak to me."

"Thank you, Sir," the Soldier said. We made an appointment for him to return the following week.

Dear reader, you may ask, "What is sacred about a Soldier returning from combat? He or she has likely witnessed the death of friends as well as the death of insurgents. He or she may have participated in the taking of life and had been a part of inflicting injury.

Is your reference to the nature of what the Soldier did or did not do in combat?"

Disambiguation of "Sacred" as used in the treatment of Combat-induced PTSD

The good done by our Soldiers in 21st Century war is scantily publicized. Decades may pass before history reaches its final judgment on the wisdom and value of removing dictators.

The Soldiers who built schools and hospitals in Iraq can't wait for the judgment of history. Our Soldiers provided food and drinking water for the starving and the parched. Medical aid for the enemy was often given priority to that of our own Soldiers.

Our Soldiers need to know now that the good they did in Iraq and Afghanistan is acknowledged and appreciated.

The concern I have for Soldiers is like that of the father described in the Book of Luke, written in 60 A.D., chapter 15:20 "And he got up and came to his father. But while he was still a long way off, his father saw him and had compassion for him, and ran and embraced him, and kissed him."

I neither feel pity for the Soldier, nor do Soldiers, as I have said, want that response from anyone, nor do I kiss Soldiers. My response is motivated by respect and admiration.

The "father" part of me, sans embracing and kissing, unlike the father in the Middle East, the setting of the story told by the physician, Luke, the setting of our 21st Century war, feels he is on sacred ground because it is a special returning home from a tough and dangerous journey.

I tell the Soldier returning from combat, infused with emotional suffering unique to our current military operations, that I feel I am on "Sacred Ground" because they are highly valued and respected. They deserve great admiration. They are dedicated to their mission and to each other.

I identify their sense of humility.

They need to know they are cherished. They need to know that what is told to them is solemn.

These Soldiers know that my pronouncement is not religious veneration. They know they are not worthy of nor desirous of religious veneration.

They know I convey no intention that they are "special" because they were traumatized. Our Soldiers are not victims. They are volunteers who courageously invested their life in whatever sacrifice was required in defense of our nation, not weighing the threats to life and limb but obediently executing their mission.

The word "sacred" spontaneously spoken to Soldiers with combat-induced PTSD came from a depth of respect that leapt from my soul, touched by the retelling and re-experiencing of combat trauma.

I am reminded of one of the verses of Rudyard Kipling's 1897 poem, "Recessional:"

"Far called, our navies melt away;
On dune and headland sinks the fire:
Lo, all our pomp of yesterday
Is one with Nineveh and Tyre!
Judge of the Nations, spare us yet,
Lest we forget, lest we forget!"

The Value and Limitations of Objectivity

The "therapeutic alliance," a term describing the relationship between therapist and patient, is the most important dimension of psychotherapy. It is sometimes called the "working alliance." It is defined by boundaries that must not be violated and by explicit and implicit rules that define the relationship.

In psychotherapy, one party agrees to be the patient. The other party agrees to be the therapist.

Legally, it is understood that the therapist, by virtue of education, training and experience, is vested with authority and responsibility. In a court of law, the therapist-patient relationship is comparable to a parent-child relationship.

Ethically, therapists are held to a high standard of conduct. The safety, wellbeing and welfare of the patient must continuously be the therapist's chief concern.

Ordinarily, the therapist is expected to be objective. Think in terms of an artful perspective, an early morning scene of a verdant spring meadow from which the fog has lifted.

One sees it clearly. There are no obstacles. Although the most distant split-rail fence, marking its back boundary, is 100 yards away, one feels as if, by reaching out, the smooth texture of the chestnut, the sturdy survivor, could be easily touched.

It is not easy to objectively describe the lush, green meadow without the subjective sensations, tender memories and cognitive appreciation the objective scene itself stimulates or "triggers."

In a word, both the objective and subjective aspect of every observation are intertwined. Both the objective and the subjective have their value and their limitations.

The mere objective reporting of an observation, in some situations, may be all that is required.

Subjectivity run amok is little more than emotional drivel.

Aristotle on virtue reminds us that the habit of choosing the mean between extremes is the most virtuous that one may choose.

"Will America get it right?"

Readers of the above section of <u>Sacred Ground</u>, "It was akin to a discovery, an important discovery," or other sections of <u>Sacred Ground</u>, may find cause to ask the doctor has he lost his objectivity. "My dear God," a reader might comment, "how can he sit there and be so emotional? He is a therapist. Where is his objectivity?"

At the unwanted risk of sounding defensive, I respond. "How can he sit there and not be affected by the anguish our Soldiers come to know?"

This is a book of questions provoked by 21st Century war and its psychological costs.

An important question for the story-teller of our Soldiers' stories: "has the story-teller reached the ancient Greek's "golden mean" expressed by Aristotle on virtue?" "Has he gotten the mixture right?"

Has truth found its way?

Will these true stories move the American public as they move the story-teller of our Soldier's stories?

Will America get it right? Will America develop, sustain and express its deep gratitude for our Soldiers?

"We can't show our feelings, Sir"

In <u>Sacred Ground</u>, the story-teller does not look at a lush, green meadow.

His visual field is populated with people, a young SGT from Mississippi, a 35-year-old SFC (Sergeant First Class) brought as a child by his parents to America from Mexico, a CPT from Colorado longing to fish for salmon in refreshing, swift, far western streams.

Snorting, powerful equinesque emotions are trapped in self constructed, sturdy stables from which they dare not escape. "We can't show our feelings, Sir…not in front of our men, Sir…not in combat, Sir."

"Agreed, but when and where does a Soldier express feelings?" I ask.

"I don't know when I can show my feelings, Sir…not in front of my wife, Sir.

My wife tells me I have no feelings, Sir. If she only knew!

I'm afraid what would happen if I ever showed my feelings, Sir. I believe I would lose control, Sir."

"What would it be like if you showed your feelings," I asked, "and you lost control?"

A long silence followed my inquiry. The Soldier looked around my office suspiciously, as if someone may hear and reject him.

"Control is very important to me, Sir."

Another long silence dwells in my office.

"Sir, I'm afraid if I lost control of my feelings I would never get control back again. I'm afraid, Sir."

"Have you ever lost control of your feelings?

"No, Sir."

"Have you ever seen someone lose control of their feelings?"

"No, Sir."

"Where does your fear of the loss of control of your feelings come from?"

"I don't know, Sir." Our session ended in uncertainty, but it is okay. We will meet again and again.

"I love animals"

LTC (Lieutenant Colonel) Jim Thomas is a handsome 40 year old man.

Standing 6 feet tall, this athletic-appearing Army officer has a full head of thick, wavy dark-brown hair, penetrating dark-brown eyes, high cheek bones and a strong military bearing.

He is surprisingly gentle. His voice is soft-spoken. A grim, serious and sad look defines his face.

LTC Thomas, as a battalion commander, has 7 company commanders, all captains, report directly to him. Each company commander may have 200-400 Soldiers, or more, under his or her command, organized into platoons and squads.

LTC Thomas knows war. He knows the cost of war. He knows the feeling of losing his Soldiers to death and to injury. He personally knows the psychological cost of 21st Century war.

"Combat stress doesn't pick and choose," the LTC said, slowly shaking his head. "It doesn't pick and choose by race, rank, gender, age or religious preference."

The LTC is a good man and a good Soldier.

He is also a good husband and a good father to their two small children. His love and faithfulness to his wife is easily learned by the way he talks about her. It was her idea that he come in for help for his textbook-case of PTSD.

"There is something different about me now…I don't know exactly what it is…but I know this, you can only cope if you want to cope.

I've had a pretty good two weeks, but I had one episode.

I took my 3 year old son out for a walk yesterday. I really want to get to know my neighbors. Some of my neighbors were out, too. I was a beautiful day. It felt like the snow was over at last.

Suddenly, I saw a large, unleashed dog. It looked like a mixed breed. It was part German Shepherd. The dog was running towards my son. I must have frozen or something.

The dog went up to my son, licked his hand and played with him. The dog's warm wet tongue made my son laugh. I was relieved. Moments before, I was terrified.

My neighbor, a woman, must have noticed something…she witnessed a sudden change in me… and she was puzzled. I could see it on her face as she looked at me.

I commented that I had to kill a lot of animals in Iraq.

I didn't want to kill them, I said.

I love animals.

We had to standup our camp from scratch. It was in the midst of piles of trash and debris.

The dogs were starving. All were scavengers and most had rabies. We had to control disease.

I did not actually do the shooting. I had to supervise it. I had to order it.

We had to shoot 15-20 dogs.

It was stressful. I can still hear their barking and growling.

Getting back to the incident with my son, I think I was paralyzed for a second…the dog frightened me.

I commented to the woman that memories from combat are activated by different reminders.

Suddenly, I realized that not all dogs are bad.

The puzzled woman seemed to understand.

Visits to the Vet

We have two cats. I don't like to go to the vet. You can always hear dogs barking there. I think my wife sensed it…that I didn't like to go to the vet. I never went alone. She usually had to go with me."

"How is it," I asked the LTC, "that you did not tell your wife that going to the vet was stressful for you?" "

"I didn't understand it at that time," the LTC said, matter of factly.

It was encouraging to observe how rapidly this brave leader of Soldiers in combat was discovering the truth of his situation.

"Every PTSD symptom you experience, LTC Thomas," I said, "has a logical explanation.

I call it the truth.

Your brain is highly efficient. First, before all else, your brain wants to keep you alive.

It is by no means simplistic. However, the PTSD symptoms are remarkably like a hot stove touched once by a child, but never touched again.

Soldiers with PTSD have a lot of hot stove memories from combat. The Soldier's brain does not want him or her to be burned again.

The Soldier's perception of danger becomes so efficient from combat trauma that it is almost like ESP (Extra Sensory Perception).

An important goal of effective treatment of Soldiers with PTSD, once trust and attachment develops between the Soldier and the therapist, is the discovery that understanding the truth of their combat memories is liberating."

"Doughnuts for Dad"

LTC Thomas said, "I'm watching the DVDs you gave me. My wife is watching with me. It has already helped her understand me better.

I'm also reading your book. I was pleased that it is an easy read...no jargon...no complicated psychiatric language. It is helping me understand myself. I'm just getting started...finished the first 4 chapters...about how you got started in this work."

I was touched by his sincerity.

We sat quietly before the LTC spoke again.

"My daughter's school had a special event last FRI, called 'Doughnuts for Dad.' I was happy to be there with my 6 year old daughter. Other dads were there, too.

We chatted. It was a nice time to be her dad."

When the LTC said, "It was a nice time to be her dad," his smile told me the sweetness of the doughnuts paled in comparison to the sweetness of the father/daughter relationship. These were the precious moments he so often missed when deployed. He is discovering that life had not lost its taste.

"The bell rang as I left.

Walking out of the school, I wondered how many people I served with in combat that will never have the opportunity to enjoy 'Doughnuts with Dad' with their children at school.

The thought brought tears to my eyes.

I tried to deal with the thought…I can only do what I can do."

"LTC Thomas," subdued, quietly I said, "may I ask you a question related to your thought?"

The LTC nodded his head in assent.

"How many Soldiers you served with in combat will have the opportunity to attend 'Doughnuts for Dad,' with their children at school because of your leadership in combat?"

His was the smile of gratitude seen on the face of someone who found, after a long search, something of value that had been lost.

"What does the sign say, Daddy?"

LTC Thomas, a man prone to be taciturn, was atypically openly self disclosing today. It was good to find him talkative, I thought.

"I had a pretty good day yesterday with the kids. I stopped for a traffic signal at an intersection. Two homeless people stood at the intersection holding up signs. Crudely written in black paint on white cardboard, one sign begged: 'Help Homeless Vets.'

The second sign, fashioned out of a discorded Keystone Beer 12-pack carrying case, held up by trembling hands, simply stated: 'Will work for food.'

My daughter is inquisitive. She asks questions. 'What does the sign say, Daddy?' She can read some.

'Why is he homeless?' she asked.

I started bawling…almost bawling…but I held it back. I don't want my kids to see that part of me.

My thought…it could have been me out there on the street or someone in my organization…or someone I'm connected with."

Tears filled the LTC's eyes.

Looking bewildered, the LTC said, "At times, I feel so incredibly connected with people…I'm almost overpowered with a strong need to serve.

Last week, you asked about my plans after I retire from the Army. I have a calling to help vets or work in a nonprofit organization. I want to feel close to a community.

When I'm awakened at night by a phone call, it's always bad news.

It will never be over. The leader is the one called. There will always be reminders. People will always need help. It is like I will never be free."

I chose not to challenge the LTC's thought, "I will never be free." Imagine how this thought must make him feel if he believes it 100%. However, this is only his third therapy session.

His progress in just two weeks is pleasing.

Soon we will discuss Dr. Aaron Beck's CBT (Cognitive Behavioral Therapy).

As our attachment strengthens, the LTC, already a bright and motivated patient, will learn to arm himself with skills to identify his ATs (Automatic Thoughts), like the "hot automatic thought," "I will never be free."

Then he will learn how to take his automatic thoughts into the court room of his mind, searching for the evidence for and the evidence against his thought.

By repeating this process until it becomes natural, the LTC will lessen the distortions in his thinking. His search for the truth of his situation will succeed.

Written between 900-750 B.C., the Book of Proverbs describes the down-to-earth objectives I find applicable to our Soldiers who grapple with combat-induced PTSD and its associated thoughts. Proverbs 3:13 reads, "How blessed is the man who finds wisdom, and the man who gains understanding."

What Soldiers with PTSD have taught me?

Two years after I started writing <u>Sacred Ground</u>, the number of my treatment sessions with Soldiers increased significantly from 12,500.

I want to describe what the Soldiers with PTSD in my practice have in common as people…the important human features of these brave people… other than their symptoms of PTSD.

The reader will judge which of these common traits is the most important, the most damaging and the most resistant to change.

The reader will determine which of these emotions is the most understandable.

Perhaps the reader, provided with these observations, will gain insight sufficient to act in supportive and understanding ways to our Soldiers.

I cannot deny that I often felt the deep sense of shame that burdens these brave Soldiers. It contributes to their strong need to isolate themselves, avoiding interacting with others whenever possible.

Their sense of guilt is closely allied to their sense of shame. So often, their sense of guilt is irrational but deeply rooted, resistant to change. This is not solely "survival guilt," a familiar term applied to Soldiers wondering "Why did I survive when my best friend gave his life?"

Many of our Soldiers returning home with PTSD have feelings of guilt. Their guilt is more moral and spiritual in nature, more ill-defined. It is not only about surviving. Their guilt is about nature of War on Terror, about the effects of trauma on their imagination.

What at first appears to family members as narcissistic self-centeredness, turns out to be thinly veiled self-loathing.

Sadness, apart from depression, bewilders these Soldiers. "Why do I feel so sad watching TV comics with my son? It makes no sense to me, doc. Honestly, I just want to be happy again. Everything is blah. I used to enjoy things…I have no joy in my life now. I wish I had a re-set button that I could use to go back to what I enjoyed before I deployed."

Many of the best trained, best equipped Soldiers in the world return from combat devoid of a sense of pride. The sense of the heroic is surprisingly missing. "I've gone from hero to zero," is their familiar thought.

These Soldiers share a strong sense of secretiveness, not because their combat missions required it. Should their "secrets" become disclosed, they imagine, complete rejection by their family, particularly by their children, would be devastating.

Shame, guilt, self-centeredness, joylessness, inexplicable sadness and secretiveness are not listed as symptoms of PTSD…but these are powerful, frightening emotions in which many Soldiers with PTSD are deeply mired. When these feelings become intolerable, the need for relief is sensed as urgent. Unfortunately, relief is often sought in desperation, too often in the context of impaired judgment.

Fortunately, these preventable critical moments can be reduced and prevented with effective treatment. The highly infrequent episodes of Soldiers going beyond their capacity to regulate and control their negative affect is dramatized by members of the media whose best interests are not in the best interests of our Soldiers and their families.

Our Soldiers feel betrayed by those members of the media who attempt to scandalize the majority of brave Soldiers by exploitation of the very few whose conduct is unacceptable.

A Change in World View

Everyone has a world view or "a particular philosophy of life or conception of the world." It's not something we get up in the morning thinking about consciously. We rarely articulate our world view. We don't greet our neighbors asking, "How's your world view today?"

Ordinarily, while we may not knowingly profess a particular philosophical perception of our world, nonetheless it is present in all of us reared in a similar culture and in a particular historical period.

One's world view, similar to one's attachment style, is relatively stable over time under relatively stable conditions. Major life events, however, may radically change one's world view.

From the 17th Century to the mid-20th Century, scholars held an optimistic world view regarding the perfectibility of mankind.

From John Locke's "tabula rasa," or blank sheet concept of the mind at birth, scholars reasoned that it would only be a matter of time before the ideal education or the ideal society or the ideal whatever would be discovered and implemented. Mankind's perfection was soon to be achieved.

Until Locke, it was accepted as factual that "kings begat kings" and "common folk begat common folk." Locke's world view challenged the "divine rights of kings." Locke's world view started the search for the best ways to influence the mind "not yet affected by experience or impressions."

Locke's world view influenced both the French and the American Revolutions.

Since Locke's time, the notion that the influence of experience determines one's destiny, as well as one's world view, has largely been unquestioned.

Locke's philosophy led the search for experiences that would perfect human nature.

For nearly 400 years, the hope that sprang from Locke's philosophy remained positively enthusiastic. It came to a crashing halt, however, when the stench of Nazi Concentration Camps was detected and when mushroom shadows of nuclear weapons were developed before mankind was perfected.

If the people of the world had a positive and hopeful world view, two 20th century historical events, anti-Semitic extremism and nuclear weaponry, dashed the hope that mankind could be perfected.

Mankind's capability for destruction exceeds its capability for understanding…and yet we survive…so far.

The World View of Soldiers with Combat-induced PTSD

The psychological influence of 21st Century war on our Soldiers is the central theme of this manuscript.

No Soldier deployed to Iraq or Afghanistan escapes its influence on his or her world view. The magnification of its influence on their world view is undeniable in our Soldiers returning from combat with PTSD.

Lieutenant Colonel Mack O'Quinn co-leads our Post-Deployment Traumatic Grief Group. A bibliophile and reflective Licensed Clinical Social Worker, LTC O'Quinn remarked that traumatic experiences may alter one's world view if the events are profound.

"I can lose my car keys and it's disturbing, but not profound. A major automobile accident with serious injuries may change one's world view if the experience was profound. It may be difficult for the injured party to grasp that he or she has a different post-accident world view.

The terror of today's combat is utter terror. The losses are profound. Innocence is lost. It is a form of rape of the mind. The world view of Soldiers is changed. The world is ugly. The ugliness is unprecedented. Their attention is focused on the here and now. They can't think about the future.

Combat trauma also reawakens the forgotten traumas of childhood.

Affinity for closeness to people is affected. They want to be close and, at the same time, they don't want to be close. They feel alone, shy and withdrawn."

What does Combat-induced PTSD look like?

Staff Sergeant (SSG) Roy Stanford is a 32 year old married Caucasian man. He is new to the TUES Afternoon Post-deployment Group. Like other Soldiers, he had "first day jitters," a pretty bad case of anxiety.

Athletic and fit, he sat calmly, successfully disguising his uneasy feelings.

Group therapists agree that, as a general rule, the most anxious member of the group is the first to speak.

One by one, the 7 members of the TUES Afternoon Post-deployment Group, all active duty Soldiers with combat-induced PTSD, came in, taking their seats in the chairs arranged in a semi-circle.

SSG Stanford spoke first. "I had a very unpleasant encounter today with a doctor at a nearby Military Treatment Facility.

He told me it was 'criminal' that no doctor had given me a profile (medical rating, temporary or permanent, for a physical or mental disorder that may impair performance of duty) for my severe asthma.

'You have had asthma for 5 years. You take 4 different medications for asthma every day. It is not only criminal,' he said. 'It is also fraudulent that you have not been placed on a profile.'"

Profiles are avoided by Soldiers who want to remain in the Army. Some profiles, for example, prevent deployment to a combat zone.

"I explained to the physician, a retired full Colonel, that some providers will accommodate a Soldier by not giving a profile when the Soldier is highly motivated to serve.

He could not believe it, he said. He got real angry with me.

I stood up for myself. The doctor said, 'I'm entering a note in your medical records that you need a profile for asthma.'

Funny thing. He didn't give me a profile, either.

I don't know about you guys, but I spend a lot of time trying to prove that I have a medical condition. In some cases, I spend a lot of time trying to prove I don't have a medical condition."

The group, permitting its newest member to have the floor, mumbled and nodded, knowingly.

The SSG continued. "Asthma and PTSD are like each other in several ways.

What does asthma look like?

What does PTSD look like?

To the average person, the Soldier with asthma looks like the average person...unless he or she is having an asthmatic attack.

To the average person, the Soldier with PTSD looks like an average person...unless he or she is having PTSD symptoms he or she cannot hide."

The group responded in general agreement with SSG Stanford. That's why PTSD is called the "invisible wound" or the "invisible injury," said one member of the group.

SSG Stanford thus introduced himself to his new fellow group members. He was warmly welcomed. No longer jittery, his anxiety level was all but invisible now...even to the trained eyes of his psychiatrist.

"War is easy. Coming home is Hell"

We end this story of the psychological cost of 21st Century war with a closer look at an earlier observation of Master Sergeant (MSG) Keith L. Johnson, "War is easy. Coming home is Hell."

The depth of insight and the truth of the meaning of MSG Johnson's statement were finally made clearer to me today. I pondered over this manuscript for the past 2 years, the 8th and 9th years of my treatment of active duty combat Soldiers, the most rewarding experience of a long career.

By now, it has been my distinct honor and privilege to provide psychiatric treatment, combining individual and group psychotherapy, in about 12,500 doctor/patient encounters.

Dear reader, you may well ask, "Why has it taken you so long, Dr. Brown, to finally begin to understand the real psychological price our American Soldiers have paid conducting 21st Century war?"

Rather than speculate, make excuses or otherwise completely dodge your question, I will simply say I must not have been ready.

My lack of readiness, unconsciously communicated to my patients, cautioned them to wait until my psychological maturity was sufficient to contain the truth in the delicate balance required by their thoughts and feelings.

It happened in the TUES Afternoon Post-deployment Psychotherapy Group. My son, Clinton, a musical artist, has perfect pitch and an equally perfect ear for music. "That's C sharp," he will say when the tea pot steams out its warning to turn off the stove. I, too, love music and, of course, I love my son, but I have no ear for musical notes, a great disappointment for me, and an even greater disappointment for my dear mother whose single ambition for me was to be a country music singer.

My ear listens for words. Shriller than a hot tea pot, the words of SGT Bill Snyder would have awakened me had I been in a deep sleep.

At first, I could not believe what I thought I heard him say. "Could you repeat that?" I requested.

He could have been speaking to a priest. "I'd be better off KIA (Killed in Action) than come home with PTSD."

Looking around the group of 7 Soldiers, all with combat-induced PTSD, I was surprised that, unlike me, no one appeared surprised, not the least bit shocked by SGT Snyder's casually delivered announcement.

I shifted in my chair.

"Group," I said solemnly, "how many of you feel the same way SGT Snyder feels?"

One by one, every member of the group agreed 100%.

I stared at SGT Snyder as if to ask him again to repeat his sentence.

As if he had he been swearing with his left palm on the Holy Bible and his right hand raised high in the air, he said, "I'd be better off KIA (Killed in Action) than come home with PTSD."

I was shocked, but not surprised. It was the feeling dreaded by a prize fighter who is stunned by one blow to the chin and the second blow to the jaw. He is staggered.

I needed to go to my corner of the ring.

I was bowled over.

Is this the way a Soldier's wife feels when he says, "I should have stayed over there?"

The SGT's words, "I'd be better off KIA than come home with PTSD," pierced my heart. I've known that these Soldiers suffer, but did I actually know the extreme severity of their suffering? Did I know actually that Soldiers with PTSD would rather be killed in action than return home with combat-induced PTSD?

Trying to Understand the Experience of Suffering

The following description of suffering is limited to suffering experienced by Soldiers under my care for the treatment of combat-induced PTSD incurred in 21st Century war. It is not intended to be an exhaustive or comprehensive discussion of suffering. It is a summary of the principles of suffering unique to combat-induced PTSD I learned from suffering Soldiers.

At the core of suffering is the fear of loss of control.

At the core of the fear of the loss of control is the fear of the greatest of all unknowns, death itself.

Suffering is worse at night. Night is a universal symbol of death. Robert Louis Stevens, in his <u>Travels with a Donkey</u>, reminds us that "Night is a dead monotonous period under a roof... ." It is a time when what can be detected is remarkably reduced, and needed distractions are unavailable.

Commonly, Soldiers with PTSD spend their nights miserably. Nightmares are not the only nocturnal disturbance dreaded by Soldiers with PTSD. The physical aches and pains of warfare, ignored during the day, make their painful reality exquisitely known under the cover of black, sleepless nights.

Daylight itself, and intentionally staying very busy, help keep unwanted, intrusive combat trauma memories out of the awareness of our Soldiers. Night brings with it a slower pace and reduced distractions, permitting the invisible air traffic control tower to land, not one after another, but jumbled dreaded, frightening, unspeakably realistic combat trauma memories. Before the last trauma memory lands, the Soldier cannot shrug off thoughts of insanity.

What Causes Soldiers with PTSD to Suffer?

Soldiers with combat-induced PTSD, incurred in 21st Century war, were in danger every day and every night for seemingly endless months. The enemies were indistinguishable from friendly or indifferent women and children. Death and injury resulted primarily from unmanned explosive devices.

Many of the symptoms of combat-induced PTSD, life-saving in combat, are anachronistic at home. Soldiers sensitized to dangerous combat are equally sensitive to the reactions of others to their behavior under stress back home from war. They sense rejection and devaluation by witnesses who, lacking understanding and appreciation of combat, laugh at their exaggerated startle response or appear puzzled by their hypervigilant, repetitive checking of doors and windows.

Much of the suffering is experienced silently and alone. These Soldiers are too ashamed to share their deeply held belief that the world is dangerous, that more frequent and worse attacks on the US will happen in time.

Learning is a change in behavior as a result of experience.

Soldiers with combat-induced PTSD have learned to be prepared for danger. They have made the honor roll, the best students in the Army, the most precisely perceptive of even the minutest signification of the need for alarm.

How have these scholars of perception of danger acquired their remarkable skills? Have Soldiers with combat-induced PTSD sat down in huge libraries or classrooms of the world's greatest universities and spent decades studying that which is universally known about danger?

Far from the tranquility of classrooms of universities, Soldiers have acquired vast amounts of knowledge from combat. They have become human owners of life-saving information that is unsurpassed. No camera or any form of artificial intelligence can match what a Soldier learns and retains in a single life-threatening moment of combat.

Any element in common with the original combat trauma possesses the power to recreate the astonishingly vivid memory of the original trauma. It is ingenious how the mind stores and instantaneously responds to the tiniest fragment of the original trauma. The speed with which the response occurs is beyond the limitation of awareness, making it disquieting, further confounding the Soldier's emotional state.

Brain MRI

LTC Thomas, the battalion commander with multiple combat deployments introduced above, was referred by his primary care provider for an MRI of the brain. "I didn't think much about it," LTC Thomas said. "I had an MRI of my shoulder 2 years ago. It was not a problem.

For some reason, I felt out of control. I had to come out of the machine. I am very claustrophobic. The technician was kind and understanding, but I had to come out of the machine. She gave me 5 mg of Valium. After a while, I was able to get back into the machine.

Can you help me understand, doctor, why I became claustrophobic?"

This was easy, I thought. It was not the first time a Soldier with PTSD told me the same story.

"Was it a closed MRI machine?" I asked.

"Yes, Sir. It was a closed tube."

"When you had an MRI 2 years ago, LTC Thomas, did you have to slide all the way into the tube?"

"No, Sir. I was able to keep my head out of the machine."

"Can you tell me what came to your mind when you were placed inside the tube?"

"I panicked, Sir. I had to get out of the tube. Nothing came to my mind but getting out of the tube. The technician was talking to me the whole time. I told her I had to get out. I had to get out now."

"Later, LTC Thomas, when you got home, did anything come to mind?"

"Yes, Sir. We were sent to Basra in the southern part of Iraq to relieve the Brits. They didn't leave the Post very often. They lived near a section called 'Mortar Road,' meaning they were under constant attack.

They slept in concrete enclosures that reminded me of caskets. We had to get down on our hands and knees to enter the structure. Once we crawled inside the concrete enclosures we stretched out to sleep. I never really got used to it. It still reminds me of caskets.

As I think about it now, the MRI tube reminded me of those concrete caskets in Basra, Iraq. Enclosed spaces make me feel very uncomfortable."

Almost in passing, the LTC said, "I don't like seeing gravel any more. I saw gravel everywhere we were deployed. Gravel was everywhere in Afghanistan."

Continuing in a casual tone, the LTC said, "I'm sleeping better now since I started treatment. I don't check my phone calls after 8 PM. I have one beer or a glass of wine with dinner. I get 7 or 8 hours of sleep. I limit my intake of fluids after a certain time in the evening.

Most of all, I feel comforted when I go to bed with my wife when she goes to bed…not staying up late and going to bed after she has already been asleep."

Before LTC Thomas started therapy, he wanted no one in his personal space, not even his wife, and he believed he'd be happier in combat, not at home. We were both encouraged by his progress.

Another Dimension of Suffering

The Mental Status Examination in psychiatry, analogous to the Physical Examination in family medicine, includes questions regarding the patient's orientation to time, place and person. Basically, the patient is asked to give (1). The date and time of day (without consulting a calendar or clock), (2). The address or the name of the place in which the patient is being examined, and (3). The patient's full name.

The sense of time, the last orientation to develop, is sensitive to stress. It may be the first orientation to become impaired under extreme stress. Imagine the influence of nightmares, flashbacks and intrusive memories of combat trauma, for example, on the Soldier's sense of time.

Combat trauma, often reported "as if it were happening in slow motion," is an example of an alteration in one's sense of time under stress. The adaptive value of viewing a traumatic event in slow motion assures that no important detail of the trauma is unobserved. The rich, full view of the trauma afforded by mental slow-motion photography is a two-sided sword. It assures complete recall, but it cuts deeply and painfully into the minds of Soldiers burdened by haunting trauma memories.

Mental health professionals advise us to live in the moment. When asked what the most important thing in the world is, the Dalai Lama simply and unhesitatingly replied, "now."

We are told that successful people are good at multi-tasking, a complex cognitive exercise only possible when one is fully living in the "now" or present.

Soldiers with combat-induced PTSD live neither in the "now" nor in the past or future. Combat trauma robs deserving Soldiers of the normality of the sense of time.

Imagine the enormity of chronic disorientation of the sense of time.

A Soldier with PTSD, having dinner with his family in a non-threatening restaurant in his hometown, is instantaneously transported to an unthinkably hideous scene of helping a seriously injured Soldier in Iraq. It was the farthest thing from his mind until his wife's steak knife produced drops of a red substance from her rare steak. Trying not to embarrass his family, hand over his mouth, he ran from the restaurant, so that he could vomit unobserved.

Many of the combat trauma memories over-ride the Soldier's sense of time, just as real today or tonight as they were when they occurred years earlier.

Perhaps the worst part of the disorientation of the sense of time is its impact during the midst of a flashback, nightmare, intrusive recollection or panic attack. It is the depressing and frightening sense that it is lasting without ever ending.

Shame and Suffering

It is difficult to separate shame and suffering. Today, in the TUES Afternoon Post-deployment group therapy I learned something new about shame. Soldiers suffering with PTSD bear an additional burden, the heavy burden of shame. What were new to me were the extent and the power of shame in the daily lives of Soldiers with PTSD.

The Soldiers in the TUES group, their statement confirmed by Soldiers in the WED Morning group, are not primarily ashamed for what they had to do in combat. They are ashamed of having combat-induced PTSD.

Sergeant First Class Stillwell, a 37 year old divorced male with a fair complexion, a mild mannered Soldier, was recently visited by his mother and aunts. "I told my mother that I have PTSD. My mother said, 'Your Uncle Bob had something like PTSD from Vietnam and now he is crazy.'

I felt ashamed. I've never met Uncle Bob, but I have heard about him all my life. What my mother said about her own brother reinforced the doubts I already have about myself. Am I going to be another Uncle Bob?

Our shame comes from being asked about PTSD."

Another Soldier said, "My kids think I'm a super dad. I don't want to let them down. I'm so ashamed I have PTSD. I fear that someday they will find out how weak I am."

"Shame is why I keep to myself," said another Soldier.

"The shame of having PTSD is why I tried to hide my issues for so long before I came for help."

"I don't want other Soldiers see where I come for help. I won't push the 3rd floor elevator button if others are on the elevator. Scotty wouldn't take the elevator for the first 3 months...but now he does."

"I don't want my unit to see me come here for help. I'm embarrassed. I feel ashamed of having PTSD. I'm afraid my unit will reject me if they know. They will see me as weak."

Looking dejected, a Sergeant First Class told his fellow group members about an incident that captures the pain of shame. "My dad and my uncles were about to watch a movie on TV. It was a war movie. In front of everybody, my dad asked me, 'Is this going to mess you up?' I was very embarrassed. It's the kind of thing that makes me ashamed of having PTSD."

Attempting to lighten the TUES group mood, I sang the Mills Brothers 1944 hit, "You always hurt the one you love." Admittedly, I was singing to a captive audience, but I was pleased by their thoughtful and careful listening to words that seem to uniquely fit their plight:

You always hurt the one you love, the one you shouldn't hurt at all.

You always take the sweetest rose and crush it 'till the petals fall.

You always break the kindest heart with a hasty word you can't recall.

So if I broke your heart last night, it's because I love you most of all.

Failing to understand the psychological cost of 21st Century war, too many relatives and friends hurt the ones they love, the ones with PTSD. Thoughtless comments imply that combat-induced PTSD is a degenerative disorder for which there is no hope, are patently heartbreaking and boldly wrong.

"I'd be better off KIA than come home with PTSD"

This book is not about Soldiers who paid the ultimate price in 21st Century war. It is not about the unbearable grief of mothers, fathers, spouses and children, relatives and friends of our Soldiers who gave their lives for us. May God be merciful to those who have come to know the meaning of the loss of a precious Soldier.

Combat-induced PTSD is a disorder caused by the trauma of combat. It has recognizable symptoms. At least 4 methods of treatment are approved by the Department of Defense. Its prognosis is strongly influenced by the Soldier's attitudes and beliefs about the disorder. Critically, the Soldier's attitudes and beliefs about the disorder, perhaps more than the disorder itself, are overwhelmingly influenced by society's attitudes and beliefs about the Soldier with PTSD.

Historians, centuries from now, might compare present attitudes toward PTSD with ancient attitudes about leprosy. Our lepers, however, are not seen as unclean and sinful, as lepers were in the Middle Ages, but as dangerous, unpredictable and as persons to be avoided.

Society's condemnation of combat-induced PTSD, like earlier society's condemnation of leprosy, is based on ignorance of the disorder. The public's lack of knowledge of combat-induced PTSD is polluting the very air our Soldiers breathe.

If even one of our Soldiers with combat-induced PTSD prefers to have been killed in action (KIA) rather than come home with dreaded PTSD, then something important is missing in our understanding, more accurately our misunderstanding, of a disorder that is affecting thousands of our Soldiers.

The suffering of Soldiers with combat-induced PTSD must be nearly intolerable. A major force driving much of the unnecessary suffering of PTSD is the shame of having the disorder. The shame of PTSD requires an audience of a condemning public. Without condemnation, there is no lasting shame.

The power of shame is vividly seen in the behavior of the losing team of the world's best athletes. You have seen the television camera focus, for example, on the dejected losing players following an important basketball tournament: they cover their face with shame hidden by large white towels draped over their bowed heads.

We may not treat our Soldiers with combat-induced PTSD as lepers. Too often, however, they are regarded as weak, losers, failures, characters to be feared, and best shunned. This unnecessarily causes the shame that increases their suffering.

Understanding the Psychological Cost of 21st Century War

This book is a collection of true stories of Soldiers, by Soldiers, for you. Nothing has been added. Nothing has been exaggerated. It is told in their own words.

I am the psychiatrist to whom these Soldiers told their stories. Whenever it was possible, the Soldiers have read each section of the book in which their stories are told. If they wanted corrections or clarifications, they were made.

Neither the Soldiers nor their author seek fame or fortune. All net proceeds from the sale of the book will be donated to the

American Red Cross whose close relationship with the US Army has a long and sound history.

The stories are told in book form with a single purpose in mind. America needs to know what price our Soldiers pay for fighting in 21st Century war.

Combat-induced PTSD can only be understood when 21st Century war is understood…but as MSG Keith L. Johnson reminds us, "War is easy. Coming home is Hell."

In a word, the psychological cost of 21st war is suffering, the kind of suffering that is intense, all-encompassing and long-lasting. No aspect of the Soldier's life is unaffected by suffering. The Soldier and the Soldier's family enter a life known only by those who know 21st Century war.

The Soldier is changed by combat. There is no prosthesis for an amputated spirit, we are told by an officer with PTSD, and several other comorbid disorders, in the movie, "Scent of a Woman." The observation also aptly describes our Soldier's amputated attachment style, amputated unique pre-combat sense of self, amputated sense of time, amputated sense of safety, amputated sense of security, amputated sense of joy, amputated refreshing sleep and amputated capacity for intimacy.

Ten psychological costs of 21st Century war are described in detail in Chapter 21, beginning on page 453. That summary includes descriptions of the damage to sleep, personhood, memory, intimacy, spiritual domain, sense of self, temperament, trust, capacity to relate to others and the presence of persistent emotional turmoil.

America, you, like me, can learn a lot about war and about coming home from war with combat-induced PTSD by listening to these remarkable Soldiers tell their stories. Listen with your heart. Listen with your head.

America, we must learn all we can about combat-induced PTSD if we are going to remove the major barrier to full recovery. That major barrier is an unhealing culture in which the lack of knowledge of PTSD causes Soldiers to suffer more needlessly here at home than in combat.

Robert S Brown
    Charlottesville
    15 NOV 2014

Military Acronyms

A
- AAR – After action report
- AAR – After action review
- ABCS – Army battle command system
- ABD – Airbase defense
- AFMC – Armed forces medical college
- AHA – Ammunition holding area
- AIPD – Army Institute For Professional Development
- AOL – Area of operations
- APO– Army Post Office
- APRT – Army Physical Readiness Test (U.S. Army)
- ASAP – Army substance abuse program (U.S. military)
- AWOL – Absent without leave

B
- BAH – Basic Allowance for Housing
- BAR – Browning Automatic Rifle
- BCD - Bad Conduct Discharge (aka Big Chicken Dinner)
- BCG – Birth Control Glasses (U.S. Military Slang)
- BCT – Basic Combat Training (U.S. Army)
- BDU – Battle Dress Uniform (U.S. Military)
- BFT – Blue Force Tracker (U.S. Military)
- BG – Bodyguard
- BGHR – By God, He's Right (U.S Military)
- BLUF – Bottom Line Up Front (US Military)

- CDAT – Computerized Dumb Ass Tanker (M1 Abrams Crewmen)
- CENTCOM – Central Command (U.S. Military)
- CIA – Central Intelligence Agency
- CIWS – Close-In Weapon System
- CO – Commanding Officer
- COA – Course of Action
- COCOM – Combatant Commander
- COMINT – Communications Intelligence
- COMSEC' – Communication Security
- CONUS – Continental United States (U.S. military, pron. "cone-us")
- COP – Combat Out Post
- CPL – Corporal (U.S. Army and Marine Corps E-4)
- CPT – Captain (US Army O-3)
- CPX – Command Post Exercise
- CQB – Close Quarters Battle
- CSM – Command Sergeant Major (U.S. Army E9 highest Army enlisted rank))
- CT – Counter-terrorism Team

D

- DFAC – Dining Facility (U.S. Military)
- DFAS – Defense Finance and Accounting Service (U.S. Military) * D.I.A – Defensive Intelligence Agency
- DOP – Drop-Off Point
- DPMs – Disruptive Pattern Material
- DTO – Daily Tasking Order
- E&E – Escape and Evade
- ECP – Entry Control Point
- EOD – Explosive Ordnance Disposal
- EOS - End of Service
- EPW – Enemy Prisoner of War
- EUCOM – European Command (U.S. Military)

- EW - Electronic Warfare (comprises EA, EP)
- FA – Field Artillery
- FEBA – Forward Edge of the Battle Area
- FLOT – Forward Line of Troops
- FM – Field Marshal
- FMC – Fully Mission Capable
- FO – Forward Observer
- FOB – Forward Operating Base
- FUBAR – Fucked Up Beyond All Recognition
- FYSA - For Your Situational Awareness

G

- G1 – General Staff Level office for Personnel and Manpower (Division and Above)
- G2 – General Staff Level office for Military Intelligence (Division and Above)
- G3 – General Staff Level office for Operations and Plans (Division and Above)
- G4 – General Staff Level office for Logistics (Division and Above)
- G5 – General Staff Level office for Military/Civil Affairs (Division and Above)
- G6 – General Staff Level office for Signal and Communication (Division and Above)
- G7 – General Staff Level office for Training and Exercises (Division and Above)
- G8 – General Staff Level office for Force Development and Analysis (Division and Above)
- G9 – General Staff Level office for Civil Operations (Division and Above)
- GBU – Guided Bomb Unit
- GEN – General
- GI – Government Issue
- GIGO – Garbage In Garbage Out
- GO – General

H

- HE – High Explosive
- HMMWV – High Mobility Multipurpose Wheeled Vehicle (U.S. Military) (Pronounced Humvee)
- HOMSEC – Homeland Security
- HQ – Headquarters
- HUMINT – Human Intelligence
- ICBM – Intercontinental Ballistic Missile

I

- ICE – Individual Carrying Equipment
- ID – Identification
- IED – Improvised Explosive Device
- IG – Inspector General (US Military)
- IFV – Infantry Fighting Vehicle
- INSCOM – United States Army Intelligence and Security Command
- Interpol – International Criminal Police Organization
- ISR – Intelligence, Surveillance, and Reconnaissance

J

- JA – Judge Advocate [General]
- JAG – Judge Advocate General
- J.S.F – Joint Strike Fighter
- JATO – Jet-assisted Take Off
- JEEP - Just Enough Essential Parts

K

- KIA – Killed In Action
- KISS – Keep It Simple, Stupid – USAF
- KP – Kitchen Police or Kitchen Patrol
- KBO – Keep Buggering On

L

- LAAD – Low Altitude Air Defense
- LCDR – Lieutenant Commander (US Navy)
- LCPL – Lance Corporal (US Marines)
- LES – Leave and Earnings Statement

- LP – Listening Post
- LGOP – Little Group Of Paratroopers
- LT – Lieutenant
- LTC – Lieutenant Colonel
- LTG – Lieutenant General
- LZ – Landing Zone

M

- MBT – Main Battle Tank
- MG – Machine Gun
- MG – Major General
- MI – Military Intelligence
- MIA – Missing In Action
- MedEvac – Medical Evacuation
- MICV – Mechanized Infantry Combat Vehicle
- MLRS – Multiple Launch Rocket System
- MOA – Military Operating Area (USAF Airspace)
- MOAB – Massive Ordnance Air Blast bomb, also known as "Mother of All Bombs". (U.S. military)
- MOAC - Mother of All Coffee (Green Bean Coffee)
- MOB – Main Operating Base
- MOBCOM – Mobile Command
- MOPP – Mission Oriented Protective Posture
- MRAP – Mine Resistant Ambush Protected
- MRE – Meal Ready to Eat (U.S. Military)
- MRX – Mission Rehearsal Exercise
- MTOE – Modified Table Of Organizational Equipment
- MTS+ – Movement Tracking System Plus

N

- NAFTA – North American Free Trade Agreement
- NATO – North Atlantic Treaty Organization
- NCI - National Cancer Institute
- NCO – Non-Commissioned Officer
- NCOIC - Non-Commissioned Officer in Charge

- ND – Negligent Discharge
- NIBC National Interagency Biodefense Campus
- NICBR - National Interagency Confederation for Biological Research
- NMC – Not Mission Capable
- NNMSA – Non-Nuclear Munitions Storage Area
- NS – Network Services
- NSA – National Security Agency

O

- OBE – Overcome By Events
- OCONUS – Outside Continental United States
- OCS – Officer Candidate School
- OIC - Officer in Charge
- OM – On the Move (Normally just spelled out Oscar Mike)
- OODA – Observe, Orient, Decide, Act
- OP – Observation Post
- ORM – Operational Risk Management
- OSP – On Site Procurement
- OPORD – Operations Order
- OPSEC – Operations Security
- OTS – Officer Training School
- OTV – Outer Tactical Vest

P

- PACOM – Pacific Command
- PCS – Permanent Change of Station
- PDS – Permanent Duty Station (U.S. Military)
- PDT – Pre-Deployment Training
- PE – Plastic Explosive
- PFC – Private First Class (U.S. Military)
- PFM – Pure Fuckin Magic (U.S. Military)
- PFT – Physical Fitness Test
- PII - Personally Identifiable Information or Personal Identity Information
- PL – Platoon Leader (U.S. Army)

- PLT – Platoon (U.S. Army)
- PMC – Partially Mission Capable
- PME – Professional Military Education
- PNG – Passive Night Goggles
- PO – Post Office
- POC – Point Of Contact
- POG – Person Other than Grunt (All non-combat arms job fields i.e. any MOS or CMF other than infantry, cavalry, armor, and artillery; among infantrymen, refers to anyone other than infantry or Special Forces)
- POW – Prisoner Of War
- POV – Privately Owned Vehicle
- PRP – Pretty Retarded Program
- PRT – Provincial Reconstruction Team
- PRT – Physical Readiness Training (U.S. Army)
- PT – Physical Training
- PTB - Powers That Be
- PV2 – Private 2nd class (U.S. Army E-2)
- PVT – Private (U.S. Army and Marine Corps E-1)
- PX – Post Exchange (U.S. Army)

R

- RATO – Rocket Assisted Take Off
- REMF – Rear Echelon Mother Fucker
- RFL – Response Force Leader
- ROE – Rules Of Engagement
- ROMA Data, Right Out of My Ass Data. Unverifiable created data (different from SWAG)
- ROWPU – Reverse Osmosis Water Purification Unit
- RPG – Rocket-Propelled Grenade
- RPM – Rounds per minute
- RSS – Regional Security System (Caribbean)
- RTB – Return to Base
- RV – Rendezvous
- RTO - Radio Telephone Operator

S

- SAAS – Standard Army Ammunition System (U.S. Army)
- SAM – Surface-to-air Missile
- SCPO – Senior Chief Petty Officer (USCG/USN E-8)
- SD - "Status Destroyed" or "Salty Dog". Equipment that is written off as unrepairable and unsalvageable.
- SEAL – Sea, Air and Land (US Navy SEALs)
- SERE – Survival, Evasion, Resistance and Escape
- SFC – Sergeant First Class (U.S. Army E7)
- SGM – Sergeant Major (U.S. Army E9 – Sometimes referred to as Staff Sergeant Major)
- SGT – Sergeant (U.S. Army E5) (U.S. Marines uses SSgt)
- SITREP – Situation Report
- SJA – Staff Judge Advocate
- SLAM – Standoff Land Attack Missile
- SMA – Sergeant Major of the Army (U.S. Army E9 – Senior Enlisted Member)
- SNAFU – Situation Normal: All Fucked Up
- SOCOM – United States Special Operations Command
- SOFA – Status of Forces Agreement
- SOP – Standard Operating Procedures
- SOS – Shit On a Shingle, or creamed chipped beef on toast.
- SPC – Specialist (U.S. Army E-4)
- SSDD – Same Shit Different Day
- SSDDBS – Same Shit Different Day Bigger Shovel
- SSG – Staff Sergeant (US Army E-6)
- SOL – Shit Out of Luck (US Army)
- SOLJWF – Shit Out of Luck and Jolly Well Fucked (U.S. Marines)
- STOVL – Short Takeoff, Vertical Landing
- SUSFU – Situation Unchanged, Still Fucked Up
- SWAG – Scientific Wild Ass Guess

T

- TAD – Temporary Additional Duty (U.S. Military)
- TBD – To Be Determined

- TDY – Temporary Duty (U.S. Military)
- TF – Task Force
- TFOA – Things Falling Off Aircraft
- TOC - Tactical Operations Center
- TIC – Troops in Contact
- TU – Tits Up (Dead, Inoperable), a.k.a. "tango uniform"
- TARFU – Things Are Really Fucked Up, or Totally and Royally Fucked Up

U

- UA – Unauthorized Absence
- UAS – Unmanned Aerial System
- UAV – Unmanned Aerial Vehicle
- UCAV – Unmanned Combat Air Vehicle
- US – Unserviceable
- USSS – United States Secret Service
- USAFE – United States Air Forces in Europe
- USAMRICD - United States Army Medical Research Institute of Chemical Defense
- USAMRIID - United States Army Medical Research Institute of Infectious Disease
- USAMRMC - United States Army Medical Research and Materiel Command
- USAMRAA - United States Army Medical Research Acquisition Activity
- USA PATRIOT Act – Uniting and Strengthening America by Providing Appropriate Tools Required to Intercept and Obstruct Terrorism Act
- USAREC – US Army Recruiting Command
- USAREUR – US Army European Command
- USMC – United States Marine Corps
- USN – United States Navy
- USO – United Service Organizations (U.S. Military)
- USR – Unit Status Report
- UUV – Unmanned Underwater Vehicle
- UXB – Unexploded Bomb (bomb disposal; British)

- UXO – Unexploded Ordnance

V

- VBIED – Vehicle-borne Improvised Explosive Device
- VDM – Visual Distinguishing Mark
- VFD – Volunteer Fire Department
- VFR – Volunteer Fire and Rescue

W

- WIA – Wounded In Action
- WO1 – Warrant Officer 1
- WSA – Weapons Storage Area
- WMD – Weapons of Mass Destruction
- WILCO – Will Comply

X

- XO – Executive Officer

www.ingramcontent.com/pod-product-compliance
Lightning Source LLC
Chambersburg PA
CBHW071351170526
45165CB00001B/5